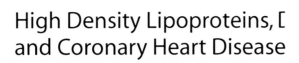

High Density Lipoproteins, [
and Coronary Heart Disease

Ernst J. Schaefer

Editor

High Density Lipoproteins, Dyslipidemia, and Coronary Heart Disease

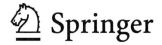 Springer

Editor
Ernst J. Schaefer, MD
Tufts University School of Medicine
Boston, MA
USA
ernst.schaefer@tufts.edu

ISBN 978-1-4419-1058-5   e-ISBN 978-1-4419-1059-2
DOI 10.1007/978-1-4419-1059-2
Springer New York Dordrecht Heidelberg London

Library of Congress Control Number: 2009943544

Printed on acid-free paper

Springer is part of Springer Science+Business Media (www.springer.com)

Preface

In this book and atlas entitled High *Density Lipoproteins, Dyslipidemia, and Coronary Heart Disease*, I am indebted to the many chapter authors who have contributed their writing as well as their insights. The work grew out of a meeting on high density lipoproteins (HDLs), chaired by me and Dr. Vassilis Zannis of Boston University, and held on June 19 and 20, 2009 in Newport, Rhode Island, as a satellite meeting following the 15th International Symposium on Atherosclerosis, held in Boston. In the introduction our understanding of overall lipoprotein metabolism is reviewed, as well as the common genetic lipoprotein disorders associated with premature coronary heart disease (CHD). These familial disorders include lipoprotein(a) excess, dyslipidemia (high triglycerides and low HDL), combined hyperlipidemia (high cholesterol and high triglycerides often with low HDL), hypoalphalipoproteinemia (low HDL), and hypercholesterolemia. We discuss the management of these disorders. We also review other disorders including cerebrotendinous xanthomatosis, phytosterolemia, deficiency of apolipoprotein B, and severe hypertriglyceridemia. The latter disorder can be associated with pancreatitus.

Thereafter, the focus is on HDL, beginning with chapters on the regulation of apolipoprotein (apo) A-I gene expression, the composition, remodeling, and the metabolism of HDL particles, as well as HDL structure, function, and its anti-inflammatory properties. Then the focus shifts to chapters on disease states characterized by apoA-I deficiency, apoA-I variants, Tangier disease due to lack of ABCA1 function, the ABCG1 transporter, the interaction of HDL particles with transporters and receptors, human lecithin:cholesterol acyl transferase (LCAT) deficiency, human cholesteryl ester transfer protein (CETP) deficiency, and scavenger receptor-B1 (SR-B1) and HDL metabolism. Then the focus shifts again to topics of greater interest to the practicing physician including chapters on the genetics of HDL in the general population, the role of nutrition, alcohol, and exercise in modulating HDL metabolism, and the effects of estrogens, niacin, statins, fibrates, CETP inhibitors, and HDL infusion therapy on HDL metabolism and CHD risk reduction. We end with a concluding chapter focusing on the current and future status of the management of lipoprotein disorders, with a special focus on HDL. In our view, HDL raising is the next frontier in CHD risk reduction.

I would like to express my indebtedness and gratitude to my father Karl for stimulating me to enter the field of medicine and science, to Solomon Berson of Mount Sinai Hospital for his encouragement to do research, and to Howard Eder and Paul Roheim at Albert Einstein College of Medicine, and Paul Schreibman at Rockefeller University for allowing me to do research in their laboratories. I am especially grateful to Robert I. Levy for providing me with a staff fellowship at the National Institutes of Health (NIH) and for teaching me about human lipoprotein metabolism, as well as for bringing me to the Human Nutrition Research Center on Aging at Tufts University. I would also like to thank Bryan Brewer for his guidance, support, and collaboration at NIH. I would also like to thank Jose Ordovas, Stefania Lamon-Fava, Alice Lichtenstein, Margaret Brousseau, and Bela Asztalos for their collaborations with me at Tufts University, as well as my institute directors Hamish Munro, Irwin Rosenberg, and Robert Russell for their support and guidance. Finally, I am extremely grateful to my wife Mary and my three children Caroline, Christopher, and Peter for their many years of love, patience, and support.

Boston, MA   Ernst J. Schaefer, MD

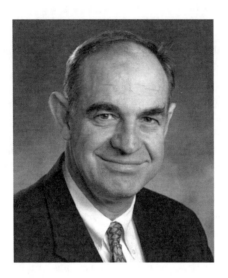

Ernst J. Schaefer received his education at Phillips Academy, Andover, Harvard College (BA), Dartmouth Medical School, and Mount Sinai School of Medicine (MD). He did research rotations at Albert Einstein College of Medicine and Rockefeller University. He did a medical residency at Mount Sinai Hospital in New York, and an endocrinology fellowship at the National Institutes of Health, where he also served as a staff associate and senior investigator in the Molecular Disease Branch. He is currently a distinguished university professor at Tufts University School of Medicine and the Friedman School of Nutrition Science and Policy at Tufts University, and a senior scientist and director of the Lipid Metabolism Laboratory at the Human Nutrition Research Center on Aging at Tufts University, as well as the director of the lipid and heart disease prevention clinic. He served on the first and second adult treatment panels of the National Cholesterol Education Program. He also was the editor of the journal Atherosclerosis between 1997 and 2007 and served as the co-chairman of the 15th International Symposium on Atherosclerosis held in Boston in 2009. He is the author of over 500 publications in the area of lipoproteins, genetics, nutrition, pharmacology, and coronary heart disease (CHD) risk reduction. His primary interest is on human high density lipoprotein metabolism and CHD.

Contents

Contributors

Bela F. Asztalos, PhD
Lipid Metabolism Laboratory, Tufts University, Boston, MA, USA

P.H.R. Barrett, PhD
Metabolic Research Centre, School of Medicine and Pharmacology,
University of Western Australia, Perth, Australia

Philip J. Barter, MBBS, PhD
Lipid Research Group, The Heart Research Institute, Sydney, NSW,
Australia and Department of Medicine, University of Sydney, NSW, Australia

H. Bryan Brewer, MD
Cardiovascular Research Institute, Lipoprotein and Atherosclerosis Research Group,
Medstar Research Institute, Washington, DC, USA

Eliot A. Brinton, MD
Metabolism Section, Division of Cardiovascular Genetics, University of Utah Medical
Center, Salt Lake City, UT, USA

Margaret E. Brousseau, PhD
Novartis Institutes for Biomedical Research, Inc, Cambridge, MA, USA

John Brunzell, MD
Department of Medicine, University of Washington, Seattle, WA, USA

Laura Calabresi, PhD
Center E. Grossi Paoletti, Department of Pharmacological Sciences,
Università degli Studi di Milano, Milano, Italy

Dick C. Chan, PhD
Metabolic Research Centre, School of Medicine and Pharmacology,
University of Western Australia, Perth, Australia

Margarita de la Llera-Moya, PhD
Department of Pediatrics, Children's Hospital of Philadelphia, Philadelphia, PA, USA

Konstantinos Drosatos, PhD
Whitaker Cardiovascular Institute, Boston University School of Medicine,
Boston, MA, USA

Adelina Duka, BSc
Whitaker Cardiovascular Institute, Boston University School of Medicine,
Boston, MA, USA

Guido Francheschini, PhD
Center E. Grossi Paoletti, Department of Pharmacological Sciences,
Università degli Studi di Milano, Milano, Italy

Akihiro Inazu, MD
The Second Department of Internal Medicine, School of Medicine,
Kanazawa University, Kanazawa, Japan and Department of Laboratory Science,
School of Health Sciences, Kanazawa University, Kanazawa, Japan

Dimitris Kardassis, PhD
Department of Biochemistry, Division of Basic Sciences,
Institute of Molecular Biology and Biotechnology,
University of Crete Medical School, Crete, Greece

Ginny Kellner-Weibel, PhD
Department of Pediatrics, Children's Hospital of Philadelphia,
Philadelphia, PA 10104, USA

Georgios Koukos, PhD
Whitaker Cardiovascular Institute, Boston University School of Medicine,
Boston, MA, USA

Monty Krieger, PhD
Department of Biology, Massachusetts Institute of Technology, Cambridge, MA, USA

Stefania Lamon-Fava, MD, PhD
Lipid Metabolism Laboratory, Tufts University, Boston, MA, USA

Hiroshi Mabuchi, MD
Department of Lipidology, School of Medicine, Institute of Medical,
Pharmaceutical and Health Sciences, Kanazawa University, Kanazawa, Japan

M. Nazeem Nanjee, PhD
Metabolism Section, Division of Cardiovascular Genetics,
University of Utah Medical Center, Salt Lake City, UT, USA

Attilio Rigotti, MD
Departamento de Gastroenterologia, Facultad de Medicina,
Pontificia Universidad Catolica, Santiago, Chile

George H. Rothblat, PhD
Children's Hospital of Philadelphia, Philadelphia, PA, USA

Kerry-Anne Rye, PhD
Lipid Research Group, The Heart Research Institute, Sydney, Australia,
Faculty of Medicine, University of Sydney, NSW, Australia and
Department of Medicine, University of Melbourne, Victoria, Australia

Sandhya Sankaranarayanan, PhD
Department of Pediatrics, Children's Hospital of Philadelphia, Philadelphia, PA, USA

Despina Sanoudou, PhD
Molecular Biology Division, Biomedical Research
Foundation of the Academy of Athens, Athens, Greece

Raul D. Santos, MD, PhD
Heart Institute (INCOR), University of Sao Paulo Hospital, Sao Paulo, Brazil

Ernst J. Schaefer, MD
Lipid Metabolism Laboratory, Tufts University, Boston, MA, USA

Alan R. Tall, MD
Department of Medicine, Columbia University, New York, NY, USA

Gerald F. Watts, MD
Metabolic Research Center, School of Medicine and Pharmacology
University of Western Australia

Eleni Zanni, PhD
Whitaker Cardiovascular Institute, Boston University School of Medicine, Boston, MA, USA

Vassilis I. Zannis, PhD
Whitaker Cardiovascular Institute, Boston University School of Medicine, Boston, MA, USA

Introduction to High-Density Lipoprotein, Dyslipidemia, and Coronary Heart Disease

Ernst J. Schaefer

Introduction

Coronary heart disease (CHD) is caused by atherosclerosis, a process which clogs the coronary arteries supplying the heart, as well as other arteries in the body. The hallmark of this process in the artery wall is the presence of cholesterol-laden macrophages or foam cells, proliferation of smooth muscle cells with excess connective tissue, calcification, and, sometimes, thrombosis as the terminal event occluding the artery. In Fig. 1 one can see a normal aorta and coronary arteries, as well as a diseased aorta and a coronary artery occluded with atherosclerosis. A heart attack or myocardial infarction (MI) occurs when one or more of the three major coronary arteries (left anterior descending, circumflex, and right) is occluded. A stroke occurs when one or more of the arteries supplying the brain is occluded. CHD and stroke together are known as cardiovascular disease, which accounts for about half of all mortality in developed societies including the United States.

It is known that aging, high blood pressure, diabetes, and smoking (elevated carbon monoxide levels in the blood) can damage the lining of the artery wall. Moreover, it is known that low-density lipoprotein (LDL) cholesterol can be deposited in the artery wall, especially at sites of damage. Therefore, high levels of LDL cholesterol (>160 mg/dl or 4.2 mmol/l) associated with high total cholesterol values (>240 mg/dl or 6.2 mmol/l) are a significant risk factor for CHD. In addition, high-density lipoproteins (HDLs) serve to remove cholesterol from the artery wall. Therefore, high levels of HDL cholesterol (>60 mg/dl or 1.6 mmol/l) are protective of CHD, and low levels (<40 mg/dl or 1.0 mmol/l) are a significant CHD risk factor [1, 2]. Diets high in animal fat, dairy products, eggs, sugar, and salt have been associated with excess obesity, elevated blood cholesterol, and high age-adjusted CHD mortality rates [3]. Replacement of animal fats with vegetable oils and omega-3 fatty acid supplementation has resulted in significant reduction in CHD morbidity and mortality [3]. The use of statins has also been associated with significant reductions in heart disease and stroke morbidity and mortality [4]. The focus of lipid management has been on lowering of LDL cholesterol [1].

Cholesterol Production

Cholesterol is a waxy substance of molecular weight 387 daltons, and is by far the most abundant sterol in plasma. Cholesterol is synthesized in cells in the body, and this source accounts for about 75% of the cholesterol in the bloodstream. Cholesterol serves as a precursor for bile acids, and steroid hormones including estrogen, testosterone, and cortisol. Cholesterol is found in cell membranes. Precursors of cholesterol include lathosterol and desmosterol, which can be measured in plasma or serum and serve as markers of cholesterol production. Subjects who overproduce cholesterol have elevated absolute levels of these constituents as well as increased values normalized to blood cholesterol levels. Cholesterol production is increased in patients with obesity and metabolic syndrome.

There are many steps in the cholesterol synthesis pathway from acetate to cholesterol. The rate-limiting enzyme in cholesterol synthesis is 3-hydroxy 3-methyl glutaryl CoA reductase or HMG CoA reductase. Statins competitively inhibit this enzyme, thereby lowering cholesterol production in the body, and decreasing cellular cholesterol synthesis by up to 80%. The cells in the body respond by increasing the level and activity of LDL receptors on their surface, and enhancing the clearance of LDL particles from the bloodstream, and lowering LDL cholesterol levels in plasma [5]. However, in intestinal cells statins can also increase the amount of cholesterol absorbed. Statins are especially effective in subjects who have elevated markers of cholesterol production, and are least effective in patients with elevated plasma markers of absorption [6]. Statins also lower the

E.J. Schaefer(✉)
Lipid Metabolism Laboratory, Tufts University,
711 Washington Street, Boston, MA 02111, USA
e-mail: ernst.schaefer@tufts.edu

E.J. Schaefer (ed.), *High Density Lipoproteins, Dyslipidemia, and Coronary Heart Disease*,
DOI 10.1007/978-1-4419-1059-2_1, © Springer Science+Business Media, LLC 2010

Fig. 1 Photographs at autopsy of a totally normal abdominal aorta (**a**) and normal coronary arteries (**b**), an abdominal aorta with severe atherosclerosis (**c**), and a coronary artery totally occluded with atherosclerosis (**d**)

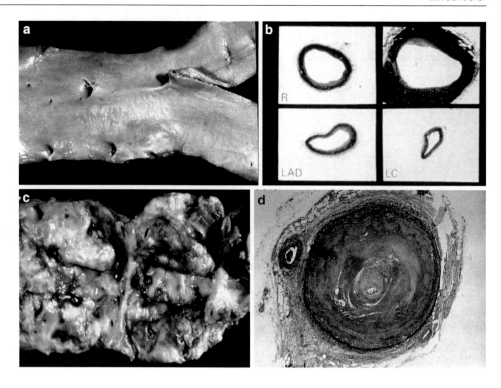

production of coenzyme Q10 which is important for muscle metabolism, and supplementation with coenzyme Q10 may reduce the muscle symptoms that many patients experience when they are taking statins.

Cerebrotendinous Xanthomatosis

There are a rare group of patients with cerebrotendinous xanthomatosis who develop cholestanol deposits in their tendons and brain tissue, despite having only modest elevations in plasma cholesterol levels. They are at increased risk of developing severe neurologic disease, and cannot convert cholesterol to chenodeoxycholate, one of the major bile acids, due to defect in the sterol 27 hydroxylase gene [7, 8]. The diagnosis is established by the finding of markedly elevated plasma cholestanol levels as measured by gas chromatogra-

phy. The treatment of choice is 250 mg orally three times daily of chenodeoxycholate, which prevents them from getting severe neurologic disease [8].

Familial Combined Hyperlipidemia

The most common familial cause of elevated LDL cholesterol is known as familial combined hyperlipidemia, found in about 15% of patients with premature CHD [9]. These patients have been shown to have increased production of very-low-density lipoprotein (VLDL) apolipoprotein (apo) B-100. Affected family members have elevated triglyceride levels, elevated LDL cholesterol levels, or both. Moreover, affected family members often have low HDL cholesterol [9]. The final steps in the cholesterol synthesis pathway are shown in Fig. 2. Here squalene is converted into lanosterol and then either into desmosterol or lathosterol, both of which are converted into cholesterol. Recently, we have documented that patients with familial combined hyperlipidemia have normal squalene levels, but elevated lathosterol and cholesterol levels indicating altered sterol metabolism and enhanced conversion of squalene into lathosterol [10]. This pattern can easily be detected by measuring sterol levels in plasma using gas chromatography. The ideal therapy for these patients in addition to dietary modification is statin therapy.

Cholesterol Absorption

Cholesterol is also absorbed in the intestine. About 25% of the cholesterol found in the bloodstream is from dietary sources. The cholesterol found in the intestine is derived both from the diet and also made by the liver, secreted into the bile, and reabsorbed. Major dietary sources include eggs, butter, whole milk, and animal fats as found in meat [3]. It is now known that almost all of the cholesterol and plant sterols from plants (beta-sitosterol and campesterol) are transported into the intestine via the Niemann Pick C like protein 1 or NPC1L1 transporter [11]. This process is blocked about 50% by ezetimibe, a specific inhibitor of NPC1L1 [12]. Cholesterol in the intestine is either placed onto chylomicrons or HDL for entry into the bloodstream, stored in the intestine as either free cholesterol or cholesteryl ester (cholesterol with a fatty acid attached), or transported back out into the intestinal lumen via the action of the two transporters ATP-binding cassette transporters G5 and G8 (ABCG5 and ABCG8). About 50% of the intestinal cholesterol and more than 95% of the intestinal beta-sitosterol and campesterol are transported back out into the intestinal lumen via these ABC transporters (see Fig. 3).

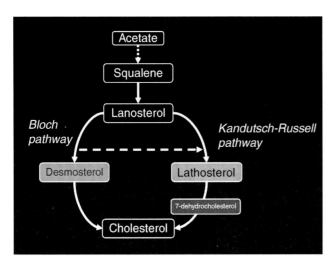

Fig. 2 A diagram showing the final steps in cholesterol synthesis from squalene to lanosterol then to either desmosterol or lathosterol, both of which can be converted to cholesterol. Elevated lathosterol and desmosterol levels in plasma serve as markers of increased cholesterol synthesis in the body

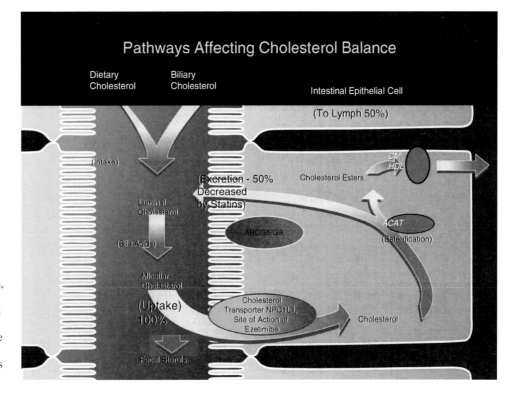

Fig. 3 A diagram showing intestinal cholesterol absorption, with cholesterol entering the intestinal cell via Niemann Pick C1 Like 1 Protein (NPC1L1), and being excreted back into the lumen of the intestine via the ATP binding cassette transporters (ABC) ABCG5 and ABCG8

Phytosterolemia

Patients with rare defects in the ABCG5 and ABCG8 transporters have markedly elevated plasma levels of plant sterols or phytosterols (specifically beta-sitosterol and campesterol), tendinous xanthomas, and premature CHD [13]. The definitive diagnosis in these patients is made by the measurement of plasma sterols by gas chromatography. Such subjects are at increased risk for developing CHD, and the most effective treatment for them is ezetimibe, which lowers their levels of plant sterols by 50%.

There are subjects in the normal population who have moderately increased levels of plasma phytosterols, and are at increased risk of CHD, because they have increased intestinal cholesterol absorption [14, 15]. Their LDL cholesterol and plasma phytosterols are very effectively reduced by ezetimibe, and these patients are less responsive to statins than those that do not have elevated levels. On average ezetimibe lowers plasma markers of intestinal absorption (beta-sitosterol and campesterol) by 50% and levels of LDL cholesterol by 18%, but increases markers of cholesterol synthesis [16, 17]. Therefore, the combination of a statin and ezetimibe is highly effective in LDL lowering especially in patients with evidence of increased intestinal absorption. Statins, of course, have the opposite effect in that they lower cholesterol synthesis markedly, but can increase cholesterol absorption [6, 15]. The average person absorbs about 50% of their intestinal cholesterol, but the range is about 20–80%. In patients on statins, ezetimibe will lower LDL cholesterol on average by 23–27% [17].

Plasma Lipids

About 70% of the cholesterol in plasma is in the esterified form, except in patients with a deficiency of lecithin:cholesterol acyl transferase (LCAT) due to severe liver disease or on a genetic basis (see chapter by Dr. Calabresi). Cholesteryl ester is cholesterol with a fatty acid attached to it, and has a molecular weight of about 650 daltons. Another major plasma lipids are triglycerides, which are molecules in which three fatty acids are attached to a glycerol backbone. The molecular weight of triglyceride is 885 daltons. Fatty acids are chains of carbon with hydrogens attached, with a methyl group (CH_3) at the omega end of the carbon chain, and a carboxylic acid group (COOH) at the alpha end of the carbon chain. All the fat stored in the fat depots in the body is triglyceride, as is much of the fat that is eaten. In the intestines the fatty acids are cleaved off of the glycerol by the action of lipases including pancreatic lipase, and then the fatty acids enter the intestine after binding to a fatty-acid-binding protein.

About 95% of all the fat that is eaten is absorbed as fatty acid by the intestine, and is converted back into triglyceride and packaged into large triglyceride-rich chylomicrons and released into the lymph and then into the bloodstream. The fatty acid content of triglyceride in chylomicrons is determined by the type of fat that is eaten.

Phospholipids are the other major class of lipids in the bloodstream. They are comprised of a phospholipid polar head group with two fatty acids attached. The major phospholipid in plasma is phosphatidylcholine or lecithin. Phospholipids are the major building blocks of cell membranes, which are bilayers of phospholipids with the fatty acids oriented toward the interior of the membrane. Therefore, the type of fatty acids attached to membrane phospholipids can have a significant effect on membrane function and fluidity [3].

Fatty Acids

Saturated fatty acids are found in foods of animal origin as well as in some vegetable oils like coconut oil and palm oil. The major saturated fatty acids are palmitic acid (16:0) and stearic acid (18:0). Neither of these fatty acids has any double bonds, and they are solid at room temperature (i.e., fat in meats such as beef, pork, lamb, or poultry). Saturated fatty acids, especially 12:0, 14:0, and 16:0 (lauric, myristic, and palmitic acids) raise LDL cholesterol levels [3].

Monounsaturated fatty acids or fats are found in vegetable oils like olive oil and canola oil, as well as in meat, and tend to be relatively neutral with regard to LDL cholesterol. The major monounsaturated fatty acid is oleic acid, which has one double bond at the 9 position from the omega end of the carbon side (18:1n9) (see Fig. 4.).

The polyunsaturated fats are those that contain more than one double bond. These are divided into the n6 fatty acids, mainly linoleic acid (18:2n6) and its derivative arachidonic acid (AA, 20:4n6), and the n3 fatty acids, namely alpha linolenic acid (ALA, 18:3n3) and its derivatives eicosapentaenoic acid (EPA, 20:5n3) and docosahexaenoic acid (DHA, 22:6n3). Linoleic and alpha linolenic acid are found in vegetable oils such as soybean oil, corn oil, sunflower seed oil, and canola oil, while EPA and DHA are found in fish or fish oil. The polyunsaturated fatty acids are essential fatty acids because humans have to obtain them from the diet, since the body cannot place a double at omega 3 or n3 position or the omega 6 or n6 position. However, the body can convert linoleic acid to AA, and alpha linolenic acid to EPA or DHA. Each double found in the carbon chain of fatty acids confers a 37° bend or kink in the carbon chain, which causes polyunsaturated fatty acids in the membrane to confer more disordered structure and greater fluidity to the membrane [3].

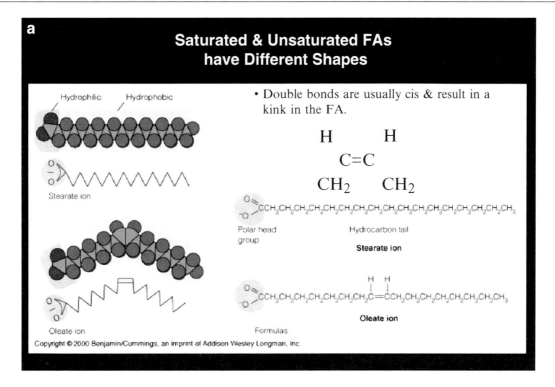

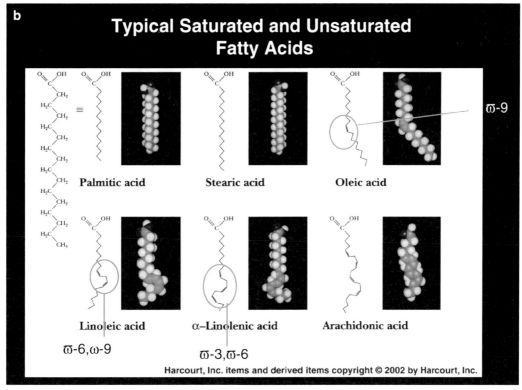

Fig. 4 Diagrams of saturated, monounsaturated, and polyunsaturated fatty acids are shown in (**a**) and (**b**).

Apolipoproteins

The protein components of lipoproteins are called apolipoproteins.

Apolipoprotein A-I

Apolipoprotein (apo) A-I is the most abundant of plasma apolipoprotein in normal subjects, with a concentration of

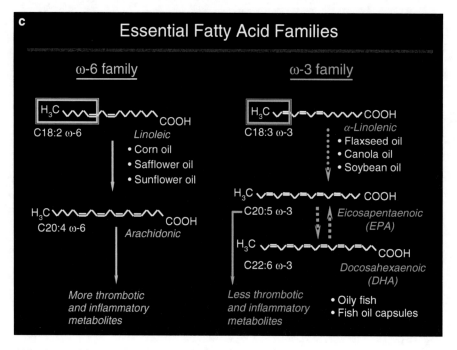

Fig. 4 (continued) The conversion of linoleic acid to arachidonic acid and linoleic acid to eicosapentaenoic and docosahexaenoic acids are shown in (**c**)

approximately 130 mg/dl. ApoA-I has a molecular weight of 28,016 daltons, and is the major protein of HDL. It is made in both the liver and the intestine. ApoA-I is an activator of lecithin:cholesterol acyltransferase or LCAT. LCAT transfers a fatty acid from lecithin to cholesterol to form cholesteryl ester and lysolecithin. ApoA-I is also an important structural protein of HDL, and serves as an acceptor of free cholesterol and phospholipids from cells via the action of the ATP-binding cassette transporter A1 (ABCA1) [3]. A model of lipid-free apoA-I is shown in Fig. 5 [18].

Apolipoprotein A-II

ApoA-II is another protein found in HDL, with a plasma concentration of about 40 mg/dl. It has a molecular weight of 17,414 daltons as a dimer linked by a disulfide bond, and is synthesized in the liver. ApoA-II has been reported to enhance the activity of both hepatic lipase and cholesteryl ester transfer protein.

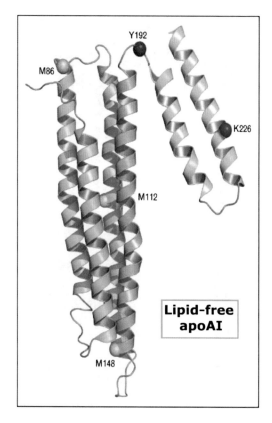

Fig. 5 The structure of lipid free apolipoprotein A-I is shown in this figure

Apolipoprotein A-IV

ApoA-IV is found in both chylomicrons and HDL, with a plasma concentration of about 5 mg/dl. It has a molecular weight of 44,465 daltons. ApoA-IV is made in both the liver and the intestine; however, its major function appears to be in the facilitation of intestinal fat absorption, as well as to increase LCAT activity. It also plays a structural role since it is found on its own HDL particle.

Apolipoprotein A-V

ApoA-V is found on both triglyceride-rich lipoproteins and HDL, and has very low plasma concentrations and a molecular weight of 39,566 daltons. ApoA-V plays an important role in modulating the activity of lipoprotein lipase, and mutations in apoA-V are a major cause of significant hypertriglyceridemia.

Apolipoprotein B-100

ApoB-100 is the integral protein of VLDL, IDL, and LDL, with a plasma concentration of about 80 mg/dl in a normal person, and a molecular weight of 512,723 daltons (550,000 if one includes the carbohydrate). Unlike other apolipoproteins which tend to have an alpha helical structure, apoB-100 has a beta-pleated sheet structure, which causes the protein to bind very tightly to the lipid in lipoprotein particles and not let go. It functions as a structural protein for VLDL and LDL particles. ApoB-100 is the major binding protein for the B/E or LDL receptor.

Apolipoprotein B-48

ApoB-48 is the major form of apoB produced by the small intestine in humans. Its molecular weight is 248,000 daltons including the carbohydrate. ApoB-48 is the integral protein in chylomicrons particles. It is produced by alternate splicing or editing of the apoB-100 mRNA, which only occurs in the human intestine.

The C Apolipoproteins

ApoC-I is mainly found on HDL, but small amounts are also found on triglyceride-rich lipoproteins (TRLs). It has a plasma concentration of about 5 mg/dl in normal subjects, and its molecular weight is 6,630 daltons. It increases the activity of LCAT, while inhibiting that of hepatic lipase and CETP. ApoC-II is found on both TRL and HDL. Its plasma concentration is about 5 mg/dl and its molecular weight is 8,900 daltons. It functions as the sole known activator of

lipoprotein lipase. ApoC-III is found on both TRL and HDL. Its plasma concentration is about 10 mg/dl, and its molecular weight is 8,800 daltons. Its serves to increase LCAT and CETP activity, while inhibiting LPL activity.

Apolipoprotein E

ApoE is found on both TRL and HDL. Its plasma concentration is about 10 mg/dl, and its molecular weight is 34,145 daltons. Its major function is to serve as a ligand for the B/E or LDL receptor. ApoE is a 299 amino acid protein that can exist in three different forms in human plasma: apoE3, the common form with cysteine at residue 112 and arginine at residue 158, as apoE4, a somewhat less common form, with arginines at both residues 112 and 158, and apoE2 the least common form with cysteines at both these positions. ApoE is essential for the liver uptake of remnants of TRL particles. ApoE2 binds significantly less well to the B/E receptor than do the other isoforms of apoE [3].

Plasma Lipoproteins

Cholesterol and triglyceride along with phospholipids are carried in plasma or serum on lipoproteins. Lipoproteins have a surface layer of phospholipids (each phospholipid has two fatty acids attached to it) with the fatty acids directed toward the core of the particle, as well as proteins known as apolipoproteins, and free cholesterol. The hydrophobic components of lipoproteins, namely cholesteryl ester and triglyceride, are carried within the core of generally spherical lipoprotein particles. A model of a plasma lipoprotein, specifically large HDL, is shown in Fig. 6, and an overview of human lipoprotein metabolism is shown in Fig. 7.

Chylomicrons

These lipoproteins are made in the intestine. They vary greatly in molecular weight ($50–1,000 \times 10^6$ daltons) and size (diameter 75–1,200 nm), have a plasma density of <0.93 g/ml, and migrate at the origin on lipoprotein electrophoresis. These particles are very rich in triglyceride (about 85% by weight in the core of the particle) and contain about 3% cholesteryl ester. These particles can also carry significant amounts of fat-soluble vitamins in their core, namely vitamin A as retinyl palmitate, carotenoids, vitamin D, vitamin E as alpha or gamma tocopherol, and vitamin K. On their surface,

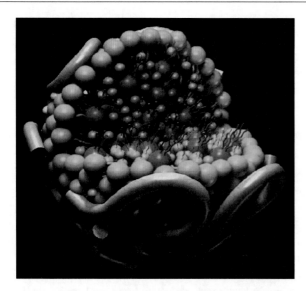

Fig. 6 A model of a large spherical alpha migrating HDL lipoprotein particle is shown with the surface phospholipids shown in *blue* with two fatty acids attached to each polar head group of phospholipid. Also on the surface are molecules of free cholesterol (*light green*) and apolipoprotein A-I (*yellow*). In the core of this spherical lipoprotein are cholesteryl esters with one fatty acid attached (*green*), and triglyceride with three fatty acids (*purple*). Created by Mr. Martin Jacob. Courtesy of Boston Heart Lab Corporation, Framingham, MA, USA

these particles contain about 2% protein, 2% free cholesterol, and 7% phospholipids. The major protein of these particles is known as apolipoprotein (apo) B-48. After chylomicrons are released into the lymph they pick up apo A-I, apo A-IV, and the C apolipoproteins (C-I, C-II, and C-III) on their large surface. The average daily production of apoB-48 in humans is about 2 mg/kg/day.

Once chylomicrons enter the bloodstream, much of the triglyceride is rapidly removed via the action of lipoprotein lipase or LPL. LPL is activated by apoC-II, and cleaves the fatty acid off the glycerol backbone. The fatty acids bind to albumin and are taken up by fat tissue or transported to a variety of other tissues in the body. In the fat, the fatty acids are converted back into triglyceride for long-term energy storage. ApoC-III inhibits this process of lipolysis. When much of the chylomicron triglyceride has been removed, the particles pick up cholesteryl ester from HDL in exchange for triglyceride via the action of cholesteryl ester transfer protein (CETP). They then are much smaller particles and are called chylomicron remnants. In this process of being metabolized to remnants, chylomicrons have lost virtually all of their surface apoA-I, apoA-IV, and C apolipoproteins to HDL, but have retained all of their apoB-48, and have picked apoE from HDL.

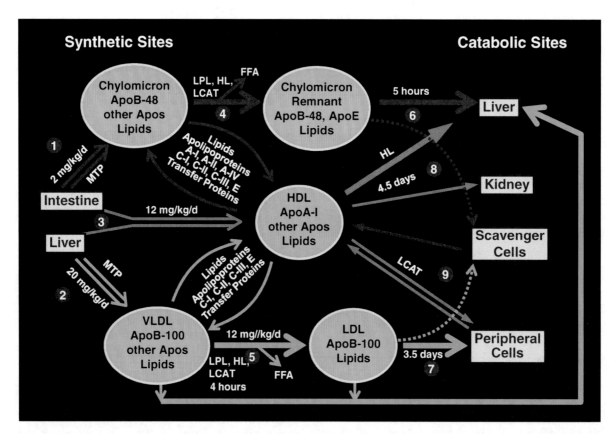

Fig. 7 A model of human lipoprotein metabolism is shown in which chylomicrons are converted to chylomicron remnant particles, which are then taken up by the liver via binding of apoE to the LDL receptor over a 4–5 h period. The liver makes very-low-density lipoproteins which can be converted to large and small LDL, which is cleared from the plasma over about 4 days. LDL is removed from the plasma by the liver and other tissues over about 3.5 days. HDL are made in both the liver and intestine, and the HDL apoA-I has a plasma residence day of about 4.5 days

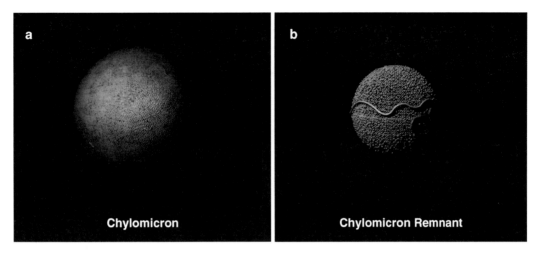

Fig. 8 A model of a chylomicron (**a**) and a chylomicron remnant (**b**) are shown. The *yellow protein* on the surface of remnants is apoB-48 and the *orange protein* is apoE. Created by Mr. Martin Jacob. Courtesy of Boston Heart Lab Corporation, Framingham, MA, USA

While the plasma residence time of chylomicron triglyceride is about 5 min, that of chylomicron apoB-48 is about 5 h [3]. Chylomicron remnants are taken up by the liver, a process that is mediated by the binding of apoE to the LDL receptor. Models of chylomicrons and their remnants are shown in Fig. 8.

Abetalipoproteinemia

Patients who cannot secrete apoB-48 into the bloodstream cannot make chylomicrons. They are rare and generally have mutations in microsomal transfer protein (MTP). MTP allows for the combining of apoB-48 with triglyceride for the secretion of chylomicron particles in the intestine and apoB-100 with triglyceride for secretion of very-low-density lipoprotein (VLDL) by the liver. If MTP is defective no apoB containing particles are present in plasma, only high-density lipoproteins. Average plasma cholesterol and triglyceride values are about 50 and 10 mg/dl, respectively, and the HDL cholesterol level is about 50 mg/dl. The diagnosis is established by the finding of undetectable levels of apoB in their plasma. They also have very low levels of vitamin A and E in their plasma. These patients tend to present with fat malabsorption in childhood, with atypical retinitis pigmentosa by about age 10 years, and if not detected at that point with spino-cerebellar ataxia in their third and fourth decades of life. The treatment of choice is with supplementation with fat-soluble vitamins (15,000 units of vitamin A per day, 1,000 mg of vitamin E per day, daily use of one tablespoon of vegetable oil as salad dressing on salad, two fish oil capsules per day, and use of vitamin K prior to surgery to support adequate clotting (one can also infuse one unit of fresh frozen plasma prior to major surgery) [19].

Hypobetalipoproteinemia

Patients with these rare disorders have truncations in apoB, resulting in mild fat malabsorption, and very low levels of total cholesterol and triglyceride of about 80 and 40 mg/dl, respectively, with an HDL cholesterol of about 40–50 mg/dl, hence their LDL cholesterol is very low. No treatment is required and they appear to have enhanced longevity. The diagnosis is made by the finding of detectable, but very low levels of plasma apoB, and the finding of an abnormally low molecular weight of apoB isolated from LDL by gel electrophoresis, as well as apoB gene mutations [20, 21].

Severe Hypertriglyceridemia

Patients with this disorder generally present in childhood with plasma triglyceride values over 1,000 mg/dl. They usually have defects in lipoprotein lipase, but may also have apoC-II deficiency, or mutations in the ApoA-V gene [22]. Plasma cholesterol levels are usually around about one-fifth to one-tenth of the triglyceride levels, with remnant lipoprotein cholesterol levels that are about twofold increased, direct LDL cholesterol levels that are less than 50 mg/dl, with HDL cholesterol levels that are usually around 20 mg/dl. These patients have marked elevations in chylomicrons and VLDL, and their plasma or serum is usually white. When lipoprotein lipase activity is measured in post-heparin plasma (plasma obtained 10 min after injecting 100 units of heparin/kg of body weight, and promptly separated and frozen at −80°), it is usually very low or absent. Some patients, however, may have a deficiency of the activator protein of lipoprotein lipase, namely apoC-II. The treatment of choice is dietary fat restriction to less than 15% of calories

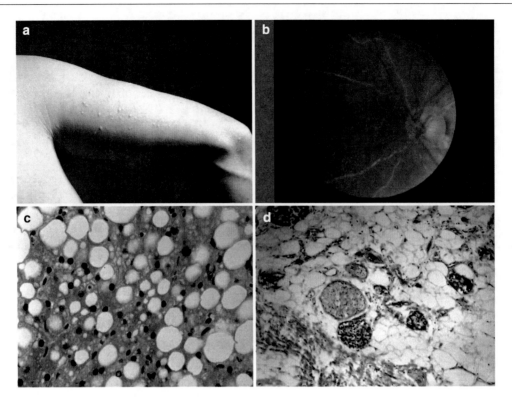

Fig. 9 Signs of severe hypertriglyceridemia (>1,000 mg/dl) are shown with eruptive xanthomas on the skin surface (**a**), lipemia retinalis in the fundus of the eye (**b**), as well as triglyceride deposition in the liver (**c**) and pancreas (**d**), where it can cause pancreatitis

from fat, but to ensure some intake of essential fatty acids by using vegetable oil and fish oil capsules (1–2 per day). These patients can develop recurrent pancreatitis and enlarged livers because of triglyceride deposition in these organs. They can also develop transient eruptive xanthomas. In Fig. 9, the eruptive xanthomas, the lipemia retinalis (milky plasma which can be visualized in retinal veins), and the triglyceride deposition in the liver and pancreas are shown. Sometimes, fenofibrate will help those who have decreased LPL activity, since fibrates are known to increase LPL gene expression and activity. In children, the dose of generic micronized fenofibrate is 67 mg/day, while in adults the dose is 200 mg/day.

When such patients present in adulthood, they are usually heterozygous for LPL deficiency or apoC-II deficiency, and are often obese, and diabetic. Treatment with a low calorie, low-saturated fat, low refined carbohydrate diet is indicated in such patients. along with weight loss if indicated, exercise, tight control of blood glucose levels if they are diabetic, and the use of 200 mg/day of generic micronized fenofibrate. If after treatment with the fibrate their triglyceride are below 300 mg/dl, and their LDL cholesterol is elevated, a statin may need to be added to control their LDL cholesterol levels [22].

Dysbetalipoproteinemia

Patients with these disorders have elevations in total plasma cholesterol and triglyceride that are both in the range of 300–400 mg/dl. Their remnant lipoprotein cholesterol levels are markedly elevated (>50 mg/dl), their direct LDL cholesterol levels are usually decreased, and their HDL cholesterol levels are usually relatively normal. As previously stated, these patients have elevations in chylomicron and VLDL remnants, and may develop tubo-eruptive xanthomas and premature CHD. They are also at increased risk of developing gout and diabetes. They usually have the apoE2/2 genotype, but may occasionally have apoE deficiency (undetectable plasma apoE) or hepatic lipase deficiency. In the latter situation their HDL cholesterol levels may be elevated. The diagnosis is established by apoE genotyping, and when the genotype is normal (i.e., apoE3/3) and apoE is present, by the measuring of hepatic lipase activity in post-heparin plasma (obtained 10 min after the injection of 100 units/kg body weight of heparin). The plasma must be promptly isolated and frozen at −80° [23–26]. Treatment consists of a diet low in cholesterol, saturated fat, and sugar, and these patients are very responsive to micronized fenofibrate 200 mg/day, a statin, and extended release niacin. These agents can also be used in combination [23–26].

Lipoproteins Containing Apolipoprotein B-100

The lipoproteins that contain apoB-100 are made in the liver, and these include very-low-density lipoprotein, large low-density lipoproteins, and small dense low-density lipoproteins. Models of these lipoprotein particles are shown in Fig. 10.

Very-Low-Density Lipoproteins

Very-low-density lipoproteins (VLDLs) are made in the liver. VLDLs vary in molecular weight ($10–80 \times 10^6$ daltons) and in size (diameter 30–80 nm), have a plasma density of 0.93–1.006 g/ml, and migrate in the pre-beta region on lipoprotein electrophoresis. These particles are rich in triglyceride (about 60% by weight in the core of the particle) and contain about 10% cholesteryl ester. On their surface, these particles contain about 8% protein, 7% free cholesterol, and 15% phospholipids. The major protein of these particles is known as apolipoprotein (apo) B-100, and other surface proteins include apoC-I, apoC-II, and apoC-III. In the fed state, the average daily production of VLDL apoB-100 in humans is about 20 mg/kg/day.

Once VLDL enters the bloodstream, much of the triglyceride is rapidly removed via the action of lipoprotein lipase or LPL, similar to intestinal chylomicron particles. LPL is activated by apoC-II, and cleaves the fatty acid off the glycerol backbone. The fatty acids bind to albumin and are taken up by fat tissue or transported to a variety of other tissues in the body. In the fat, the fatty acids are converted back into triglyceride for long-term energy storage. ApoC-III inhibits this process of lipolysis. When much of the VLDL triglyceride has been removed, the particles pick up cholesteryl ester from HDL in exchange for triglyceride via the action of cholesteryl ester transfer protein. They also pick up apoE from HDL. VLDL are then either removed from plasma by the liver via the LDL receptor or become low-density lipoproteins.

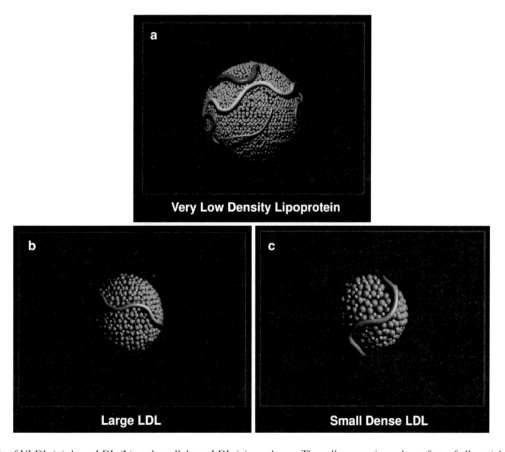

Fig. 10 Models of VLDL (**a**), large LDL (**b**), and small dense LDL (**c**) are shown. The *yellow protein* on the surface of all particles is apoB-100, with apoE (*orange*) and C apolipoproteins (smaller proteins in *yellow*) on the surface of VLDL. Created by Mr. Martin Jacob. Courtesy of Boston Heart Lab Corporation, Framingham, MA, USA

Familial Dyslipidemia

About 15% of patient with premature CHD have familial dyslipidemia, characterized by elevated triglyceride levels, and decreased HDL cholesterol levels [9]. These patients also usually have normal LDL cholesterol levels, but increased small dense LDL, and decreased large HDL particles [9]. These patients often have delayed clearance of VLDL and enhanced clearance of HDL, but some may also have overproduction of VLDL [3]. In contrast to patients with familial combined hyperlipidemia (see previous section), these patients do not have any evidence of enhanced conversion of squalene to lathosterol and cholesterol. These patients also are often overweight and may be insulin resistant or have diabetes. Restriction of calories and simple carbohydrates, along with exercise, optimization of plasma glucose levels, and either niacin or fibrate therapy [27].

Low-Density Lipoproteins

Low-density lipoproteins (LDLs) are mainly produced from the conversion of VLDLs to intermediate-density lipoproteins (IDLs) to LDLs. LDLs have a molecular weight of about 2×10^6 daltons, a diameter of 18–25 nm, a plasma density of 1.019–1.063 g/ml, and migrate in the beta region on lipoprotein electrophoresis. These particles are rich in cholesteryl ester (about 40% by weight in the core of the particle) and contain about 5% triglyceride. On their surface, these particles contain about 25% protein, 10% free cholesterol, and 20% phospholipids. The predominant protein of LDL is apoB-100. Occasionally LDL can contain trace amounts of other surface proteins, namely apoC-I, apoC-II, apoC-III, and apoE. In the fed state, the average daily conversion of VLDL apoB-100 to LDL apoB-100 in humans takes about 4–5 h, and is about 12 mg/kg/day. In normal plasma, LDL contains about 60–70% of the total cholesterol and about 80–90% of the total apoB. LDL apoB-100 has a plasma residence of about 3.5 days, and is taken up by various tissues through the action of the LDL receptor. LDL has been divided into large LDL (density 1.019–1.040 g/ml) and small dense LDL (density 1.041–1.063 g/ml). Small dense LDL is reported to more atherogenic than large LDL, and its apoB-100 also has a significantly longer residence time than that of apoB-100 in large LDL [3].

Familial Hypercholesterolemia

About 1 in 500 subjects in the general population, and about 1% of patients with premature CHD have heterozygous familial hypercholesterolemia, due to delayed clearance of LDL associated with defects in the LDL receptor or apoB genes [28–30]. These patients can develop arcus senilis, tendinous xanthomas in the Achilles tendons and on the hands, as well as xanthelasma, due to cholesterol deposition (see Fig. 11). Heterozygotes with this disorder usually have LDL cholesterol levels in excess of 300 mg/dl, while homozygotes often have value over 600 mg/dl [28–30]. Homozygotes are at high risk of developing CHD and aortic stenosis prior to age 20 years, unless treated [28]. Optimal therapy in homozygotes includes LDL apheresis, as well as ezetimibe and statin therapy. Heterozygotes usually can be effectively treated with the combination of an effective statin and ezetimibe.

Lipoprotein (a)

The final apoB-100 particle to be discussed in this section is lipoprotein (a) or Lp(a). This particle is often a small dense LDL particle, with a protein known as apo(a) attached to apoB-100. A model of Lp(a) is shown in Fig. 12 The apo(a) protein has multiple and variable copies of kringle 4-like domains (shaped like Danish pastries) and one copy of a kringle 5-like domain. These kringles have a high degree of homology with the kringle domains of plasminogen, important for clot lysis. High levels of Lp(a) >30 mg/dl are associated with an increased risk of CHD [31, 32]. Lp(a) is atherogenic because it is not only directly deposited in the artery wall, but also because it may prevent clot lysis by plasminogen. Moreover, Lp(a) serves as an acceptor of oxidized phospholipid from LDL.

Familial Lipoprotein (a) Excess

Lipoprotein (a) is in large part determined by the number of apo(a) isoforms, which are inherited. A decreased number of kringle 4-like repeats results in less intrahepatic degradation of apo(a) and more secretion. Most patients with familial Lp(a) excess have decreased kringle 4 repeats. Familial lipoprotein(a) excess is found in about 20% of familial with premature CHD [9]. The metabolism of apo(a) requires further elucidation. In our view, apo(a) attaches itself to VLDL apoB-100, and then remains with VLDL as it is converted to LDL, or if the VLDL is catabolized directly, the apo(a) is detached and recombined with a newly formed VLDL particle. Lp(a) excess is associated with both increased apo(a) and apoB-100 secretion into plasma Lp(a), as well as delayed clearance of apo(a), especially in patients with elevated LDL [33]. Lp(a) can be measured by using immunoassays specific for apo(a) or by measuring Lp(a) cholesterol using a lectin-based assay. Elevated levels of Lp(a) have been shown to be

Fig. 11 Signs of familial hypercholesterolemia are shown with arcus senilis (**a**), tendinous xanthomas on the Achilles tendons (**b**), and on the hands (**c**), and xanthelasma on the eyelids (**d**)

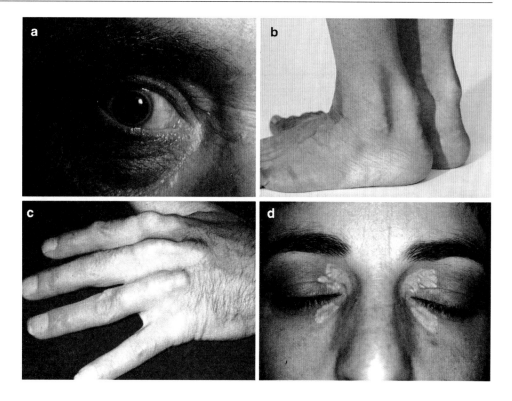

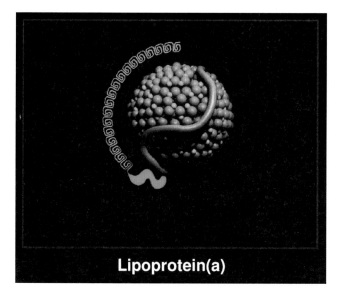

Fig. 12 A model of lipoprotein(a) (Lp(a) with the apo(a) protein attached to apoB-100 on the surface of a small dense LDL particle. High levels of Lp(a) >30 mg/dl are associated with an increased risk of heart disease and stroke, and can be lowered with niacin. Created by Mr. Martin Jacob. Courtesy of Boston Heart Lab Corporation, Framingham, MA, USA

Lp(a) levels got benefit from hormonal replacement therapy in terms of recurrent CHD risk reduction, as compared to placebo [34]. Clinical trials currently underway with niacin and a CETP inhibitor will test the hypothesis whether lowering elevated Lp(a) will reduce CHD risk.

Conclusions

Atherogenic lipoproteins include remnant lipoproteins, LDL, small dense LDL, and Lp(a), while HDL particles are protective. When dietary animal fats are replaced with vegetable oil or when subjects are given omega-3 fatty acid, significant CHD risk reduction has been noted [3]. When patients with CHD, hypercholesterolemia, diabetes, hypertension, or normal lipids with elevated C-reactive protein have been treated with statins, significant reductions in CHD morbidity and mortality have been noted [4]. The use of lipid-modifying agents including anion exchange resins, niacin, and fibrates has been associated with CHD risk reduction [34]. In the past, the focus has been on treating elevated LDL cholesterol levels; however, in the future efforts will be made to optimize the entire spectrum of lipoprotein abnormalities so frequently seen in subjects with CHD or high-risk subjects including elevated triglycerides, remnant lipoprotein cholesterol, small dense LDL, and lipoprotein(a), and low HDL cholesterol levels.

an independent predictor of CHD, and can be lowered by using estrogens in women, niacin, and CETP inhibitors. In the Hormone Estrogen Replacement Atherosclerosis Study (HERS) in women with CHD, only those with elevated

References

1. Expert Panel (2001) Executive summary of the third report of the National Cholesterol Education Program (NCEP) Expert Panel on Detection, Evaluation, and Treatment of High Blood Cholesterol in Adults (Adult Treatment Panel III). JAMA 285:2486–2497

2. Ingelsson E, Schaefer EJ, Contois JH, McNamara JR, Sullivan L, Keyes MJ, Pencina MJ, Schoonmaker C, Wilson PW, D'Agostino RB, Vasan RS (2007) Clinical utility of different lipid measures for prediction of coronary heart disease in men and women. JAMA 298:776–785

3. Schaefer EJ (2002) E.V. McCollum Award Lecture: Lipoproteins, nutrition, and heart disease. Am J Clin Nutr 75:191–212

4. Baigent C, Keech A, Kearney PM, Blackwell L, Buck G, Pollicino C, Kirby A, Sourjina T, Peto R, Collins R, Simes R (2005) Cholesterol Treatment Trialists Collaborators. Efficacy and safety of cholesterol-lowering treatment:prospective meta-analysis of data from 90, 056 participants in 14 randomised trials of statins. Lancet 366:1267–1278

5. Lamon-Fava S, Diffenderfer MR, Barrett PH, Buchsbaum A, Matthan NR, Lichtenstein AH, Dolnikowski GG, Horvath K, Asztalos BF, Zago V, Schaefer EJ (2007) Effects of different doses of atorvastatin on human apolipoprotein B-100, B-48, and A-I metabolism. J Lipid Res 48:1746–1753

6. van Himbergen TM, Matthan NR, Resteghini NA, Otokozawa S, Ai M, Stein EA, Jones PH, Schaefer EJ (2009) Comparison of the effects of maximal dose atorvastatin and rosuvastatin therapy on cholesterol synthesis and absorption markers. J Lipid Res 50:730–739

7. Lamon-Fava S, Schaefer EJ, Garuti R, Salen G, Calandra S (2002) Two novel mutations in the sterol 27-hydroxylase gene causing cerebrotendinous xanthomatosis. Clin Genet 61:185–191

8. Keren Z, Falik-Zaccel TC (2009) Cerebrotendinous xanthomatosis (CTX), a treatable lipid storage disorder. Pediatr Endocrinol Rev 7:6–11

9. Genest JJ, Martin-Munley S, McNamara JR, Ordovas JM, Jenner J, Meyers R, Wilson PWF, Schaefer EJ (1992) Prevalence of familial lipoprotein disorders in patients with premature coronary artery disease. Circulation 85:2025–2033

10. van Himbergen T, Otokozawa S, Matthan NR, Schaefer EJ, Buchsbaum A, Ai M, van Tits LJH, de Graaf J, Stalenhoef A (2009) Familial combined hyperlipidemia is associated with alterations in the cholesterol synthesis pathway. Arterioscler Thromb Vasc Biol (2010) 30:113–120.

11. Altmann SW, Davis HR Jr, Zhu LJ, Yao X, Hoos LM, Tezloff G, Iyer SP, Macquire M, Golovko A, Zeng M, Wang L, Murgolo N, Graziano MP (2004) Niemann-Pick C1 Like 1 protein is critical for intestinal absorption. Science 303:1201–1204

12. Davis HR Jr, Basso F, Hoos LM, Tezloff G, Lally SM, Altmann SW (2008) Cholesterol homeostasis by the intestine: lessons from Niemann Pick C1 Like 1 (NPC1L1). Atheroscler Suppl 9:77–81

13. Patel MD, Thompson PD (2006) Phytosterols and vascular disease. Atherosclerosis 186:12–19

14. Matthan NB, Pencina M, Larocquw JM, Jacques PF, D'Agostino RB, Schaefer EJ, Lichtenstein AH (2009) Alterations in cholesterol absorption and synthesis characterize Framingham offspring study participants with coronary disease. J Lipid Res 50(9):1927–35

15. Matthan NR, Restighini N, Robertson M, Ford I, Shepherd J, Packard C, Buckley BM, Jukema JW, Lichtenstein AH, Schaefer EJ (2009) Cholesterol absorption and synthesis in individuals with and without CHD events during pravastatin therapy: insights from the PROSPER Trial. J Lipid Res (2010) 51:202–209

16. Sudhop T, Lutjohann D, Kodal A, Igel M, Tribble DL, Shah S, Perevozskaya I, von Bergmann K (2002) Inhibition of intestinal cholesterol absorption by ezetimibe in humans. Circulation 106:1943–1948

17. Pearson TA, Ballantyne CM, Veltri E, Shah A, Bird S, Lin J, Rosenberg E, Tershakovec AM (2009) Pooled analysis of effects on C reactive protein and low density lipoprotein cholesterol in placebo controlled trials of ezetimibe or ezetimibe added to baseline statin therapy. Am J Cardiol 103:369–374

18. Ajees AA, Anantharamaiah GM, Mishra VK, Hussain MM, Murthy VK (2006) Crystal structure of human apolipoprotein A-I: insights into its protect effect against cardiovascular disease. Proc Natl Acad Sci USA 103:2136–2131

19. Zamel R, Khan R, Pollex H, Hegele RA (2008) Abetalipoproteinemia: 2 case reports and literature review. Orphanet J Rare Dis 3:19–25

20. Tarugi P, Averna M, DiLeo E, Cefalu AB, Noto D, Magnolo L, Cattin L, Bertolini S, Calandra S (2007) Molecular diagnosis of hypobetalipoproteinemia: an ENID review. Atherosclerosis 195:19–27

21. Hegele RA, Pollex RL (2009) Hypobetalipoproteinemia: phenomics and genomics. Mol Cell Biochem 326:35–43

22. Hegele RA, Joy T (2009) Novel LPL mutations associated with LPL deficiency: 2 case reports and a literature review. Can J Physiol Pharmacol 87:151–160

23. Brom DJ, Byrne P, Jopnes S, Marais AD (2002) Dysbetalipoproteinemia: clinical and pathophysiologic features. S Afr Med J 92:892–897

24. Schaefer EJ, Gregg RE, Ghiselli G, Forte TM, Ordovas JM, Zech LA, Lindgren FT, Brewer HB Jr (1986) Familial apolipoprotein E deficiency. J Clin Invest 78:1206–1219

25. Connelly PW, Hegele RA (1998) Hepatic lipase deficiency. Crit Rev Clin Lab Sci 35:547–572

26. Deeb SS, Zambon A, Carr MC, Ayyobi AF, Brunzell JD (2003) Hepatic lipase and dyslipidemia:interactions among genetic variants, obesity, and diet. J Lipid Res 44:1279–1286

27. Knopp RH, Paramsothy P, Atkinson B, Dowdy A (2008) Comprehensive lipid management versus aggressive LDL lowering to reduce cardiovascular risk. Am J Cardiol 101:48B–57B

28. Sprecher DL, Hoeg JM, Schaefer EJ, Zech LA, Gregg RE, Lakatos E, Brewer HB Jr (1985) The association of LDL receptor activity, LDL cholesterol level, and clinical course in homozygous familial hypercholesterolemia. Metabolism 34:294–299

29. Hobbs HH, Brown MJ, Goldstein JL (1992) Molecular genetics of the LDL receptor gene in familial hypercholesterolemia. Hum Mutat 1:445–466

30. Farese RV Jr, Linton MF, Young SG (1992) Apolipoprotein B mutations affecting cholesterol levels. J Intern Med 231:643–652

31. Schaefer EJ, Lamon-Fava S, Jenner JL, Ordovas JM, Davis CE, Lippel K, Levy RI (1994) Lipoprotein(a) levels predict coronary heart disease in the lipid research clinics coronary prevention trial. JAMA 271:999–1003

32. Erqou S, Kaptoge S, Perry PC, DiAngelantino E, Thompson A, White IR, Marcovina SM, Collins R, Thompson SG, Danesh J; Emerging Risk Factors Collaboration (2009) Lipoprotein(a) as a risk factor coronary heart disease and stroke. JAMA 302:412–423

33. Jenner JL, Seman LJ, Millar JS, Lamon-Fava S, Welty FK, Dolnikowski GG, Marcovina SM, Lichtenstein AH, Barrett PH, deLuca C, Schaefer EJ (2005) The metabolism of apolipoproteins (a) and B-100 within plasma lipoprotein(a) in human beings. Metabolism 54:361–369

34. Shlipak MG, Simon JA, Vittinghoff E, Lin F, Barrett-Connor E, Knopp RH, Levy RI, Hulley SB (2000) Estrogen and progestin, lipoprotein(a), and the risk of recurrent coronary heart disease events after menopause. JAMA 283:1845–1852

Regulation of ApoA-I Gene Expression and Prospects to Increase Plasma ApoA-I and HDL Levels

Vassilis I. Zannis, Adelina Duka, Konstantinos Drosatos, Despina Sanoudou, Georgios Koukos, Eleni Zanni, and Dimitris Kardassis

Abbreviations

C/EBP	CAAT/enhancer binding protein
CAT	Chloramphenicol acetyl transferase
EGR-1	Early growth response factor-1
FXR	Farnesoid X receptor
HNF-4	Hepatocyte nuclear factor-4
HDL	High density lipoprotein
HRE	Hormone response element
LRH-1	Liver receptor homolog-1
LXRs	Liver X receptors
PPARα	Peroxisome proliferator-activated receptor α
PLTP	Phospholipid transfer protein
RORα	Retinoic acid receptor-related orphan receptor α
RXRα	Retinoid X receptor α
SHP	Small heterodimer partner
SP1	Specificity protein 1
SR-BI	Scavenger receptor class B type I
SREBP	Sterol regulatory element binding protein
WT	Wild type

Transcriptional Regulation of the Human ApoA-I Gene in Cell Culture and in ApoA-I Transgenic Mice

Role of hormone nuclear receptors, SP1 and of a common enhancer on the transcriptional regulation of the human apoA-I gene in cell cultures. Earlier studies established that there is a linkage and common regulatory mechanism of the apoA-I/apoCIII/apoA-IV gene cluster (Fig. 1a). In this cluster, the distal regulatory region of the apoCIII promoter is an enhancer that increases the strength of the neighboring promoters in vitro [1–4]. When the apoCIII enhancer is joined with the proximal apoA-I promoter, then the activity of the promoter increases over tenfold [1–4]. The proximal apoA-I promoter contains two hormone response elements (HREs) that bind orphan and ligand-dependent nuclear receptors [5, 6]. The apoCIII enhancer also has two HREs which differ in their receptor specificity, and also has three SP1 binding sites [1, 7] (Fig. 1a).

Systematic in vitro mutagenesis of different sites of the promoter/enhancer cluster and determination of the promoter activity by CAT assays showed that mutations in the HRE, and the SP1 binding sites affect the activity of the apoA-I promoter/enhancer cluster in HepG2 cells [1–7]. Mutation in the proximal HREs reduced the strength of the promoter/enhancer to 6% of the WT control, whereas mutations in the HRE (I$_4$) of the enhancer reduced the activity of the promoter enhancer cluster to 18% of the WT control (Fig. 1b). Finally, the individual mutations in the SP1 binding site reduced the activity of the promoter enhancer cluster to 40–60% of the WT control (Fig. 1b).

The receptor specificity of the HREs of the apoA-I promoter and the apoCIII enhancer were determined by DNA binding gel electrophoresis assays. These analyses established that both HREs present in the proximal apoA-I promoter bind HNF-4, other orphan receptors, and a variety of ligand-dependent nuclear receptors with different affinities [6] (Fig. 1c). One of the HREs of the enhancer binds also HNF-4, other orphan nuclear receptors, and ligand-dependent nuclear receptors with different affinities, whereas the other HRE does not bind HNF-4, binds other orphan receptors, and different combinations of ligand-dependent nuclear receptors with different affinities [7] (Fig. 1c).

Transcriptional regulation of the human apoA-I gene in transgenic mice. To validate the conclusions drawn by the in vitro experiments, we generated a variety of transgenic mouse lines which express the WT A-I/CIII cluster or the same cluster with the mutations in the HREs and the binding sites of SP1 and other transcription factors. In these constructs, the apoCIII gene was replaced by the CAT gene (Fig. 2).

V.I. Zannis (✉)
Whitaker Cardiovascular Institute,
Boston University School of Medicine,
Boston, MA, USA
e-mail: vzannis@bu.edu

E.J. Schaefer (ed.), *High Density Lipoproteins, Dyslipidemia, and Coronary Heart Disease*,
DOI 10.1007/978-1-4419-1059-2_2, © Springer Science+Business Media, LLC 2010

Fig. 1 (**a**) Arrangement of the apoA-I and apoCIII genes on chromosome 11. The figure also shows the position of the HREs as well as other regulatory elements of the proximal apoA-I promoter and the apoCIII enhancer. (**b**) Diagram showing how mutations in the HNF-4 and SP1 binding sites affect the activity of the apoA-I promoter/apoCIII enhancer in HepG2 cells. The information was obtained by transient transfection assays using the wild-type promoter or promoters mutated in the sites indicated by the *arrows*. *Ovals* represent transcription factors bound to different regulatory elements. (**c**) Position of the HREs of the apoA-I promoter/apoCIII enhancer and binding specificity to these elements of orphan and ligand-dependent nuclear receptors

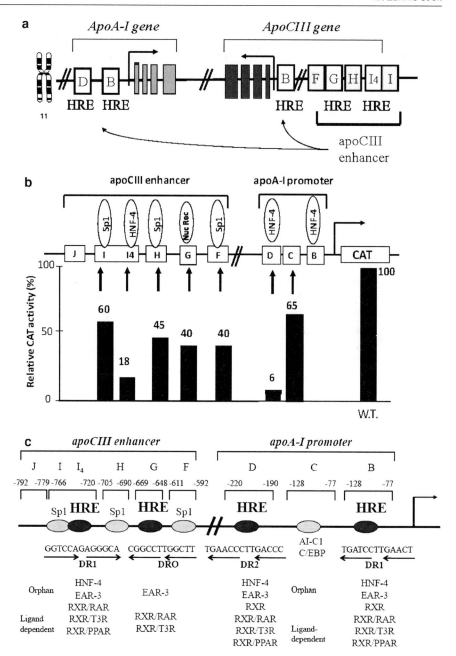

In these mice that are harboring wild-type and mutated promoter/enhancer constructs, the activity of the apoA-I promoter in vivo was assessed by the analysis of the steady state hepatic apoA-I mRNA levels using Northern blotting and phosphorimaging. Three or more mouse lines were studied for each construct. In the mutant lines we systematically altered individual HREs [8, 9], or individual SP1 binding sites [9]. Using these mouse lines, we were able to assess what is the contribution of the different HREs and the SP1 binding sites and the binding sites of other transcription factors in the strength and the tissue-specific expression of the apoA-I gene in vivo [8–10].

Analysis of mice expressing the WT apoA-I construct showed that major sites of apoA-I synthesis were the liver and the intestine (Fig. 2). Minor sites were kidney, spleen, and lung [8].

Mutations in the HREs of the proximal apoA-I promoter reduced the hepatic and intestinal expression of the apoA-I gene to 15% of the WT control (compare lanes 2,3 of the WT control with lanes 6,7 of the transgenic mice) (Figs. 2 and 3a). This finding was unexpected. The cell culture studies had shown that mutations in proximal HRE inactivate the apoA-I promoter in HepG2 cells [5]. In contrast, the in vivo data demonstrated that the promoter carrying these mutations

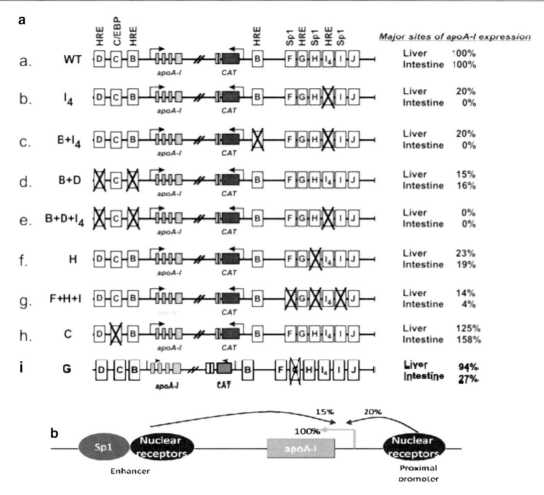

Fig. 2 (**a**) Summary of expression data in transgenic mice carrying the WT apoA-I/apoCIII locus (a) or the same locus mutated at the HREs (b–e, i) or the SP1 binding sites (f, g) or the C/EBP binding site (h). The mutation sites are indicated by *X*. The *panel* illustrates that mutations in the proximal apoA-I promoter or the apoCIII enhancer drastically reduce, but do not eliminate, the hepatic transcription whereas mutations in the apoCIII enhancer may abolish or diminish the intestinal transcription. (**b**) Simplified presentation of the apoA-I transgene containing the proximal promoter of the apoCIII enhancer and the major factors which control apoA-I gene expression

maintains 16% of intestinal expression, and approximately 15% hepatic expression.

A mutation in the HRE of the apoCIII enhancer that binds HNF-4 abolished the intestinal expression and reduced the hepatic expression to 20% of the WT control. Compare lanes 2,3 representing two WT transgenic mice with lanes 8,9 representing two mutant transgenic mice (Fig. 3c). The same result is essentially obtained when both the HREs of the apoCIII enhancer, and the proximal apoCIII promoter were mutated. In this case, the intestinal expression was lost, and the hepatic expression was reduced to approximately 20% of the wild-type control (Fig. 2).

Mutagenesis of all the three HREs of the proximal promoter and the apoCIII enhancer that bind HNF-4 abolished the hepatic and intestinal expression of the apoA-I gene (Fig. 4a). The findings demonstrate that different members of hormone nuclear receptor family are essential for the

expression of the apoA-I gene. The factors which bind to the proximal promoter alone contribute 20% to the hepatic transcription and the factors which bind to the apoCIII enhancer alone contribute 15% to the hepatic transcription. However, through synergistic interaction of the factors which bind to the promoter and the enhancer, we achieve 100% transcription (Fig. 4b).

Mutations in the other HRE on element G of the apoCIII enhancer that does not bind HNF-4 but binds other orphan- and ligand-dependent nuclear receptors, do not affect the hepatic expression, but reduced the intestinal expression to 27% of the WT control (Fig. 2).

Analysis of another transgenic line that carries mutations in the SP1 binding site on element H of the enhancer showed that it reduced the hepatic expression to 23% and intestinal expression to approximately 19% of the WT control (Fig. 2). Mutations in all three SP1 binding sites of the apoCIII

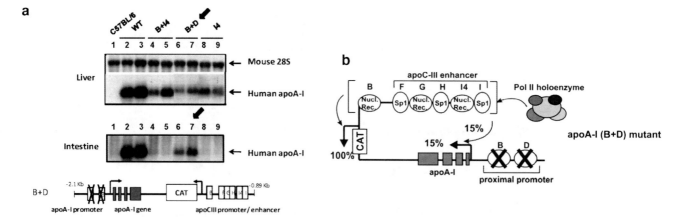

a

Mutations in the two HREs of the apoA-I promoter reduced the hepatic, intestinal and renal expression of the apoA-I gene to approximately 15% of the WT control.

b

Reduction in hepatic expression (15%) and intestinal expression (16%) of the apoA-I gene. No effect on apoCIII expression

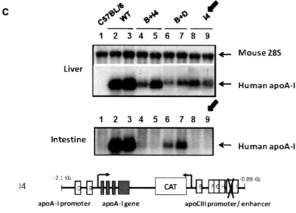

c

Mutations in the HRE of the apoCIII enhancer abolished the intestinal expression and reduced the hepatic expression of the apoA-I gene to 20% of the control

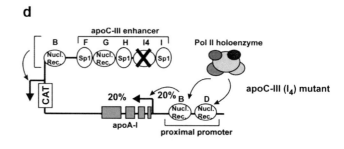

d

Reduction in hepatic expression (20%) of the apoA-I gene. Complete inhibition of the intestinal expression of the apoA-I gene.

Fig. 3 (**a**) Northern blotting of hepatic and intestinal RNA highlighting the changes in expression in the transgenic that carries the B&D mutation in both HREs of the proximal promoter that bind HNF-4 and other nuclear receptors. (**b**) Proposed mechanism of transcription when the proximal apoA-I promoter is inactivated as a result of the mutations in the two HREs of the proximal promoter. (**c**) Northern blotting of hepatic and intestinal mRNA highlighting the changes in expression in the transgenic that carries the I_4 mutation in the HRE of the apoCIII enhancer that binds HNF-4 and other nuclear receptor. (**d**) Proposed mechanism of transcription when the enhancer is inactivated as a result of mutations in the HRE of the enhancer that bind HNF-4 and other nuclear receptors

enhancer on elements H, I, and F reduced to 14 and 4% respectively the hepatic and the intestinal expression as compared to the WT control (Fig. 2).

Finally, mutations in the C/EBP binding site of the proximal promoter increased the hepatic and intestinal expression to 125 and 158% as compared to the WT control [11] (Fig. 2). The effects of all the mutations on different regulatory elements of the proximal apoA-I promoter and the apoCIII enhancer on the in vivo transcription of the apoA-I gene is summarized in Fig. 2.

Figures 3b, d and 4b provide putative mechanisms of the transcription of the apoA-I/apoCIII gene cluster by mutations in the different regulatory elements of the cluster and how

these mutations might affect gene transcription. The most interesting and unexpected finding was that inactivation by mutagenesis of the proximal apoA-I promoter, preserves hepatic and intestinal transcription at levels approximately 15% as compared to the WT control (Fig. 3a, b). This indicates that in the absence of the proximal promoter, the apoCIII enhancer alone can drive the hepatic and intestinal transcription of the apoA-I gene. On the other hand, the mutations in the HRE of the enhancer that binds HNF-4 abolished the intestinal expression and reduced the hepatic expression to 20% of the WT control (Fig. 3c, d). In this case, the proximal promoter alone can drive the hepatic transcription of the apoA-I gene with an efficiency of 20% as compared to the WT control.

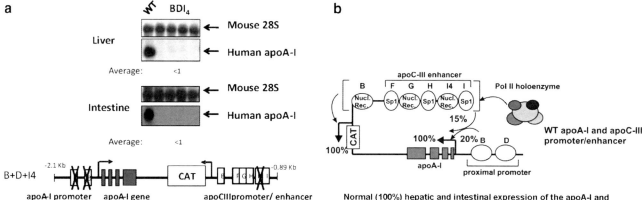

a

Liver

← Mouse 28S
← Human apoA-I

Average: <1

Intestine

← Mouse 28S
← Human apoA-I

Average: <1

B+D+I4

apoA-I promoter apoA-I gene apoCIIIpromoter/ enhancer

Mutations in the HREs of the apoA-I promoter and apoCIII enhancer (which bind HNF-4) abolished the intestinal and hepatic expression of the apoA-I gene.

b

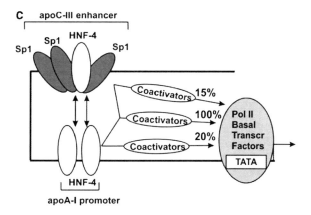

apoC-III enhancer

WT apoA-I and apoC-III promoter/enhancer

proximal promoter

Normal (100%) hepatic and intestinal expression of the apoA-I and apoC-III genes. We observe transcriptional synergism in vivo: The contribution of the promoter is 20% and of the enhancer is 15%. The result is not additive (35%) but synergistic (100%).

c apoC-III enhancer

Sp1 Sp1 HNF-4 Sp1

Coactivators 15%
Coactivators 100% Pol II Basal Transcr Factors
Coactivators 20%
TATA

HNF-4

apoA-I promoter

Fig. 4 (**a**) Northern blotting of hepatic and intestinal mRNA highlighting the changes in expression in the transgenic that carries the B&D&I$_4$ mutations in the HRE of the proximal promoter and the apoCIII enhancer that bind HNF-4 and other nuclear receptors. (**b**) Proposed mechanism of transcription of the apoA-I gene by the WT promoter and enhancer. (**c**) Schematic representation showing putative independent and the synergistic contributions of protein complexes assembled on the proximal apoA-I promoter and the apoCII enhancer on the transcription of the apoA-I gene. The diagram is based on the in vivo transcription data shown in (**a**) and Fig. 3a–c as well as on the establishment of physical interactions between HNF-4 and SP1 at the indicated sites of the apoCIII promoter and the apoCIII enhancer. The mechanism involves a simplified version of known protein–protein interactions of the promoter and enhancer complexes and coactivators, with the proteins of the basal transcription complex

Mutations in all the SP1 binding sites of the apoCIII enhancer have similar effects (Fig. 2).

Figure 4c depicts a putative simplified mechanism that may explain the synergy between the proximal promoters and the apoCIII enhancer in the transcription of the genes of the apoA-I/apoCIII/apoA-IV gene cluster. The transcription factors SP1 and HNF-4 are involved in the transcriptional activation of the genes of the cluster. Inactivation of the proximal promoter still allows the factors bound to the enhancer to interact with coactivators and proteins of the basal transcription complex, and drive the transcription of the apoA-I gene at levels of 15% of the WT control. Inactivation of the enhancer allows the factors bound to the proximal promoter drive the transcription at levels of 20% of the WT control. However, when both the factors that recognize the proximal promoter and the apoCIII enhancer are allowed to bind to their cognate sites, then we speculate that they can cooperate via protein–protein interactions and this leads to transcriptional synergism that drives the transcription at levels of 100% [12–14] (Fig. 4c).

Genetic mutations in apoA-I and other genes of the HDL pathway influence the stability and the concentration of HDL and apoA-I in plasma. Following synthesis and secretion by the liver and other tissues, apoA-I interacts with a variety of other proteins present in the surface of cells or in plasma to form the HDL particle (Fig. 5).

More precisely, secreted apoA-I via interactions with ABCA1 (Fig. 3, step 1) receives phospholipids and cholesterol from cells. Absence of ABCA1 decreases dramatically plasma apoA-I levels despite the normal synthesis and

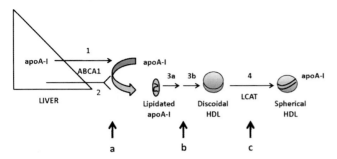

Fig. 5 Schematic representation of interaction of the secreted apoA-I with various membrane and plasma proteins that lead to the biogenesis of HDL. a–c and the corresponding *arrows* indicate defects in different steps of the pathway that reduce the plasma apoA-I and HDL levels

secretion of apoA-I [15]. The lipidated apoA-I produced goes through one or more steps (Fig. 5, steps 3a, 3b) that are not fully understood, and reaches the stage of discoidal HDL particles. The esterification of cholesterol present on these particles by the action of the plasma enzyme lecithin:cholesterol acyltransferase (LCAT) converts the discoidal HDL into spherical particles (Fig. 5, step 4). Mutations in ABCA1 and LCAT in humans have profound effects on plasma apoA-I and HDL levels. Using adenovirus-mediated gene transfer of apoA-I mutants in apoA-I-deficient mice, we have shown that mutations in apoA-I can disrupt different steps of the pathway and result in low plasma HDL and apoA-I levels. These mutations generate the following phenotypes that are indicated by arrows in Fig. 5: (a) do not synthesize HDL due to apoA-I mutations that prevent apoA-I/ABCA1 interactions [16–18]; (b) generate unstable lipidated apoA-I intermediates that are catabolized fast by the kidney [19]; (c) accumulate discoidal HDL [20, 21]. Some other apoA-I mutations cause hypertriglyceridemia or other forms of dyslipidemia and may also affect low plasma HDL and apoA-I levels and distribution in different lipoprotein fractions [22]. An example of detailed analyses on how apoA-I mutations disrupt the pathway of biogenesis of HDL and lead to low HDL levels is provided for the naturally occurring apoA-I(Leu141Arg)$_{Pisa}$ and the apoA-I(Leu159Arg)$_{Fin}$ mutants [19].

Cell culture studies showed that both the apoA-I$_{Pisa}$ and apoA-I$_{Fin}$ were secreted efficiently from cells [20].

In vitro assays showed that both mutants had near-normal capacity to promote ABCA1-mediated cholesterol efflux but had diminished capacity to activate LCAT. The in vitro experiments thus suggested that these mutants might have affected the activity of LCAT in vivo. To confirm this finding, we performed adenovirus-mediated gene transfer of the apoA-I(Leu141Arg)$_{Pisa}$ and apoA-I(Leu159Arg)$_{FIN}$ mutants in apoA-I-deficient (apoA-I$^{-/-}$) mice. The gene transfer resulted in greatly decreased total plasma cholesterol and decrease in the cholesteryl ester to total cholesterol ratio (CE/TC) in mice expressing the apoA-I(Leu141Arg)$_{Pisa}$ and apoA-I(Leu159Arg)$_{FIN}$ as compared to mice expressing the

WT apoA-I. The plasma apoA-I levels were greatly reduced (see table on top of panels A–E of Fig. 6). FPLC fractionation of plasma showed diminished HDL cholesterol peaks (Fig. 6K, L). Electron microscopy showed the presence of only few spherical particles (compare Fig. 6B, D representing the two mutants with Fig. 6A representing WT apoA-I). The mutations caused accumulation of preβ1-HDL and small size α4-HDL particles in mice expressing the two mutants (Fig. 6G, I), as compared to mice expressing wild-type (WT) apoA-I (Fig. 6F).

In an attempt to correct the low apoA-I and HDL levels, we treated apoA-I-deficient mice with adenoviruses expressing either of the two mutants and human LCAT. This treatment normalized the plasma apoA-I levels (see table on top of panels A–E of Fig. 6), as well as the HDL cholesterol levels (Fig. 6K, L). The total cholesterol ester to cholesterol ratio of HDL containing the mutant proteins was low (<0.3) and increased to normal levels (~0.75) following LCAT treatment (Fig. 6K, L). The treatment also restored normal preβ- and α-HDL subpopulations (Fig. 6H, J) and generated spherical HDL as determined by EM (Fig. 6C, E). Figure 6M is a schematic representation that is consistent with the experimental finding. The mutations appear to create LCAT insufficiency in plasma that prevents cholesterol esterification of an early nascent HDL precursor and slows down its conversion to discoidal and then spherical HDL. As a result, this cholesteryl ester-poor intermediate is catabolized fast by the kidney, resulting in low apoA-I and HDL levels.

Regulation of the apoA-I gene in cell cultures and in animal models deficient in specific transcription factors. A series of in vivo studies have highlighted the importance of the HREs for the transcriptional activity of apoA-I as well as the other genes of the cluster. The expression of the apoA-I/apoCIII/apoA-IV genes is abolished in fetal liver of mice in which the HNF-4 is inactivated by homologous recombination [23] or in hepatic cell cultures infected with recombinant adenoviruses expressing a dominant negative form of HNF-4 [24].

Inactivation of PPARα in mice is associated with reduced levels of hepatic apoA-I mRNA and reduced plasma apoA-I and HDLc levels [25]. On the other hand, liver-specific inactivation of the RXRα gene in mice is associated with reduced expression of the apoA-I gene [26]. Finally, inactivation of the orphan receptor retinoic acid receptor-related orphan receptor α (RORα) in mice decreased intestinal apoA-I mRNA levels [27]. Consistent with this observation, it was found that the orphan receptor RORα binds to the TATA box of the rat and mouse apoA-I gene and increases apoA-I transcription in CaCo-2 cells [27].

Plasma apoA-I and HDLc levels as well as apoA-I gene transcription increase in mice with experimental nephrotic syndrome, and these changes were associated with a fivefold increase in the levels of early growth response factor (EGR-1).

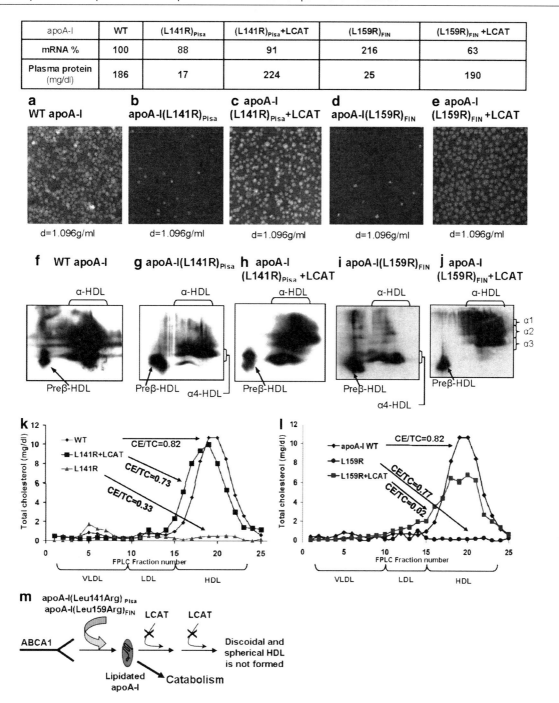

apoA-I	WT	(L141R)$_{Pisa}$	(L141R)$_{Pisa}$+LCAT	(L159R)$_{FIN}$	(L159R)$_{FIN}$ +LCAT
mRNA %	100	88	91	216	63
Plasma protein (mg/dl)	186	17	224	25	190

Fig. 6 *Top table*: ApoA-I mRNA levels expressed as percent of WT (control) and the plasma apoA-I levels when apoA-I$^{-/-}$ mice were infected with adenoviruses expressing the mutant apoA-I forms. *Panels A–E*: EM picture of HDL isolated from apoA-I$^{-/-}$ 4 h postinfection with the adenoviruses expressing the indicated apoA-I mutants alone or the apoA-I mutants and human LCAT. *Panels F–J*: Analysis of the plasma of mice infected with the same adenoviruses as those used in *Panels A–E* by 2D electrophoresis. *Panels K–L*: FPLC profile of mice infected with adenoviruses expressing the indicated mutants alone or the apoA-I mutants and LCAT. The phenotypes observed are similar for low or high dose of adenovirus (data not shown). *Panel M*: Schematic representation showing the pathway of biogenesis of HDL and how the two mutations contribute to the catabolism of the lipidated apoA-I particles

In contrast, EGR-1$^{-/-}$ mice had reduced plasma HDLc, apoA-I and hepatic apoA-I mRNA levels [28]. These findings suggest that EGR-1, which binds to the regulatory element D, contributes to the basal as well as inducible transcription of the human apoA-I gene [28].

Bile acids, which are natural ligands for the nuclear receptor farnesoid X receptor (FXR) inhibit apoA-I gene expression in vitro and in vivo [29, 30]. It was shown that FXR and the monomeric nuclear receptor LRH-1 bind to the apoA-I promoter next to the previously characterized regulatory element B (Fig. 1c). FXR inhibits and LRH-1 activates the apoA-I promoter. It was proposed that FXR downregulates the apoA-I gene transcription both by binding to the apoA-I promoter as well as by inducing small heterodimer partner (SHP) which, in turn, represses the activity of LRH-1 [31].

In vivo regulation of expression of the human apoA-I gene in apoA-I transgenic mice. Earlier studies in transgenic mice and rabbits indicated that fibrates increase the human apoA-I gene transcription as well as apoA-I and HDL plasma levels [32–34]. It was suggested that the increase was mediated by activating PPARα [35], which binds to the regulatory element D of apoA-I (Fig. 1c). The rodent apoA-I gene expression is repressed by fibrate treatment [35]. It has been proposed that the repression is caused by nucleotide differences in element D of the rodent gene which prevent binding of PPARα, as well as due to the binding of Rev-Erbα adjacent to the TATA box of the rat apoA-I promoter [35].

The transgenic mice depicted in Fig. 2B that carry the human apoA-I gene under the control of the apoA-I promoter and apoCIII enhancer have been bred with apoA-1$^{-/-}$ mice to generate apoA-I transgenic mice in apoA-I-deficient background. These mice synthesize HDL, which contains human apoA-I as its main apolipoprotein. As indicated, these mice are expected to record faithfully changes in human apoA-I gene transcription in vivo in response to extracellular stimuli such as diet, exercise, and administration of various drugs designed to increase plasma apoA-I and HDL levels. We have treated a group of female apoA-I transgenic mice with a powder diet containing equivalent of 160 mg fenofibrate/65 kg/day. The fenofibrate treatment did not increase the hepatic apoA-I mRNA or the plasma apoA-I levels (Fig. 7a, b) but increased 1.95-fold the total cholesterol levels in the treated group as compared to the control group. The FPLC analysis showed that all plasma cholesterol following fenofibrate treatment was distributed in the HDL region, and the HDL cholesterol peak was shifted toward lower densities (Fig. 7c).

The differences between our study and in previous studies [32–34] can be explained on the basis of the mechanism of transcriptional regulation of the human apoA-I gene in vitro and in vivo described above. In the transgenic mice and rabbits used in previous studies [32–34], the transgene lacks the apoCIII enhancer, and the transcription of the apoA-I gene was driven by the proximal apoA-I promoter alone [36, 37]. As demonstrated in Fig. 3d in the absence of apoCIII enhancer, the intestinal transcription of the apoA-I gene is abolished, and the hepatic transcription is reduced to 20% as compared to mice that carry both the proximal promoter and the apoCIII enhancer [8, 10].

It is expected that in the fenofibrate-treated mice the expression of the human *apoA-I* gene will be controlled by synergistic interactions between RXRα/PPARα heterodimers bound to the proximal promoter and the distal enhancer as well as the interactions of the distantly bound RXRα/PPARα heterodimers and SP1 [8] (Fig. 4b, c). These interactions are not possible in the transgenic mice that lack the apoCIII enhancer, and this may explain the altered expression of the human *apoA-I* transgene lacking the apoCIII enhancer that was observed previously [32–34].

Microarray analysis of hepatic mRNA of untreated and treated mice showed the fenofibrate treatment upregulated greatly (5.86-fold) the phospholipid transfer protein (*Pltp*) and the lipoprotein lipase (*Lpl*) (8.85-fold) [38] genes expression as

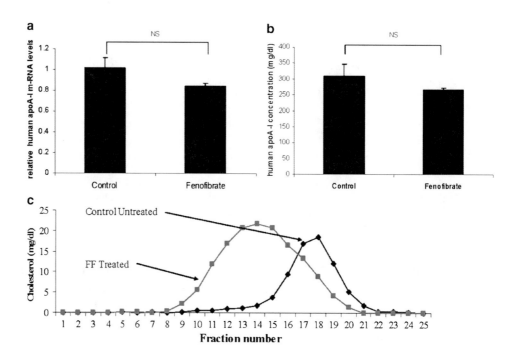

Fig. 7 Hepatic human apoA-I mRNA and plasma apoA-I levels and FPLC profiles of apoA-I transgenic mice treated with either a control or a fenofibrate containing diet. (**a**) Hepatic apoA-I mRNA levels. (**b**) Plasma apoA-I levels. (**c**) FPLC profiles of total cholesterol

reported previously [38, 39]. The increased *Pltp*-mediated phospholipid transfer cannot explain the observed increase and the shift of the HDL peak to the lower density region in response to fenofibrate treatment. The fenofibrate treatment caused 1.51-fold reduction in Sr-Bi gene expression, and this change may have contributed to some extent to the increase in the size and the levels of HDL [40]. Previous studies have also indicated that fenofibrate promotes the degradation of Sr-Bi [41]. The fenofibrate treatment also downregulated greatly (9.75-fold) the expression of *Apoa4* gene as described previously [42]. In addition, the fenofibrate treatment caused small but not statistically significant changes in the expression of mouse *Apoc3*, *Apoa2*, and apoA-V genes as well as in other genes that are involved in the biogenesis and maturation of HDL such as *Abca1, Lcat, Abcg1 and Apoe* (Table 1). Overall, the increase in HDL could not be accounted for by upregulation of apoA-I and Apoa2 genes as suggested previously [32–34] or due to changes in several other genes implicated in the biogenesis of HDL. However, significant increases were observed in the expression of genes involved in triglyceride hydrolysis (Table 1) and in phospholipid biosynthesis that are important for HDL formation [43].

Currently, there is an intense interest to increase HDL levels in humans by affecting either apoA-I synthesis or any other protein involved directly or indirectly in the biogenesis of HDL. The new apoA-I transgenic mouse model that carries the apoA-I gene and the control of its proximal promoter and the apoCIII enhancer may be an optimal model to study the effect of new pharmaceuticals and other stimuli on the upregulation of the apoA-I that will lead to an increase in plasma HDL levels.

It is important in any attempt to increase plasma HDL levels not only to avoid undesirable side effects but also to produce functional HDL particles. In this regard, studies of transgenic and knockout mice have established that increased expression of apoA-I increase HDL levels and protect from atherosclerosis. This indicates that the HDL generated by overexpression of either apoA-I is functional and has car-

dioprotective effects. In contrast, inactivation of the SR-B1 gene increase HDL level but promote atherogenesis, or may have acquired new properties that are detrimental [40].

Acknowledgments This work was supported by grants from the National Institutes of Health (HL48739), the 6th Framework Programme of the European Union (LSHM-CT-2006-0376331). We thank Anne Plunkett for preparing the manuscript.

Table 1 Changes in lipoprotein related hepatic genes in the apoA-I transgenic mice (Fig. 2B) following fenofibrate treatment

Gene name	Symbol	Fold
Lipoprotein lipase	*Lpl*	8.85
Phospholipid transfer protein	*Pltp*	5.86
ATP-binding cassette, sub-family G, member 1	*Abcg1*	1.29
ATP-binding cassette, subfamily A, member 1	*Abca1*	1.10
Apolipoprotein A-V	*Apoa5*	−1.07
Apolipoprotein A-II	*Apoa2*	−1.17
Apolipoprotein E	*Apoe*	−1.19
Lecithin:cholesterol acyltransferase	*Lcat*	−1.26
Apolipoprotein C-III	*Apoc3*	−1.34
Scavenger receptor, class B, type I	*Sr-Bi*	−1.51
Apolipoprotein A-IV	*Apoa4*	−9.75

References

1. Talianidis I, Tambakaki A, Toursounova J, Zannis VI (1995) Complex interactions between SP1 bound to multiple distal regulatory sites and HNF-4 bound to the proximal promoter lead to transcriptional activation of liver-specific human APOCIII gene. Biochemistry 34(32):10298–10309
2. Kardassis D, Tzameli I, Hadzopoulou-Cladaras M, Talianidis I, Zannis V (1997) Distal apolipoprotein C-III regulatory elements F to J act as a general modular enhancer for proximal promoters that contain hormone response elements. Synergism between hepatic nuclear factor-4 molecules bound to the proximal promoter and distal enhancer sites. Arterioscler Thromb Vasc Biol 17(1):222–232
3. Ogami K, Hadzopoulou-Cladaras M, Cladaras C, Zannis VI (1990) Promoter elements and factors required for hepatic and intestinal transcription of the human ApoCIII gene. J Biol Chem 265(17):9808–9815
4. Ktistaki E, Lacorte JM, Katrakili N, Zannis VI, Talianidis I (1994) Transcriptional regulation of the apolipoprotein A-IV gene involves synergism between a proximal orphan receptor response element and a distant enhancer located in the upstream promoter region of the apolipoprotein C-III gene. Nucleic Acids Res 22(22): 4689–4696
5. Papazafiri P, Ogami K, Ramji DP, Nicosia A, Monaci P, Cladaras C et al (1991) Promoter elements and factors involved in hepatic transcription of the human ApoA-I gene positive and negative regulators bind to overlapping sites. J Biol Chem 266(9):5790–5797
6. Tzameli I, Zannis VI (1996) Binding specificity and modulation of the ApoA-I promoter activity by homo- and heterodimers of nuclear receptors. J Biol Chem 271(14):8402–8415
7. Lavrentiadou SN, Hadzopoulou-Cladaras M, Kardassis D, Zannis VI (1999) Binding specificity and modulation of the human ApoCIII promoter activity by heterodimers of ligand-dependent nuclear receptors. Biochemistry 38(3):964–975
8. Kan HY, Georgopoulos S, Zannis V (2000) A hormone response element in the human apolipoprotein CIII (ApoCIII) enhancer is essential for intestinal expression of the ApoA-I and ApoCIII genes and contributes to the hepatic expression of the two linked genes in transgenic mice. J Biol Chem 275(39):30423–30431
9. Georgopoulos S, Kan HY, Reardon-Alulis C, Zannis V (2000) The SP1 sites of the human apoCIII enhancer are essential for the expression of the apoCIII gene and contribute to the hepatic and intestinal expression of the apoA-I gene in transgenic mice. Nucleic Acids Res 28(24):4919–4929
10. Zannis VI, Kan HY, Kritis A, Zanni EE, Kardassis D (2001) Transcriptional regulatory mechanisms of the human apolipoprotein genes in vitro and in vivo. Curr Opin Lipidol 12(2):181–207
11. Kan HY, Georgopoulos S, Zanni M, Shkodrani A, Tzatsos A, Xie HX et al (2004) Contribution of the hormone-response elements of the proximal ApoA-I promoter, ApoCIII enhancer, and C/EBP binding site of the proximal ApoA-I promoter to the hepatic and intestinal expression of the ApoA-I and ApoCIII genes in transgenic mice. Biochemistry 43(17):5084–5093

12. Kardassis D, Falvey E, Tsantili P, Hadzopoulou-Cladaras M, Zannis V (2002) Direct physical interactions between HNF-4 and Sp1 mediate synergistic transactivation of the apolipoprotein CIII promoter. Biochemistry 41(4):1217–1228

13. Lemon B, Tjian R (2000) Orchestrated response: a symphony of transcription factors for gene control. Genes Dev 14(20):2551–2569

14. Chen JL, Attardi LD, Verrijzer CP, Yokomori K, Tjian R (1994) Assembly of recombinant TFIID reveals differential coactivator requirements for distinct transcriptional activators. Cell 79(1):93–105

15. Zannis VI, Lees AM, Lees RS, Breslow JL (1982) Abnormal apoprotein A-I isoprotein composition in patients with Tangier disease. J Biol Chem 257(9):4978–4986

16. Chroni A, Liu T, Gorshkova I, Kan HY, Uehara Y, von Eckardstein A et al (2003) The central helices of apoA-I can promote ATP-binding cassette transporter A1 (ABCA1)-mediated lipid efflux. Amino acid residues 220-231 of the wild-type apoA-I are required for lipid efflux in vitro and high density lipoprotein formation in vivo. J Biol Chem 278(9):6719–6730

17. Zannis VI, Chroni A, Krieger M (2006) Role of apoA-I, ABCA1, LCAT, and SR-BI in the biogenesis of HDL. J Mol Med 84(4):276–294

18. Chroni A, Koukos G, Duka A, Zannis VI (2007) The carboxy-terminal region of apoA-I is required for the ABCA1-dependent formation of alpha-HDL but not prebeta-HDL particles in vivo. Biochemistry 46(19):5697–5708

19. Koukos G, Chroni A, Duka A, Kardassis D, Zannis VI (2007) LCAT can rescue the abnormal phenotype produced by the natural ApoA-I mutations (Leu141Arg)Pisa and (Leu159Arg)FIN. Biochemistry 46(37):10713–10721

20. Chroni A, Duka A, Kan HY, Liu T, Zannis VI (2005) Point mutations in apolipoprotein a-I mimic the phenotype observed in patients with classical lecithin:cholesterol acyltransferase deficiency. Biochemistry 44(43):14353–14366

21. Koukos G, Chroni A, Duka A, Kardassis D, Zannis VI (2007) Naturally occurring and bioengineered apoA-I mutations that inhibit the conversion of discoidal to spherical HDL: the abnormal HDL phenotypes can be corrected by treatment with LCAT. Biochem J 406(1):167–174

22. Chroni A, Kan HY, Kypreos KE, Gorshkova IN, Shkodrani A, Zannis VI (2004) Substitutions of glutamate 110 and 111 in the middle helix 4 of human apolipoprotein A-I (apoA-I) by alanine affect the structure and in vitro functions of apoA-I and induce severe hypertriglyceridemia in apoA-I-deficient mice. Biochemistry 43(32):10442–10457

23. Li J, Ning G, Duncan SA (2000) Mammalian hepatocyte differentiation requires the transcription factor HNF-4alpha. Genes Dev 14(4):464–474

24. Fraser JD, Keller D, Martinez V, Santiso-Mere D, Straney R, Briggs MR (1997) Utilization of recombinant adenovirus and dominant negative mutants to characterize hepatocyte nuclear factor 4-regulated apolipoprotein AI and CIII expression. J Biol Chem 272(21):13892–13898

25. Peters JM, Hennuyer N, Staels B, Fruchart JC, Fievet C, Gonzalez FJ et al (1997) Alterations in lipoprotein metabolism in peroxisome proliferator-activated receptor alpha-deficient mice. J Biol Chem 272(43):27307–27312

26. Wan YJ, An D, Cai Y, Repa JJ, Hung-Po CT, Flores M et al (2000) Hepatocyte-specific mutation establishes retinoid X receptor alpha as a heterodimeric integrator of multiple physiological processes in the liver. Mol Cell Biol 20(12):4436–4444

27. Vu-Dac N, Gervois P, Grotzinger T, De Vos P, Schoonjans K, Fruchart JC et al (1997) Transcriptional regulation of apolipoprotein A-I gene expression by the nuclear receptor RORalpha. J Biol Chem 272(36):22401–22404

28. Zaiou M, Azrolan N, Hayek T, Wang H, Wu L, Haghpassand M et al (1998) The full induction of human apoprotein A-I gene expression by the experimental nephrotic syndrome in transgenic mice depends on cis-acting elements in the proximal 256 base-pair promoter region and the trans-acting factor early growth response factor 1. J Clin Invest 101(8):1699–1707

29. Srivastava RA, Srivastava N, Averna M (2000) Dietary cholic acid lowers plasma levels of mouse and human apolipoprotein A-I primarily via a transcriptional mechanism. Eur J Biochem 267(13): 4272–4280

30. Claudel T, Sturm E, Duez H, Torra IP, Sirvent A, Kosykh V et al (2002) Bile acid-activated nuclear receptor FXR suppresses apolipoprotein A-I transcription via a negative FXR response element. J Clin Invest 109(7):961–971

31. Delerive P, Galardi CM, Bisi JE, Nicodeme E, Goodwin B (2004) Identification of liver receptor homolog-1 as a novel regulator of apolipoprotein AI gene transcription. Mol Endocrinol 18(10): 2378–2387

32. Hennuyer N, Poulain P, Madsen L, Berge RK, Houdebine LM, Branellec D et al (1999) Beneficial effects of fibrates on apolipoprotein A-I metabolism occur independently of any peroxisome proliferative response. Circulation 99(18):2445–2451

33. Berthou L, Duverger N, Emmanuel F, Langouet S, Auwerx J, Guillouzo A et al (1996) Opposite regulation of human versus mouse apolipoprotein A-I by fibrates in human apolipoprotein A-I transgenic mice. J Clin Invest 97(11):2408–2416

34. Duez H, Lefebvre B, Poulain P, Torra IP, Percevault F, Luc G et al (2005) Regulation of human apoA-I by gemfibrozil and fenofibrate through selective peroxisome proliferator-activated receptor alpha modulation. Arterioscler Thromb Vasc Biol 25(3):585–591

35. Vu-Dac N, Chopin-Delannoy S, Gervois P, Bonnelye E, Martin G, Fruchart JC et al (1998) The nuclear receptors peroxisome proliferator-activated receptor alpha and Rev-erbalpha mediate the species-specific regulation of apolipoprotein A-I expression by fibrates. J Biol Chem 273(40):25713–25720

36. Rubin EM, Ishida BY, Clift SM, Krauss RM (1991) Expression of human apolipoprotein A-I in transgenic mice results in reduced plasma levels of murine apolipoprotein A-I and the appearance of two new high density lipoprotein size subclasses. Proc Natl Acad Sci USA 88(2):434–438

37. Walsh A, Ito Y, Breslow JL (1989) High levels of human apolipoprotein A-I in transgenic mice result in increased plasma levels of small high density lipoprotein (HDL) particles comparable to human HDL3. J Biol Chem 264(11):6488–6494

38. Schoonjans K, Peinado-Onsurbe J, Lefebvre AM, Heyman RA, Briggs M, Deeb S et al (1996) PPARalpha and PPARgamma activators direct a distinct tissue-specific transcriptional response via a PPRE in the lipoprotein lipase gene. EMBO J 15(19): 5336–5348

39. Bouly M, Masson D, Gross B, Jiang XC, Fievet C, Castro G et al (2001) Induction of the phospholipid transfer protein gene accounts for the high density lipoprotein enlargement in mice treated with fenofibrate. J Biol Chem 276(28):25841–25847

40. Rigotti A, Trigatti BL, Penman M, Rayburn H, Herz J, Krieger M (1997) A targeted mutation in the murine gene encoding the high density lipoprotein (HDL) receptor scavenger receptor class B type I reveals its key role in HDL metabolism. Proc Natl Acad Sci USA 94(23):12610–12615

41. Lan D, Silver DL (2005) Fenofibrate induces a novel degradation pathway for scavenger receptor B-I independent of PDZK1. J Biol Chem 280(24):23390–23396

42. Staels B, van Tol A, Verhoeven G, Auwerx J (1990) Apolipoprotein A-IV messenger ribonucleic acid abundance is regulated in a tissue-specific manner. Endocrinology 126(4):2153–2163

43. Jacobs RL, Devlin C, Tabas I, Vance DE (2004) Targeted deletion of hepatic CTP:phosphocholine cytidylyltransferase alpha in mice decreases plasma high density and very low density lipoproteins. J Biol Chem 279(45):47402–47410

High Density Lipoprotein Particles

Bela F. Asztalos

Introduction

HDL was first measured as a subclass of lipoproteins in the early 1950s, but garnered wide interest only after the publication by Barklay and Barklay in Nature in 1963 documented gender differences in HDL cholesterol levels [1]. Additional interest in HDL was generated by Fredrickson's association of HDL deficiency with Tangier disease in 1964 [2]. In the following decades, HDL was associated with many important physiological functions (including reverse cholesterol transport, anti-inflammatory processes, and lipoprotein controlled anti-oxidation). Despite the accumulation of evidence for the patho-physiological importance of HDL, it has been relegated to a status below that of LDL for the last several decades. The reasons for this are that: (1) increased LDL-C has been clearly linked to increased cardiovascular disease risk, (2) reductions in LDL cholesterol with statins have been clearly associated with significant reductions in coronary heart disease (CHD) risk, and (3) even though low HDL cholesterol is associated with CHD, the number of studies clearly documenting the benefits of raising HDL are limited. Many leading experts in the lipoprotein field have recognized the importance of HDL-C in CVD-risk assessment, but there is a lack of effective and well-tolerated strategies for raising HDL-C. As a result, only LDL-C target levels were included in the ATP/AHA guidelines. Recent data on raising HDL and its effects on CVD progression [3] have, however, raised the interest level in HDL research. With the promise, albeit as of yet undelivered, of increasing HDL-C by CETP inhibition, administration of small apoA-I-mimetic peptides, or by new more tolerable niacin drugs, HDL has moved into the mainstream of clinical lipid management.

Separation of HDL Subclasses

HDL comprises a heterogeneous group of lipoprotein particles, whose common characteristic is that they all float in the $d > 1.063$ and $d < 1.21$ g/ml fraction after 48 h ultracentrifugation (UC) with a 100,000 G-force. By the traditional nomenclature, HDL contains apolipo-proteins, charged lipids, and neutral lipids. The major apolipoproteins (apo) of HDL are apoA-I and apoA-II. Minor apolipo-proteins include apoA-IV, A-V, C-I, C-II, C-III, D, E, F, H, J, L, M, O, and P. HDL can be separated into subclasses containing different apolipoproteins. The first separations were capable of isolating HDL into an apoA-I- and apoA-II-containing fraction (LpA-I:A-II) and a fraction containing only apoA-I but no apoA-II (LpA-I) [4]. Alaupovic, using immuno-absorption chromatography, separated several distinct HDL subclasses, each containing a variety of different apolipo-proteins [5].

HDL can be separated by its electrophoretic mobility into preβ-, α- and preα-mobility subclasses based on an RF relative to albumin, which marks α-mobility [6, 7]. HDL can also be separated based on size by size exclusion chromatography and nondenaturing (nd) gradient polyacrylamide gel electrophoresis (PAGE). Size exclusion chromatography has lower resolution than ndPAGE. However, it is relatively fast and preparative. In addition to its low resolution, the disadvantage of this method is the fact that charged lipids on the surface of HDL tend to desorb, leading to alterations in composition and the disintegration of large HDL particles. One-dimensional (1D) nondenaturing (nd) polyacrylamide gel electrophoresis (PAGE) separates HDL particles first by surface charge and later – when the gel pore-size is comparable to particle size – by size. In practice, the disadvantage of 1D ndPAGE is its inability to separate preβ-migrating subclasses from α-mobility particles. Moreover, the measurements of HDL particles with similar size are troublesome: α-1 comigrates with the similarly sized preβ-2 and α-4 comigrates with preβ-1 particles. With two-dimensional separation of HDL particles, these problems can be avoided.

B.F. Asztalos (✉)
Lipid Metabolism Laboratory, Tufts University,
Boston, MA 02111, USA
e-mail: bela.asztalos@tufts.edu

E.J. Schaefer (ed.), *High Density Lipoproteins, Dyslipidemia, and Coronary Heart Disease*,
DOI 10.1007/978-1-4419-1059-2_3, © Springer Science+Business Media, LLC 2010

Fig. 1 The apoA-I-containing
HDL subpopulation profile of an
apparently healthy subject (**a**), of a
CHD patient (**b**), schematic
representation of the routinely
determined apoA-I-containing
HDL particles (**c**) and an integration
curve of the α-mobility HDL
particles (**d**). α-2 and α-3,
highlighted with a darker shade,
comprise the LpA-I:A-II
sub-fractions (containing both
apoA-I and apoA-II), while the
other particles are LpA-I
sub-fractions (containing apoA-I,
but no or only trace amount of
apoA-II). *Asterisks*, marks the
serum albumin or α-front

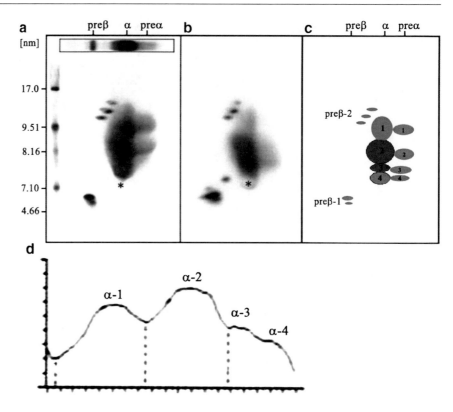

Two-dimensional (2D) separation of HDL particles – by electrophoretic mobility in the first dimension and by size in the second dimension – was first published by Fielding and colleagues in the late 1980s. Subsequently, Asztalos and Roheim adopted and improved this method for HDL particle assessment in the early 1990s (Fig. 1) [7]. The introduction of immunoblotting and image-analysis allowed for the quantization of results. Moreover, assessment of HDL subpopulations in epidemiological studies has lead to the characterization of the HDL subpopulation profile in large numbers of both normal subjects and patients with cardiovascular disease. Investigation of cohorts with genetic disorders influencing HDL metabolism have led to a theory of in vivo HDL remodelling which is currently still evolving (see chapter "The Kinetics and Remodeling of HDL Particles; Lessons from Inborn Errors of Lipid Metabolism") [8]. Recently, characterization of HDL subpopulations has also been developed as a diagnostic tool. Here, we focus on the complexity of HDL particles in the normal population.

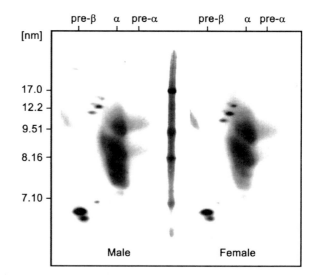

Fig. 2 The apoA-I-containing HDL subpopulations of an apparently healthy male (HDL-C=51.2 mg/dl) and a female subject (HDL-C =69 mg/dl) separated by nondenaturing, two-dimensional gel electrophoresis and recognized by 125I-labeled antibody monospecific to human apolipoprotein A-I

HDL Structure

We have quantitatively determined ten distinct apoA-I-containing HDL subpopulations (see Fig. 1a, in chapter "The Kinetics and Remodeling of HDL Particles; Lessons from Inborn Errors of Lipid Metabolism") and have established that the proportion of these particles is different between healthy

males and females (Fig. 2). Moreover, we have documented that the percent distributions of apoA-I-containing HDL particles are significantly different in subjects with various HDL deficiency states and/or cardiovascular disease than from gender matched subjects and healthy controls (see Fig. 1b). Figure 3 represents our working theory of the physico-chemical structure and.

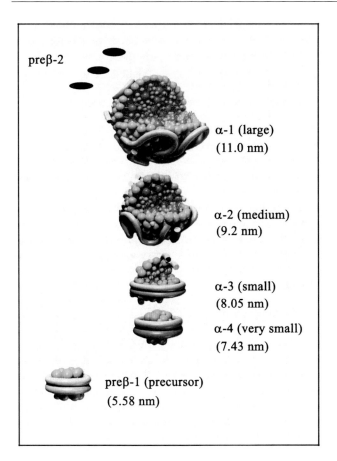

Fig. 3 Our working theory of the physico-chemical structure and size of the major apoA-I-containing HDL subpopulations. *Light yellow cylinders* represent apoA-I and *darker yellow cylinders* represent apoA-II molecules. *Blue, green,* and *purple spheres* represent PL, free-cholesterol, and TG, respectively. The chemical composition of preβ-2 has not been investigated, therefore it is labeled as *solid black*. Created by Mr. Martin Jacob. Courtesy of Boston Heart Lab Corporation, Framingham, MA, USA

Please refer to chapter 10 "The Kinetics and Remodeling of HDL Particles; Lessons from Inborn Errors of Lipid Metabolism" for detailed steps of HDL metabolism/remodeling.

ApoA-I is secreted by the liver and small intestine as a monomer in lipid-free form with a molecular weight of about 28 KD. ApoA-I self associates to form a dimer by specific mechanisms when its concentration reaches >10 μg/ml in the circulation. Two apoA-I molecules form a belt-shaped disc, in which the two apoA-I molecules have opposite orientations: one apoA-I's N-terminal lies proximal to the other apoA-I's C-terminal. The two apoA-I molecules are secured with salt bridges [9, 10]. This apoA-I-belt migrates at the preβ-1 position on nd-2D PAGE with an estimated molecular size between 4.5 and 5.6 nm. By electron microscope, these particles look like flattened discs in stacks ranging from a couple of stacked discs to a rope-like structure containing tens of stacked discs. Compositionally, the only protein present in preβ-1 HDL is apoA-I. In addition, the apoA-I belt

harbors some phospholipids (PL), and there may be trace amounts of free-cholesterol on the particle as well [12]. There are several different hypotheses, none of which are supported by solid direct measurements, about the lipid/protein ratio in this particle. Estimates range from less than 10 PL/apoA-I to more than 100 PL/apoA-I. This apoA-I-lipid disc is a good acceptor of cellular cholesterol via the ATP binding cassette transporter A1 (ABCA1) pathway [11, 12]. When free cholesterol and phospholipid are added to preβ-1 HDL via ABCA1, the particle is converted into the smallest α-mobility HDL particle, α-4 HDL [8]. In the presence of lecithin cholesteryl acyltransferase (LCAT), lipases, and lipid-transfer proteins, the small discoidal α-4 HDL mature into the larger spherical α- and preα-mobility HDL particles.

In addition to HDL modeling enzymes and lipid-transfer proteins, HDL particle distribution and composition is influenced in a number of different ways. It is well known, although not well documented, that HDL particle distribution (and therefore overall HDL particle size) has a stronger correlation with triglyceride (TG) levels than with HDL-C or apoA-I levels [13]. HDL particle distribution is also significantly influenced by several inflammatory conditions. For example, serum amyloid A replaces apoA-I in HDL particles in inflammatory states, resulting in size and functional changes in HDL [13–16].

How other inflammatory markers like C-reactive protein (CRP), lipoprotein associated phospholipase A2 (LpPLA2), secretory phospholipase A2 (sPLA2), endothelial lipase (EL), or the cell master inflammatory regulator NFκB influence HDL metabolism is not well studied and is poorly understood. There is data indicating that diabetes, insulin resistance, and uncontrolled high blood-glucose levels also significantly influence HDL metabolism. The accompanying hypertriglyceridemia only partially explains the substantial differences in HDL size between normal and affected subjects. It is worth noting that it is not TG levels, but the mechanism of TG-rich lipoprotein (TRL) metabolism that influences HDL particle distribution and overall HDL size. A perfect example by which to demonstrate this phenomenon is the different effect of statins and fibrates on HDL particle distribution and overall HDL size. Both drugs decrease plasma TG levels by about the same amount (30%), but statins increase overall HDL size by selectively increasing the concentrations of the largest (α-1) HDL particles, while fenofibrate and gemfibrozil increase the concentrations of smaller HDL particles (α-2 and α-3) and (slightly) decrease the concentration of the large α-1 particles. Lipoprotein researchers believe that statins decrease catabolism of HDL (the empty CETP cycle Fig. 5 in chapter "The Kinetics and Remodeling of HDL Particles; Lessons from Inborn Errors of Lipid Metabolism") by decreasing TRL concentration. TG in turn increasing hepatic lipase (HL) activity and decreasing HDL size [18]. In a collaborative work with F. C. de Beer's group, we have demonstrated how HDL2 (the large HDL subclass) changes after incubation with purified CETP (Fig. 4). Stains also substantially decrease inflammation (as evidenced by decreased CRP level) and are associated with increased HDL size. On the other hand, fibrates work through the PPARα pathway, increasing apoA-I and apoA-II production (about 2%), but also enhance HDL apoA-I catabolism. In contrast to statins, fibrates do not decrease LDL-C; therefore, they must influence CETP activity in a different way (which is as of yet not understood). When TG-enriched LDL is present, CETP exchanges TG for cholesteryl ester (CE) between LDL and HDL at a relatively fast rate. CETP performs the same function, but at a slower rate between VLDL and HDL. This difference alone explains a large part of the discrepancy between the two drug families' effects on HDL. Another potential difference might lie in the fact that

fibrates influence lipase activity more than statins. Also, PPARα is a master regulator of hundreds of cell functions, some of which might interfere with lipoprotein metabolism.

Other key players in HDL remodeling are lipases. In preliminary studies with the DeBeer's group, we have investigated the effects of HL, EL, and EL+SPLA2 on the HDL2 subfraction. We have demonstrated that HL and EL, both of which express strong phospholipase activity, generated small α-4 particles from the large HDL2 (α-1–α-2 sized) sub-fractions (Fig. 5). In combination, EL and sPLA2 generated substantial amounts of various smaller particles from the large HDL2 sub-fraction. However, in contrast to administration of EL alone, administration of EL + sPLA2 produced a large amount of preβ1 HDL particles thereby suggesting a synergistic effect of sPLA2 and EL on preβ-1 production (Fig. 5).

We have also investigated the role of scavenger receptor B1 (SR-B1) in HDL remodeling. We have injected human HDL2 into human SRB1 transgenic mice and followed the changes between 30 and 180 min. We have observed a gradual decrease in HDL particle size, as large HDL2 concentrations decreased and small sized HDL particles increased (e.g., α-4). However, preβ1 particles were not generated (Fig. 6). This result was direct evidence for our hypothesis that selective removal of cholesterol from large HDL particles does not produce an apoA-I-phospholipid disc like preβ-1.

It is widely believed that apoA-I is necessary for lipidated HDL-particle formation in humans. The first conflicting result to emerge was the finding of large lipid-rich apoE-containing HDL particles (LpE) devoid of any apoA-I. Further corroboration that apoA-1 is unnecessary for the formation of larger spherical HDL particles presented itself when we studied a Brazilian family whose members had a mutation resulting in lack of apoA-I production, but did not affect production of other proteins in the AI/CIII/AIV gene cluster (i.e. apoA-IV

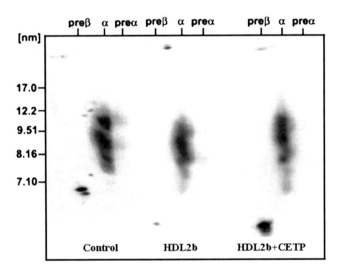

Fig. 4 Effects of in vitro incubation of HDL2 with purified CETP on particle size

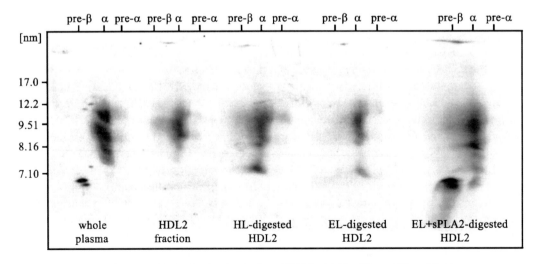

Fig. 5 HDL particle distribution before and 4 H after in vitro incubation of HDL2 with HL, EL, and EL + sPLA2

Fig. 6 SR-B1 and hSR-B1-mediated size decrease of HDL2 particles after injection into hSR-B1 transgenic mice

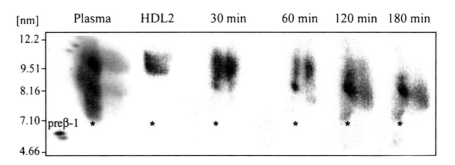

or apoC-III), unaffected. Despite the disruption in apoA-I production, they nonetheless all possessed HDL-C [19]. Homozygous family members had lipidated HDL particles with apoA-II as the major apolipoprotein. It is worth noting that the HDL of these subjects was probably dysfunctional as they presented with extensive xanthomas and premature CVD (see chapter on human apolipoprotein A-I deficiency).

HDL Proteomics

Figure 7 represents the distribution of the six most abundant apolipoproteins in a healthy male subject. This composite picture indicates that some HDL proteins such as apoA-IV and the majority of apoE are not incorporated into the apoA-I-containing HDL particles in humans. This figure also indicates that the distribution of other lipoproteins in the apoA-I-containing HDL particles are unique and vary widely between subjects [20, 21]. The presence or concentration of specific apolipoproteins on an HDL particle determines the function and metabolism of that specific particle. To discuss the effects of these apolipoproteins on HDL function and metabolism is beyond the scope of this chapter, but it is worth noting that in many cases these apolipoproteins have opposing effects on the same enzymes or lipid transfer proteins. HDL composition and function is extraordinarily complex due to the presence of proteins other than the generally accepted apolipoproteins of HDL (listed above) and the other known HDL-associated enzymes, transfer proteins, and acute phase proteins.

Even when only the aforementioned apolipoproteins had been identified, HDL was already known to be the most complex lipoprotein subfamily. Despite this, the intricacies of HDL have long been thought to be even more complex because of the theorized presence of many other proteins, but concrete data supporting this hypothesis has only recently begun to emerge. Vaisar, Heinecke, and colleagues, as well as Davidson, Chapman, and colleagues have recently published data on HDL proteomics [22, 23]. The Heinecke group found 48 different proteins in the HDL2 and HDL3 fractions, while the Chapman group found 28 different proteins in the

HDL density fraction. The large discrepancy in HDL-associated protein numbers is presumably due to the different methods the two groups utilized for HDL isolation. The Heinecke group separated whole HDL and HDL3 using horizontal rotor ultracentrifugation. The Chapman group separated five HDL subfractions (light HDL2b and HDL2a, and dense HDL3a, HDL3b, and HDL3c) by isopycnic density gradient ultracentrifugation. Both groups measured the tryptic digested peptides by LC-ESI-MS/MS, but the Chapman group used a somewhat different and less sensitive detection method. Heinecke's laboratory published 13 new HDL-associated proteins of which eight were not present in HDL3. Moreover, they illustrated that the HDL-associated proteins were participants of four physiological functions: (1) lipid metabolism, (2) proteinase regulation, (3) complement regulation, and (4) the acute-phase response. Chapman's group put emphasis on the abundance patterns of representative proteins across the HDL subpopulations: class A, limited to dense HDL3; class B, preferentially in dense HDL3 but present in all subfractions; class C, evenly distributed; class D, preferentially in light HDL2 but present in all subfractions; and class E, limited to light HDL2.

The limitation of both studies is the use of ultracentrifugal separation of HDL and its subfractions. It has been documented that even apoA-I, the basic component of HDL, is shed from HDL particles during ultracentrifugal separation [24]. Both the high salt concentration and the high G-force probably contribute to the loss of HDL-associated proteins into the lipid free fraction. Either the high salt concentration and/or the high G-force knock out even the building protein, apoA-I, from HDL. It is well known that up to 30% of apoA-I is found in the $d > 1.21$ g/ml bottom fraction. In addition to the 25% lost of apoA-I into the bottom fraction, we have observed an increase in the small preβ-1 concentration while the concentration of larger, mainly α-1 HDL fraction decreased after UC separation (Fig. 8) [24]. Moreover, the concentration of the α-2 (LpA-I:A-II) fraction was also dramatically reduced, and the concentration of the other but smaller LpA-I:A-II fraction (α-3) was increased. Throughout the particle size-range there was a shift from α-mobility to pre-α-mobility, indicating a significant change in surface charge which was most likely driven by changes in particle composition [25].

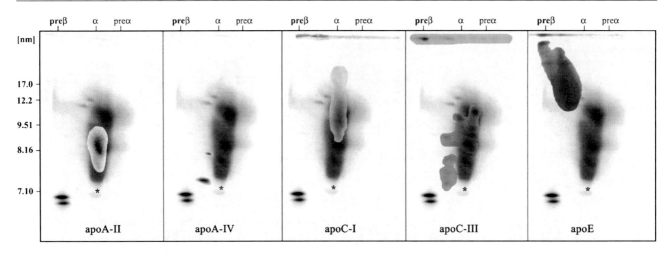

Fig. 7 The distribution of various apolipoproteins separated by nondenaturing two-dimensional PAGE and recognized by monospecific antibodies. ApoA-I-containing HDL particles are represented by *gray scale*. Each other apolipoprotein distribution is represented by different color superimposed with the apoA-I-containing particle distribution

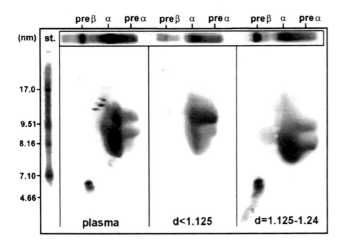

Fig. 8 Effects of ultracentrifugal separation on the physical–chemical parameters of HDL2 ($d < 1.125$ g/ml) and HDL3 ($d < 1.25–1.24$ g/ml) subfractions reseparated by two-dimensional ndPAGE

We have investigated HDL proteomics in our laboratory using 2D PAGE methodology. Three of the most abundant apoA-I-containing HDL subclasses (small α-4–α-3, medium α-2, and large α-1) were separated by 2D ndPAGE and electroeluted from the gel under nondenaturing conditions. To remove comigrating proteins, each fraction was absorbed on a monospecific anti-apoA-I column and eluted with low pH buffer after washing off the nonspecific proteins. After tryptic digestion, yielded peptides were analyzed by LC-ESI-MS/MS. We identified 92 different proteins associated with the three HDL subfractions. Of these 92 proteins, all of the previously published HDL-associated-proteins were detected in our HDL fractions. In addition, we also found 61 previously unpublished HDL-associated proteins. A total of 67 different proteins were associated with the large, LpA-I, α-1 HDL subfraction. Fifty-one of these proteins were associated with only the α-1 subfraction. Twenty-eight different proteins were associated with the large LpA-I:A-II, α-2 HDL subfraction of which 16 were associated exclusively with the α-2 fraction. Twenty-one different proteins were associated with the small combined α-4–α-3 HDL subfractions. Nine of these proteins were specific to this HDL subfraction.

In addition to the unexpectedly large number of different proteins associated with these three HDL subfractions, the concentration of complement C3 (a key player in innate immunity) was more abundant than apoA-I in α-1 HDL particles, a surprising finding. Besides lipoprotein metabolism, several of these HDL-associated proteins are involved in: (a) complement regulation $n = 21$ [the ten most abundant complement regulatory proteins were complement-3C, C4-A, C4-B, H, B, clusterin, clusterin precursors, C1, C4-binding protein, and C5 in decreasing order]; (b) plasma protease-activity regulation $n = 16$ [the ten most abundant proteases were serine protease C1-inhibitor, inter-α-trypsin inhibitor heavy chain H1, H2, and H4, plasmin, serine peptidase inhibitor, vitronectin, antithrombin III, heparin cofactor II, *N*-acethylmuranoyl-L-alanine amidase, kallikrein]; (c) blood coagulation $n = 7$ [fibrinogen β-chain, prothrombin, apoH or β2-glycoprotein 1, C-1 inhibitor vitamin K-dependent protein S, protein S100A-9, coagulation factor XII and XIII]; (d) angiogenesis $n = 3$; (e) cell adhesion $n = 5$; (f) hypertension [angiotensinogen]; (g) cell oxidation $n = 3$; and (h) hemoglobin metabolism [hemopexin].

The number and abundance of the HDL-associated proteins suggest that many of these proteins are on separate, although similar HDL particles, resulting in a high variability in protein composition within HDL subclasses. The binding of a protein, by weak or stronger forces, is presumably influenced by HDL size and by other proteins as well as lipid composition. Some proteins attach to HDL by hydrophobic forces, while others might use other anchor proteins to attach themselves to the particles.

Conclusions

Data on HDL composition confirms earlier work that HDL is more than just a lipid carrier. Moreover, new proteomics data on HDL raises questions about the major function of HDL. Recent data suggests that HDL's contributions to innate immunity, plasma protease activity, and blood coagulation might be functions of HDL that are as important as reverse cholesterol transport. We hypothesize that HDL not only carries a diverse group of proteins, but also actively regulates their metabolic fate and/or activity by not only separating them in space but also by bringing them into contact when conditions dictate. However, none of these functions of HDL have yet been studied. Further work is needed to determine HDL metabolomics (proteomics and lipidomics) and to clarify the true pathophysiologic importance of HDL.

It is however clear that very small discoidal preβ-1 precursor-HDL interacts with ABCA1 to promote cellular cholesterol and phospholipd efflux (Fig. 9a), and in so doing is converted to very small discoidal α-4 HDL (see Fig. 2c in chapter "The Kinetics and Remodeling of HDL Particles; Lessons from Inborn Errors of Lipid Metabolism"). This particle in turn is acted upon by LCAT which converts its free cholesterol into cholesteryl ester, and also serves as an acceptor for apoA-II from the liver and as an acceptor of TRL surface components and triglyceride generated during lipolysis. During this process, small spherical α-3 HDL and medium spherical α-2 HDL are formed, which not only contain apoA-I but also apoA-II. These spherical particles then go through a number of steps described in the next chapter in order to form large protective spherical α-1 HDL, which is the most effective particle for delivering cholesterol to the liver (Fig. 9b) [12]. However, as previously stated, a large number of other proteins interact with HDL particles, especially large spherical HDL, and these proteins are involved in the immune response, proteolysis, coagulation, angiogenesis, and other processes [22, 23].

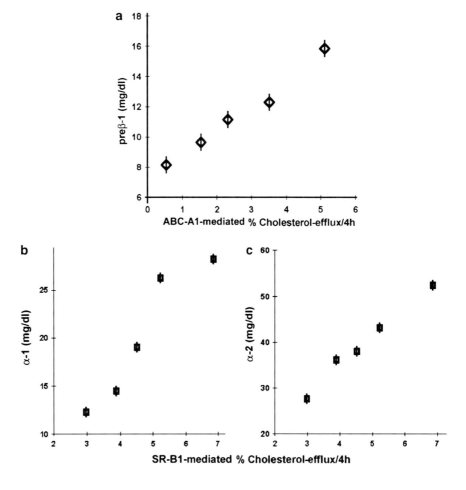

Fig. 9 (a) Correlation between preβ-1 HDL particle concentration and cell-cholesterol efflux via the ABC-A1 pathway. J774 cells were incubated with apoB-depleted sera.
(b) Correlations between α-1 and (c) α-2 HDL-particles concentration and cell-cholesterol efflux via the SR-B1 pathway. Fu5AH cells were incubated with apoB-depleted sera

References

1. Barklay M, Barklay RK, Skipski VP (1963) High-density lipoprotein concentrations in men and women. Nature 200:362–363
2. Fredrickson DS (1964) The inheritance of high density lipoprotein deficiency (Tangier Disease). J Clin Invest 43:228–236
3. Nissen SE, Tsunoda T, Tuzcu EM, Schoenhagen P, Cooper CJ, Yasin M, Eaton GM, Lauer MA, Sheldon WS, Grines CL, Halpern S, Crowe T, Blankenship JC, Kerensky R (2003) Effect of recombinant apoA-I Milano on coronary atherosclerosis in patients with acute coronary syndromes: a randomized controlled trial. JAMA 290(17):2292–2300
4. Puchois P, Kandoussi A, Fievet P, Fourrier JL, Bertrand M, Koren E, Fruchart JC (1987) Apolipoprotein A-I containing lipoproteins in coronary artery disease. Atherosclerosis 68(1–2):35–40
5. Kostner G, Alaupovic P (1972) Studies of the composition and structure of plasma lipoproteins. Separation and quantification of the lipoprotein families occurring in the high density lipoproteins of human plasma. Biochemistry 11(18):3419–3428
6. Castro GR, Fielding CJ (1988) Early incorporation of cell-derived cholesterol into pre-beta-migrating high-density lipoprotein. Biochemistry 27(1):25–29
7. Asztalos BF, Sloop CH, Wong L, Roheim PS (1993) Two-dimensional electrophoresis of plasma lipoproteins: recognition of new apo A-I-containing subpopulations. Biochim Biophys Acta 1169(3):291–300
8. Asztalos BF, Schaefer EJ, Horvath KV, Yamashita S, Miller M, Franceschini G, Calabresi L (2007) Role of LCAT in HDL remodeling: investigation of LCAT deficiency states. J Lipid Res 48(3):592–599
9. Phillips JC, Wriggers W, Li Z, Jonas A, Schulten K (1997) Predicting the structure of apolipoprotein A-1 in reconstituted high-density lipoprotein disks. Biophys J 73:2337–2346
10. Segrest JP, Jones MK, Klon AE, Sheldahl CJ, Hellinger M, De Loof HM, Harvey SC (1999) A detailed molecular belt model for apolipoprotein A-I in discoidal high density lipoprotein. J Biol Chem 274(45):31755–31758
11. Asztalos BF, de la Llera-Moya M, Dallal GE, Horvath KV, Schaefer EJ, Rothblat GH (2005) Differential effects of HDL subpopulations on cellular ABCA1- and SR-BI-mediated cholesterol efflux. J Lipid Res 46(10):2246–2253
12. Cheung MC, Brown BG, Wolf AC, Albers JJ (1991) Altered particle size distribution of apolipoprotein A-I-containing lipoproteins in subjects with coronary artery disease. J Lipid Res 32(3):383–394
13. de Beer MC, Webb NR, Whitaker NL, Wroblewski JM, Jahangiri A, van der Westhuyzen DR, de Beer FC (2009) SR-BI selective lipid uptake: subsequent metabolism of acute phase HDL. Arterioscler Thromb Vasc Biol 29(9):1298–1303
14. Jahangiri A, de Beer MC, Noffsinger V, Tannock LR, Ramaiah C, Webb NR, van der Westhuyzen DR, de Beer FC (2009) HDL remodeling during the acute phase response. Arterioscler Thromb Vasc Biol 29(2):261–267
15. Van Lenten BJ, Wagner AC, Navab M, Anantharamaiah GM, Hama S, Reddy ST, Fogelman AM (2007) Lipoprotein inflammatory properties and serum amyloid A levels but not cholesterol levels predict lesion area in cholesterol-fed rabbits. J Lipid Res 48(11):2344–2353
16. van der Westhuyzen DR, Cai L, de Beer MC, de Beer FC (2005) Serum amyloid A promotes cholesterol efflux mediated by scavenger receptor B-I. J Biol Chem 280(43):35890–35895
17. Guerin M, Lassel TS, Le Goff W, Farnier M, Chapman MJ (2000) Action of atorvastatin in combined hyperlipidemia: preferential reduction of cholesteryl ester transfer from HDL to VLDL1 particles. Arterioscler Thromb Vasc Biol 20(1):189–197
18. Santos RD, Schaefer EJ, Asztalos BF, Polisecki E, Wang J, Hegele RA, Martinez LR, Miname MH, Rochitte CE, Da Luz PL, Maranhão RC (2008) Characterization of high density lipoprotein particles in familial apolipoprotein A-I deficiency. J Lipid Res 49(2):349–357
19. Asztalos BF, Brousseau ME, McNamara JR, Horvath KV, Roheim PS, Schaefer EJ (2001) Subpopulations of high density lipoproteins in homozygous and heterozygous Tangier disease. Atherosclerosis 156(1):217–225
20. Asztalos BF, Horvath KV, Kajinami K, Nartsupha C, Cox CE, Batista M, Schaefer EJ, Inazu A, Mabuchi H (2004) Apolipoprotein composition of HDL in cholesteryl ester transfer protein deficiency. J Lipid Res 45(3):448–455
21. Vaisar T, Pennathur S, Green PS, Gharib SA, Hoofnagle AN, Cheung MC, Byun J, Vuletic S, Kassim S, Singh P, Chea H, Knopp RH, Brunzell J, Geary R, Chait A, Zhao XQ, Elkon K, Marcovina S, Ridker P, Oram JF, Heinecke JW (2007) Shotgun proteomics implicates protease inhibition and complement activation in the antiinflammatory properties of HDL. J Clin Invest 117(3):746–756
22. Davidson WS, Silva RA, Chantepie S, Lagor WR, Chapman MJ, Kontush A (2009) Proteomic analysis of defined HDL subpopulations reveals particle-specific protein clusters: relevance to antioxidative function. Arterioscler Thromb Vasc Biol 29(6):870–876
23. Asztalos BF, Roheim PS, Milani RL, Lefevre M, McNamara JR, Horvath KV, Schaefer EJ (2000) Distribution of ApoA-I-containing HDL subpopulations in patients with coronary heart disease. Arterioscler Thromb Vasc Biol 20(12):2670–2676
24. Zhang W, Asztalos B, Roheim PS, Wong L (1998) Characterization of phospholipids in pre-alpha HDL: selective phospholipid efflux with apolipoprotein A-I. J Lipid Res 39(8):1601–1607

The Kinetics and Remodeling of HDL Particles: Lessons from Inborn Errors of Lipid Metabolism

Bela F. Asztalos and John Brunzell

Introduction

An inverse relationship between HDL cholesterol level and premature cardiovascular disease has been observed in many large-scale prospective studies [1–4]. Decreased plasma HDL cholesterol levels (<40 mg/dl in men and <50 mg/dl in women) have been associated with an increased risk of coronary heart disease (CHD) [5]. HDL is thought to be protective against CHD through multiple pathways including both reverse cholesterol transport and non-cholesterol dependent mechanisms.

HDL is the smallest and densest of all plasma lipoproteins. It consists of a number of distinct particles that vary in size, shape, density, surface charge, composition, and physiological function. HDL has several potentially antiatherogenic properties. The best known of these is the ability of HDL to remove cholesterol from peripheral cells, including macrophages, in the artery wall [6]. Other HDL functions include: inhibition of LDL oxidation, improvement in endothelial function, inhibition of the binding of monocytes to the endothelium, promotion of endothelial repair, stabilization of nitric oxide synthesis, as well as antithrombotic and antiinflammatory properties. HDL is also a key player in innate immunity. At least 49 proteins have been identified in HDL by mass spectrometry, some related to lipid metabolism, some related to complement regulation, some related to acute-phase response, and a few that are proteinase inhibitors [7]. Several cell surface-bound and soluble plasma proteins influence the charge, size, shape, and composition of HDL. These factors include ATP-binding cassette transporter A1 (ABCA1), ABCG1, lecithin:cholesterol acyltransferase (LCAT), cholesteryl ester transfer protein (CETP), phospholipid transfer protein (PLTP), lipoprotein lipase (LPL), hepatic lipase (HL), endothelial lipase (EL), secretory phospholipase A2 (sPLA2), and scavenger receptor B1 (SRB1).

This article summarizes our knowledge about HDL metabolism step by step from the secreted lipid-free apoA-I to the large lipid-rich HDL particles, which both transport cholesterol to bile and recycle particles in HDL remodeling. We corroborate several of the steps within this concept with data generated on human subjects who have genetic disorders, which influence specific steps/factors in HDL metabolism/remodeling. The most commonly reported gene defects in marked HDL-deficiency states are in the genes coding for apolipoprotein A-I (apoA-I): ABCA1, LCAT, and CETP.

The various HDL particles in human plasma are classified using many different parameters dependent on the separation method utilized. In this article, we discuss only the apoA-I containing HDL particles, separated by two-dimensional, nondenaturing gel electrophoresis, and detected by immunoblotting for apoA-I (see Fig. 1a in chapter "High Density Lipoprotein Particles"). We separate 12 distinct apoA-I-containing HDL subpopulations by electrophoretic mobility (preβ-, α-, and preα-mobility particles) and size (5.4–11.7 nm) [8]. In addition to apoA-I, these HDL particles contain other lipoproteins and plasma proteins. Ten of the 12 HDL subpopulations contain no apoA-II (LpA-I particles) (lighter shade) while two of them, α-2 and α-3, contain both apoA-I and apoA-II (LPA-I:A-II particles) (darker shade) (see Fig. 1c in chapter "High Density Lipoprotein Particles").

Using the nondenaturing 2D method, we have mapped the sequence and mechanisms of many of the steps in HDL metabolism/remodeling in humans by using individuals deficient in genes influencing HDL metabolism/remodeling (Fig. 1). We have collected plasma samples from subjects carrying one (heterozygous) and two (homozygous) defective alleles encoding: apoA-I [9], ABCA1 [10], LCAT [11], CETP [12], HL, and LPL. In addition, we have carried out cell-cholesterol efflux assays via the ABCA1, ABCG1, and SRB1 [13] pathways. On the basis of the results from these studies, we have built the working hypothesis of HDL metabolism/remodeling that we present in this chapter.

B.F. Asztalos (✉)
Lipid Metabolism Laboratory, Tufts University,
Boston, MA 02111, USA
e-mail: bela.asztalos@tufts.edu

E.J. Schaefer (ed.), *High Density Lipoproteins, Dyslipidemia, and Coronary Heart Disease*,
DOI 10.1007/978-1-4419-1059-2_4, © Springer Science+Business Media, LLC 2010

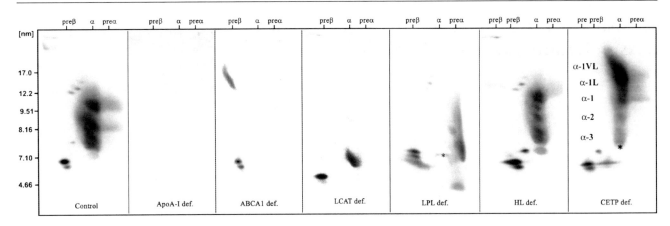

Fig. 1 ApoA-I containing HDL particles in various disorders of HDL metabolism

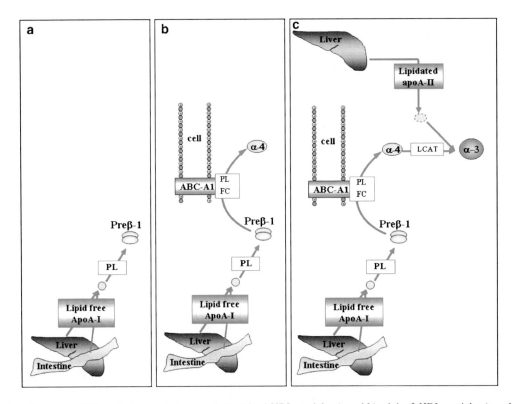

Fig. 2 Formation of precursor HDL particles (pre-beta) (panel **a**); alpha-4 HDL particles (panel **b**); alpha-3 HDL particles (panel **c**)

Step 1: ApoA-I synthesis

ApoA-I is a key molecule in the formation and function of HDL. ApoA-I is a 28 KD protein with 243 amino acid residues, which is synthesized in the liver and the intestine (Fig. 2a). Marked HDL deficiency states (HDL cholesterol <5 mg/dl) and undetectable plasma apoA-I levels have been reported in humans as a result of mutations at the APOA1/C3/A4 gene locus [9, 14–21]. These mutations have caused amino acid alteration of the carboxyl terminal region containing helices 6 (amino acid residues 145–164) and/or

7 (167–183) of apoA-I [22–24]. This region is considered to be important for protein–protein interaction between apoA-I and ABCA1 as well as LCAT activation, which is required for lipid efflux from peripheral tissues and conversion of discoidal HDL into spherical HDL particles [24]. Subjects with these mutations lack apoA-I-containing HDL in plasma, presenting with either normal or decreased triglyceride levels, normal LDL cholesterol levels, and often premature CHD [14–21]. There are also cases of isolated apoA-I deficiency. Subjects homozygous for apoA-I deficiency have no normal HDL particles irrespective of whether the apoA-I

gene only or the whole apoA-I-A-IV-C-III cluster is affected (Fig. 2). Heterozygous apoA-I-deficient subjects have all HDL particles present in plasma, but preβ-1 and α-1 concentrations are low. The low levels of preβ-1 and α-1 particles in heterozygous subjects are characteristic of this condition and can distinguish these subjects from other low-HDL subjects.

When apoA-I enters into the circulation, it promptly picks up some phospholipid (PL) and forms a discoid-shaped particle containing two apoA-I molecules (dimer). Both the lipid-free monomer and the apoA-I-PL dimer have preβ-mobility, but they differ in size. The apoA-I-PL dimer particles are considered as preβ-1 particles (modal diameter = 5.6 nm). We assume that about 6–8 PL/apoA-I molecules comprise a preβ-1 particle.

Step 2: Cellular Cholesterol Efflux via ABCA1

In the absence of functional ABCA1, only preβ-1 HDL particles are present in plasma. ABCA1 affects cellular lipid efflux in the presence of apoA-I. Cellular lipid transport from the Golgi to the plasma membrane is defective in patients with ABCA1 deficiency (Tangier disease) and in Abca1$^{-/-}$ mice, resulting in retention of caveolin-1, the main structural protein of caveolae, in the Golgi complex [25]. Over expression of caveolin-1 increases the number of caveolae and enhances HDL-mediated cholesterol efflux [26]. It has been reported that caveolin-1 and ABCA1 are expressed coordinately in differentiated THP-1 cells and that both of them promote cellular cholesterol efflux [27]. Immunoprecipitation analysis indicated an interaction between caveolin-1 and ABCA1 in the cytoplasm and in the plasma membrane after HDL incubation. It is hypothesized that the molecular interaction between caveolin-1 and ABCA1 is associated with the HDL-mediated cholesterol efflux pathway [26].

Fibroblasts in patients with Tangier disease (TD) show a marked defect in apoA-I- and HDL-mediated cholesterol efflux [28, 29]. As a consequence, only the native preβ-1 HDL is present in TD patients' plasma (Fig. 2a and Fig. 1). The preβ-1 particles are rapidly catabolized rather than matured to larger particles. This is a clear indication that cellular cholesterol efflux via ABCA1 is not essential for the formation of preβ-1 HDL particles.

On the other hand, preβ-1 is a very good substrate for ABCA1 and can promote cellular cholesterol efflux (see Fig. 9a in chapter "High Density Lipoprotein Particles"). As preβ-1 pulls phospholipids and cholesterol from the cell via ABCA1, it is transformed into α-4 (modal diameter = 7.4 nm), which is still a discoidal particle containing two apoA-I molecules, PL, and free cholesterol. Heterozygous TD patients have HDL particles with all sizes however, apoA-I is present predominantly in the smaller (preβ-1, α-4, and α-3) HDL particles when compared to unaffected individuals whose apoA-I is present predominantly in the larger, α-1 and α-2, HDL particles. Earlier, we have clearly indicated that no other HDL particle but preβ-1 is able to promote cellular cholesterol efflux via the ABCA1 pathway [13]. Cellular cholesterol efflux showed a significant and positive association with preβ-1 concentration when hepatoma cells (J774) were incubated with apoB-depleted plasma with various concentrations of preβ-1 particles (see Fig. 9a in chapter "High Density Lipoprotein Particles").

Data supporting the role of ABCA1 in the development of atherosclerosis is controversial. About 99% of cholesterol transported to the bile via the liver is carried by LDL. Therefore, the direct role of HDL in reverse cholesterol transport is negligible. Many argue that HDL removes cholesterol from macrophages in the vessel wall, which results in decreased cholesterol deposition. However, a recent publication indicated that the physiological expression of ABCA1 in the liver modulated susceptibility to atherosclerosis, but selective removal of macrophage ABCA1 did not [30]. These data indicate that ABCA1 plays a role in atherosclerosis contributing to HDL maturation.

Step 3: Cholesterol Esterification by LCAT

LCAT is a 416 amino acid long protein synthesized in the liver. After secretion, it either binds to lipoproteins or is present in lipid-free form in plasma [31]. LCAT synthesizes the majority of cholesteryl esters in plasma by transferring a fatty acid from lecithin (phosphatidylcholine) to the 3-hydroxyl group of cholesterol. It is generally believed that LCAT maintains the unesterified-cholesterol gradient between peripheral cells and HDL. Efflux of free cholesterol (FC) from cells occurs by a passive diffusion of FC between cellular membranes and acceptors and by mechanisms facilitated by ABCs and SRBI. In the presence of LCAT, the bidirectional movement of cholesterol between cells and HDL results in net cholesterol efflux [32, 33]. Therefore, LCAT plays a central role in the initial steps of reverse cholesterol transport. LCAT is activated primarily by apoA-I, but it can also be activated by apoA-IV, apoC-I, and apoE [34, 35]. Both the binding and activation of LCAT on the surface of HDL are essential for esterification of FC and accumulation of cholesteryl esters in the core of HDL particles (Fig. 2c): LCAT has two distinct substrates (activities): HDL (α) and LDL (β) [36]. Lack of α-LCAT activity alone causes fish eye disease (FED). Familial LCAT deficiency (FLD) is characterized by the absence of both LCAT activities. In affected individuals, LCAT protein maybe be present but both forms are inactive in plasma [37]. Previously, we observed that LCAT activity was not necessary for the transformation of preβ-1 HDL into α-mobility HDL [11]. Preβ-1 particles bind to ABCA1 and remove phospholipids and unesterified cholesterol from cells [13]. During this process, there are probably changes in apoA-I conformation and electrophoretic charge. We hypothesize that α-4 HDL also contains only two molecules of apoA-I as in preβ-1 HDL. Larger (~8–20 nm) α-mobility HDL particles have also been observed in subjects homozygous for LCAT deficiency. The tight bands of these particles suggest that these are poorly lipidated, discoidal HDL aggregates. We do not know whether LCAT can act on these large, stacked disks or use only the small α-4 HDL as a substrate. The apoA-I-containing HDL subpopulation profile of heterozygotes resembles that of CHD patients with low HDL-C as apoA-I distribution is shifted toward the smaller particles. ApoA-II is also dramatically reduced in homozygous LCAT-deficient subjects, probably due to fast catabolism of these particles [38]. Interestingly, apoA-II comigrates with preβ-1 HDL, which normally contains only apoA-I, in homozygous LCAT-deficient subjects.

We hypothesize that as a result of cholesteryl ester increase in the core of small HDL particles, apoA-II, which is secreted as a lipidated dimer, binds to some of the small LpA-I particle (α-4) and forms a larger LpA-I:A-II HDL particle (α-3).

Step 4: LPL-Mediated Hydrolysis

LPL hydrolyses core TG in VLDL resulting in the release of surface PL, FC, and apolipoproteins. These molecules can be used for HDL building. Via the concerted action of LCAT and LPL, HDL size increases by the transformation of α-3 into α-2-like but not normal α-2 HDL particles. However, as a result of LPL-mediated HDL-constituent release from VLDL, α-1 and larger than α-1 HDL particles form (Fig. 3). We hypothesize that α-1 particles are formed from smaller LpA-I HDL particles by fusion. We do not think that LpA-I:A-II α-3 expels apoA-II and forms α-1.

LPL activity is also necessary for the lipid composition changes that accompany α-4's acceptance of apoA-II to form α-3. ApoA-II is secreted from the liver in an already lipidated form containing two apoA-II molecules (apoA-II dimer). The newly formed LpA-I:A-II particles are α-3 particles (modal diameter = 7.9 nm). The native apoA-II-lipid disc can be detected in human plasma in preβ-position with a modal size around 3 nm – as detected on nondenaturing 3–16% linear-gradient gel, run to semi equilibrium in order to retain this small particle. About 0.5–1% of plasma total apoA-II is present in the apoA-II disc. Patients with homozygous LPL deficiency have a unique HDL subpopulation profile containing very low levels of amorphous α-mobility particles. In addition, apoA-II forms its own particle which contains only trace amounts of apoA-I.

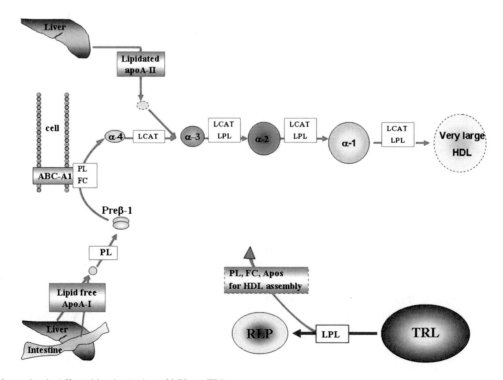

Fig. 3 HDL Maturation is Affected by the Action of LPL on TRL

Step 5: ABCG1-Mediated Cholesterol Efflux

Our preliminary data indicate that the FC pool available for efflux is increased by the expression of ABCG1 in some cells. This observation is consistent with previous studies, which proposed that the enhanced efflux observed in cells expressing ABCG1 is linked to this protein's ability to enrich the membrane pool of cholesterol that undergoes efflux [39, 40]. Further evidence that ABCG1 increases the availability of cholesterol in the plasma membrane comes from the observation that the cholesterol oxidase-sensitive pool of membrane cholesterol is expanded upon ABCG1 expression. Thus, the major role of ABCG1 in certain cell types is to enrich the plasma membrane with cholesterol, perhaps in specific pools in the membrane. The efficiency of this efflux might be dependent on the structure and concentration of the acceptor.

In addition to the efflux of cholesterol, ABCG1 expression also stimulates the release of cellular phospholipids to HDL_3 and to human serum. Kobayashi et al. [41] have shown that ABCG1 in HEK293 cells can mediate the efflux of cholesterol as well as choline phospholipids to HDL_3, and that ABCG1 differs from ABCA1 in the type of phospholipid transported . The fractional release of phospholipid is considerably less than that obtained with cholesterol. The reason for this reduced release probably reflects both the lower aqueous solubility of phospholipid compared to cholesterol, which is consistent with the aqueous diffusion mechanism [42] and the distribution of phospholipid in both plasma and internal membranes, where cholesterol is enriched in the plasma membrane and thus more available for efflux [43–47]. The extent to which ABCG1-mediated phospholipid release to lipoproteins can modify the composition of the acceptor particles remains to be determined (Fig. 4). Our preliminary data also indicate that unlike SR-BI, expression of ABCG1 has no impact on the influx of either form of cholesterol.

We have preliminary data indicating that the binding of extracellular acceptor particles are necessary for cellular-cholesterol efflux mediated by ABCA1 and SR-BI but not for ABCG1. Moreover, while the small LpA-I preβ-1 is a good acceptor for cholesterol via the ABCA1 pathway, the larger, more lipidated LpA-I:A-II α-2 promote cellular cholesterol efflux via the ABCG1 pathway [48].

Step 6: CETP Cycle

CETP mediates the CE exchange from HDL for TG from VLDL, although not stoichiometrically (Fig. 5a). Though HDL is able to carry cholesterol directly to bile via the liver SRB1 receptor (Fig. 6), this is only a minor part of reverse cholesterol transport (RCT). The majority of cholesterol is transported to the bile via LDL, which is helped by high CETP activity. As a result of CETP activity HDL becomes smaller and TG-enriched. In the presence of CETP, there is no detectable level of the larger than α-1 (α-1L and α-1VL)

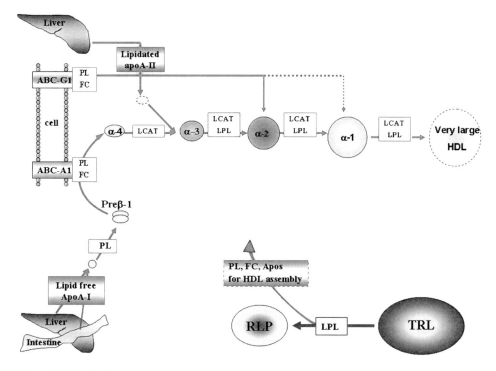

Fig. 4 Role of ABCG1 in HDL lipidation

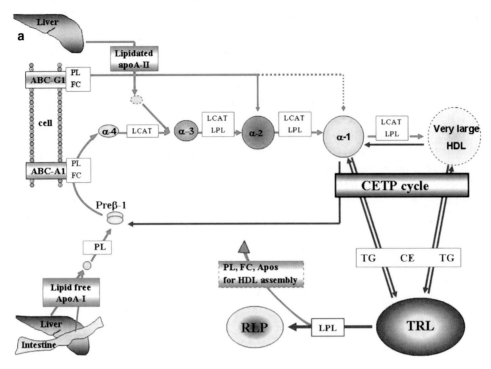

b **Metabolic reactions driven by triglycerides (VLDL)
   induce variability in LDL and HDL composition and size**

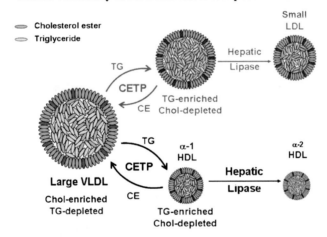

Fig. 5 The concerted action of CETP (**a**) and HL (**b**) on lipoprotein particle remodeling. Figure (**b**) is a modified version of a slide from the AHA slide library

HDL particles (Fig. 2). Moreover, the CETP-mediated TG-enrichment of α-1 makes this HDL particle a good substrate for HL (see Fig. 5a, b).

CETP is a member of the lipopolysaccharide-binding/lipid transfer protein family that transfers cholesteryl esters and triglycerides and, to lesser extent, phospholipids, between HDL, VLDL, and LDL [49]. As CETP-mediated transfers of cholesteryl esters between HDL and LDL are rapid relative to the rate at which the lipoproteins are catabolized, these cholesteryl ester pools are in equilibrium in vivo. This is not necessarily the case for CETP-mediated transfers of cholesteryl esters and triglycerides between HDL and VLDL. When VLDL levels are elevated, CETP-mediated transfers of core lipids from HDL to VLDL exceed those from VLDL to HDL, generating core cholesteryl ester-depleted, triglyceride-enriched HDL that have an excess of surface constituents and are structurally labile. This imbalance is corrected by the dissociation of lipid-free/lipid-poor apoA-I and a reduction in HDL size. CETP also can remodel HDL into small particles by a fusion process that does not involve the dissociation of lipid-free/lipid-poor apoA-I [50].

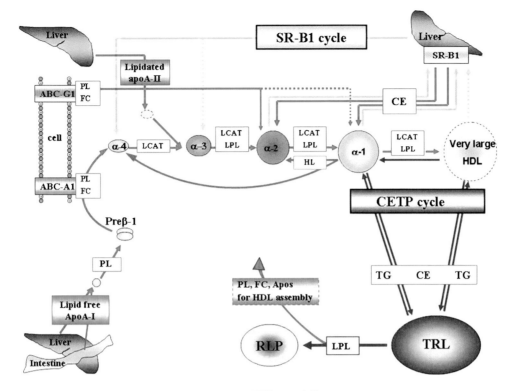

Fig. 6 The effects of SR-B1-mediated selective cholesterol uptake on HDL remodeling

Homozygous (HO) CETP deficient subjects (Fig. 1) have nearly all apoA-I in particles larger than alpha-1 HDL [12]. Compound heterozygotes have nearly all apoA-I in particles similar to α-1 but increased in size. Heterozygotes have a large amount of α-1 particles. All affected subjects we have studied have decreased concentrations of the smaller α-mobility particles. Preβ-1 level is normal in heterozygotes and elevated in the compound-heterozygotes and homozygotes. These data indicate that the effect of CETP on the HDL-subpopulation profile is dose dependent. It is worth noting that HDL in homozygotes is different from normal not only in size but also in composition. The larger than normal-sized particles contain several apolipoproteins: A-I, A-II, all the Cs, and apoE. These apos are distributed among the various HDL particles in an unaffected person. For example, in unaffected individuals, apoE mainly forms its own HDL particles (LpE).

Step 7: HL-Mediated Lypolyses

The TG-enriched α-1 and very large HDL particles are good substrates for HL (Fig. 5a, b). HL has both triglyceride and phospholipase activity with triglyceride lipase activity less than LPL and phospholipase activity less than EL. HDL particles in HL deficiency are triglyceride and phospholipid enriched [51]. Via a concerted effect of HL and CETP (Fig. 5b), the core of α-1 shrinks dividing the particles into small, α-4, and probably some still unrecognized α-1-remnants (see Fig. 5 in chapter "High Density Lipoprotein Particles"). We believe that the α-1 remnants fuse with pro-α-2 particles, which initially contain equal amounts of apoA-I and apoA-II, ultimately resulting in α-2 particles. We hypothesize that the pro apo-α-2 particles form when the newly secreted and lipidated apoA-II fuses with the α-3 particles. We also hypothesize that the LCAT-mediated cholesterol accumulation in the core of α-3 HDL is preparing this particle for accepting apoA-II to form the short-lived intermediate pro-α-2 particles. After the formation of α-2 from these two intermediate particles, α-2 probably gains more core material as a result of the concerted act of LCAT and LPL. The final result is the most abundant and stable HDL particle. Compared to unaffected subjects, homozygous HL-deficient subjects have increased preβ-1, slightly decreased α-4 and α-3, substantially decreased α-2, and normal to slightly elevated α-1 HDL particles. This pattern is exclusively unique for HL deficient subjects. The HDL subpopulation distribution (profile) of heterozygous HL-deficient subjects is normal. This unique HDL subpopulation profile indicates that HDL size increase (maturation) is not a simple linear process. This hypothesis is supported by the observation that there is a strong inverse correlation between the concentrations of the small LpA-I preβ-1 and α-4, and the large LpA-1 α-1. However, there is no correlation between the concentrations of the small LpA-I:A-II α-3 and the large LpA-I α-1. Moreover, we have observed a positive correlation between the concentrations of α-1 and α-2. All this information indicates that LpA-I (preβ-1, α-4, α-1, and all the preα-mobility HDL particles) metabolizes independently from LpA-I:A-II but that some of the LpA-I particles serve as the basis for the formation of LpA-I:A-II HDL.

Step 8: SR-B1 Cycle

The last step in HDL-mediated reverse cholesterol transport is the selective CE transfer to bile via the liver SR-B1 pathway (SR-B1 cycle) (Fig. 6). Earlier, we have demonstrated that the selective cholesterol removal from HDL, via the SR-B1 pathway, decreased concentrations of the large lipid enriched α-1 and increased the concentrations of the smaller α-3 and α-4-size particles, but preβ-1 particles were not produced via this pathway (see Fig. 6 in chapter "High Density Lipoprotein Particles") [52].

Despite the fact that HDL mediates only about 1% of direct total RCT, this step is believed to be a very significant one because HDL carries cholesterol from macrophages in the vessel wall, which directly inhibits plaque formation. The indirect action of HDL in RCT is mediated through transfer of CE to LDL, which then delivers it to liver. It has become increasingly obvious that there are a number of pathways for the flux of cholesterol between cells and serum lipoproteins. At least three protein-mediated pathways have been identified and these proteins demonstrate both similarities and differences. ABCG1 and SR-BI require cholesterol acceptors that contain phospholipids, and the efficiency of the acceptor is determined by the composition and size of the extracellular particle. Therefore, the best substrates for cell-cholesterol efflux are the large, lipid-enriched α-1 and α-2 HDL particles (see Fig. 9b in chapter "High Density Lipoprotein Particles"). In contrast, phospholipid-free or phospholipid-poor apoproteins or helical amphipathic peptides serve as cholesterol acceptors via the ABCA1 pathway. Cholesterol efflux via ABCA1 has an absolute requirement for the binding of apoprotein to the cell, with recent evidence indicating that efficient efflux requires binding both directly to the ABCA1 protein and indirectly to other membrane domains [43]. Other data indicate that acceptor binding to the donor cell is not a requirement for efflux via the ABCG1 pathway [42]. There is also evidence that some cholesterol efflux occurs via aqueous diffusion [53]. The two ABC transporters participate in unidirectional flux of cholesterol between cells and extracellular acceptors, despite differences in the nature of the acceptor. In contrast, SR-B1 expression enhances the efflux of cell FC and also the influx of both lipoprotein FC and CE.

The role of cholesterol efflux in RCT has largely focused on macrophages and macrophage-derived foam cells. All three transporters are present in macrophages, although the level of expression and the contribution to efflux of SR-B1 remains controversial. However, it is now well established that macrophages express both ABCA1 and ABCG1, and the expression of these proteins is increased in cholesterol-enriched macrophages. There is evidence that ABCA1 and ABCG1 function coordinately with ABCA1 initially providing phospholipids to lipid-poor apoproteins (preβ-HDL) that becomes further enriched with phospholipids and cholesterol through the action of ABCG1 [54, 55]. It is speculated that SR-BI, if present, could also contribute to the lipidation of newly generated HDL; however, it is apparent that SR-BI plays a major role in the flux of cholesterol between HDL and hepatocytes and endocrine cells, whereas the ABC-mediated cell cholesterol efflux might be the major pathways for the removal of excess cholesterol from macrophages.

Step 9: HDL Catabolism

In addition to LPL and HL, there are other lipases and transfer proteins participating in HDL remodeling (Fig. 7). Our preliminary data, generated in a collaboration with FC de Beer's lab, indicate that EL and sPLA2 also lipolyse PL on medium to large HDL particles and transform them to small α-4 and preβ-1 particles, respectively (see Fig. 5 in chapter "High Density Lipoprotein Particles"). EL – as HL – is a member of the triglyceride lipase family with strikingly different substrate specificities. EL has high phospholipase and very low triglyceride lipase activity. EL also differs from HL, in that it does not dissociate lipid-free/lipid-poor apoA-I from HDL [56, 57]. PLTP is a member of the same protein family as CETP. It transfers phospholipids and UC from VLDL to HDL as well as between different HDL particles. PLTP remodels HDL into large and small particles by particle fusion and the dissociation of lipid-free/lipid-poor apoA-I [58]. The role of PLTP in atherogenesis is controversial, with reports that its expression in macrophages both enhances and inhibits atherosclerosis in mice [59, 60]. So far, no subjects with EL, sPLA2, and PLTP deficiency have been identified and investigated. Therefore, we do not have direct in vivo evidence for the above mentioned steps in HDL remodeling in human.

ApoA-I, if present in lipid-poor particles, is catabolized in the kidney through the cubulin/megalin pathways [61] (Fig. 8). Larger HDL particles can be taken up whole and also catabolized by the liver [62] (Fig. 8).

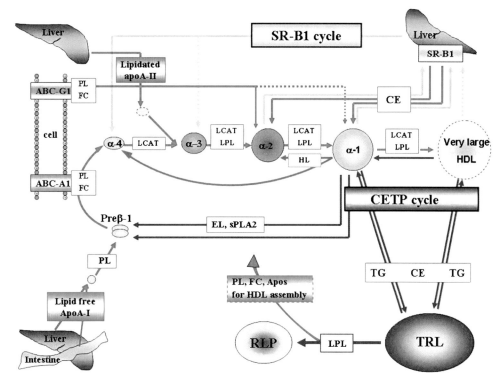

Fig. 7 The effects of phospholipases on HDL remodeling

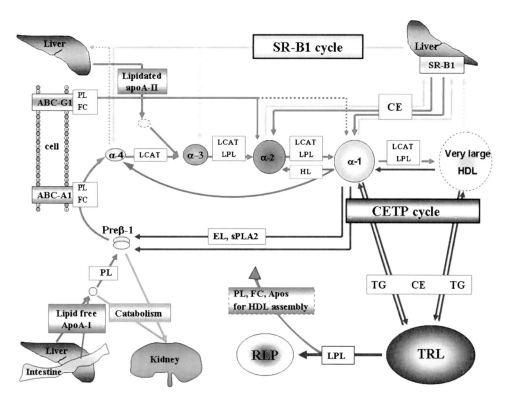

Fig. 8 ApoA-I catabolism by the cubulin/megalin pathway in the kidney

One of the key events in remodeling is the dissociation of lipid-free or lipid-poor apoA-I from spherical HDL by CETP, PLTP, and HL [63, 64]. Lipid-free/lipid-poor apoA-I accounts for up to 5% of the total plasma apoA-I and accepts cholesterol and phospholipids that efflux from cell membranes via ABCA1. Progressive lipidation of apoA-I via this pathway generate discoidal HDL and recycles apoA-I back into the HDL fraction. This reduces the rate at which apoA-I is cleared from the circulation and helps maintain circulating HDL levels. Work on reconstituted HDL indicates that apoA-II also inhibits the CETP-mediated remodeling of HDL and the dissociation of lipid-free/lipid-poor apoA-I [65]. The ability of CETP to remodel HDL and mediate the dissociation of apoA-I is also influenced by the phospholipid composition of the particles [66], while TG-enrichment enhances both HDL remodeling by PLTP and the dissociation of apoA-I. ApoA-I and apoA-II also regulate the hydrolysis of HDL phospholipids by EL and the HL-mediated hydrolysis of HDL phospholipids and triglyceride.

It is known that the kidney and liver are major sites of HDL catabolism and that structural integrity of its apolipoprotein components are major factors in determining the half life of HDL [67–70]. SR-BI has been shown to function as an HDL receptor that mediates selective cholesterol uptake [71]. However, unlike catabolism of LDL by LDL receptors, HDL catabolism by SR-BI does not involve holoparticle uptake and lysosomal degradation. This conclusion was supported by the finding that transgenic mice deficient in SR-BI display elevated levels of plasma HDL cholesterol yet exhibit no change in the level of plasma apoA-I [72].

Conclusions

The measurement of apoA-I-containing lipoproteins by two dimensional gel electrophoresis has given us insight into the synthesis, remodeling, and catabolism of HDL particles. It is clearly the small discoidal HDL particles that are essential for cellular cholesterol efflux along with subsequent cholesterol esterification. Adequate levels of lipoprotein lipase and hepatic lipase are clearly critical for the normal metabolism of triglyceride and phospholipid on all lipoproteins, including HDL. Both CETP and SRB1 are critical for the transfer of cholesteryl esters either to triglyceride-rich lipoproteins via CETP or for cellular bidirectional-transfer via SRB1. The recycling of apoA-I onto discoidal particles allows for its reutilization in the reverse cholesterol transport process, and the kidney plays a major role in the clearance of apoA-I on small discoidal HDL particles. The effects of various lipid disorders, lifestyle modifications, and pharmacologic therapies on HDL particles will be discussed in subsequent chapters. All of the nine steps

in HDL particle formation, remodeling, and catabolism mentioned in this chapter are critical for normal HDL metabolism and reverse cholesterol transport. Patients having defects in apoA-I production and cellular cholesterol efflux are clearly at increased risk for premature CHD, and are unable to form large protective HDL, a sign of normal HDL metabolism.

References

1. Miller NE, Thelle DS, Forde OH, Mjos OD (1977) The Tromsø heart-study. High-density lipoprotein and coronary heart-disease: a prospective case-control study. Lancet 1(8019):965–968
2. Gordon DJ, Probstfield JL, Garrison RJ, Neaton JD, Castelli WP, Knoke JD, Jacobs DRJr, Bangdiwala S, Tyroler HA (1989) High-density lipoprotein cholesterol and cardiovascular disease. Four prospective American studies. Circulation 79(1):8–15
3. Assmann G, Schulte H (1992) Relation of high-density lipoprotein cholesterol and triglycerides to incidence of atherosclerotic coronary artery disease (the PROCAM experience). Prospective Cardiovascular Münster study. Am J Cardiol 70(7):733–737
4. Robins SJ, Collins D, Wittes JT, Papademetriou V, Deedwania PC, Schaefer EJ, McNamara JR, Kashyap ML, Hershman JM, Wexler LF, Rubins HB; VA-HIT Study Group. Veterans Affairs High-Density Lipoprotein Intervention Trial (2001) Relation of gemfibrozil treatment and lipid levels with major coronary events: VA-HIT: a randomized controlled trial. JAMA 285(12):1585–1591
5. Barter P, Gotto AM, LaRosa JC, Maroni J, Szarek M, Grundy SM, Kastelein JJ, Bittner V, Fruchart JC (2007) HDL cholesterol, very low levels of LDL cholesterol, and cardiovascular events. N Engl J Med 357:1301–1310
6. Lewis GF, Rader DJ (2005) New insights into the regulation of HDL metabolism and reverse cholesterol transport. Circ Res 96(12):1221–1232
7. Vaisar T, Pennathur S, Green PS, Gharib SA, Hoofnagle AN, Cheung MC, Byun J, Vuletic S, Kassim S, Singh P, Chea H, Knopp RH, Brunzell J, Geary R, Chait A, Zhao XQ, Elkon K, Marcovina S, Ridker P, Oram JF, Heinecke JW (2007) Shotgun proteomics implicates protease inhibition and complement activation in the antiinflammatory properties of HDL. J Clin Invest 117(3):746–756
8. Asztalos BF, Sloop CH, Wong L, Roheim PS (1993) Two-dimensional electrophoresis of plasma lipoproteins: recognition of new apo A-I-containing subpopulations. Biochim Biophys Acta 1169(3):291–300
9. Santos RD, Schaefer EJ, Asztalos BF, Polisecki E, Wang J, Hegele RA, Martinez LR, Miname MH, Rochitte CE, Da Luz PL, Maranhão RC (2008) Characterization of high density lipoprotein particles in familial apolipoprotein A-I deficiency. J Lipid Res 49(2):349–357
10. Asztalos BF, Brousseau ME, McNamara JR, Horvath KV, Roheim PS, Schaefer EJ (2001) Subpopulations of high density lipoproteins in homozygous and heterozygous Tangier disease. Atherosclerosis 156(1):217–225
11. Asztalos BF, Schaefer EJ, Horvath KV, Yamashita S, Miller M, Franceschini G, Calabresi L (2007) Role of LCAT in HDL remodeling: investigation of LCAT deficiency states. J Lipid Res 48(3):592–599
12. Asztalos BF, Horvath KV, Kajinami K, Nartsupha C, Cox CE, Batista M, Schaefer EJ, Inazu A, Mabuchi H (2004) Apolipoprotein composition of HDL in cholesteryl ester transfer protein deficiency. J Lipid Res 45(3):448–455

13. Asztalos BF, de la Llera-Moya M, Dallal GE, Horvath KV, Schaefer EJ, Rothblat GH (2005) Differential effects of HDL subpopulations on cellular ABCA1- and SR-BI-mediated cholesterol efflux. J Lipid Res 46(10):2246–2253

14. Schaefer EJ, Heaton WH, Wetzel MG, Brewer HBJr (1982) Plasma apolipoprotein A-I absence associated with marked reduction of high density lipoproteins and premature coronary artery disease. Arteriosclerosis 2:16–26

15. Schaefer EJ (1984) The clinical, biochemical, and genetic features in familial disorders of high density lipoprotein deficiency. Arteriosclerosis 4:303–322

16. Schaefer EJ, Ordovas JM, Law S, Ghiselli G, Kashyap ML, Srivastava LS, Heaton WH, Albers JJ, Connor WE, Lemeshev Y et al (1985) Familial apolipoprotein A-I and C-III deficiency, variant II. J Lipid Res 26:1089–1101

17. Ordovas JM, Cassidy DK, Civeira F, Bisgaier CL, Schaefer EJ (1989) Familial apolipoprotein A-I, C-III, and A-IV deficiency with marked high density lipoprotein deficiency and premature atherosclerosis due to a deletion of the apolipoprotein A-I, C-III, and A-IV gene complex. J Biol Chem 264:16339–16342

18. Norum RA, Lakier JB, Goldstein S, Angel A, Goldberg AB, Block WD, Noffze DK, Dolphin PJ, Edelglass J et al (1982) Familial deficiency of apolipoproteins A-I and C-III and precocious coronary artery disease. N Engl J Med 306:1513–1519

19. Karathanasis SK, Norum RA, Zannis VI, Breslow JL (1983) An inherited polymorphism in the human apolipoprotein A-I gene locus related to the development of atherosclerosis. Nature 301:718–720

20. Karathanasis SK, Ferris E, Haddad EA (1987) DNA inversion within the apolipoprotein AI/CIII/AIV-encoding gene cluster of certain patients with premature atherosclerosis. Proc Natl Acad Sci USA 84:7198–7202

21. Forte TM, Nichols AV, Krauss RM, Norum RA (1984) Familial apolipoprotein AI and apolipoprotein CIII deficiency. Subclass distribution, composition, and morphology of lipoproteins in a disorder associated with premature atherosclerosis. J Clin Invest 74:1601–1613

22. Sorci-Thomas MG, Thomas MJ (2002) The effects of altered apolipoprotein A-I structure on plasma HDL concentration. Trends Cardiovasc Med 12:121–128

23. Zannis VI, Chroni A, Krieger M (2006) Role of apoA-I, ABCA1, LCAT, and SR-BI in the biogenesis of HDL. J Mol Med 84:276–294

24. Frank PG, Marcel YL (2000) Apolipoprotein A-I: structure-function relationships. J Lipid Res 41:853–872

25. Orso E, Broccardo C, Kaminske WE, Bottcher A, Liebisch G, Drobnik W, Gotz A, Chambenoit O, Diederich W, Langmann T, Spruss T, Luciani MF, Rothe G, Lackner KJ, Chimini G and Schmitz G (2000) Transport of lipids from golgi to plasma membrane is defective in Tangier disease patients and ABCA-1-deficient mice. Nat Genet 24:192–196

26. Lin YC, Ma C, Hsu WC, Lo HF, Yang VC (2007) Molecular interaction between caveolin-1 and ABCA1 on high-density lipoprotein-mediated cholesterol efflux in aortic endothelial cells. Cardiovasc Res 75:575–583

27. Arakawa R, Abe-Dohmae S, Asai M, Ito JI, Yokoyama S (2000) Involvement of caveolin-1 in cholesterol enrichment of high density lipoprotein during its assembly by apolipoprotein and THP-1 cells. J Lipid Res 41:1952–1962

28. Rogler G, Trumbach B, Klima B, Lackner KJ, Schmitz G (1995) HDL-mediated efflux of intracellular cholesterol is impaired in fibroblasts from Tangier disease patients. Arterioscler Thromb Vasc Biol 15:683–690

29. Rust S, Rosier M, Funke H, Real J, Amoura Z, Piette JC, Deleuze JF, Brewer HB, Duverger N, Denefle P, Assmann G (1999) Tangier disease is caused by mutations in the gene encoding ATP-binding cassette transporter 1. Nat Genet 22:352–355

30. Brunham LR, Singaraja RR, Duong M, Timmins JM, Fievet C, Bissada N, Kang MH, Samra A, Fruchart JC, McManus B, Staels B, Parks JS, Hayden MR (2009) Tissue-specific roles of ABCA1 influence susceptibility to atherosclerosis. Arterioscler Thromb Vasc Biol 29(4):548–554

31. McLean J, Fielding C, Drayna D, Dieplinger H, Baer B, Kohr W, Henzel W, Lawn R (1986) Cloning and expression of human lecithin-cholesterol acyltransferase cDNA. Proc Natl Acad Sci USA 83:2335–2339

32. Fielding CJ, Fielding PE (1995) Molecular physiology of reverse cholesterol transport. J Lipid Res 36:211–228

33. Czarnecka H, Yokoyama S (1996) Regulation of cellular cholesterol efflux by lecithin:cholesterol acyltransferase reaction through nonspecific lipid exchange. J Biol Chem 266:2023–2028

34. Jonas A, von Eckardstein A, Kezdy KE, Steinmetz A, Assmann G (1991) Structural and functional properties of reconstituted high density lipoprotein discs prepared with six apolipoprotein A-I variants. J Lipid Res 32:97–106

35. Steinmetz A, Kaffarnik H, Utermann G (1985) Activation of phosphatidylcholine-sterol acyltransferase by human apolipoprotein E isoforms. Eur J Biochem 152:747–751

36. Santamarina-Fojo S, Hoeg JM, Assmann G, Brewer HBJr (2001) Lecithin cholesterol acyltransferase deficiency and fish eye disease. In: Scriver CR, Beaudet AL, Sly WS, Valle D (eds) The metabolic and molecular bases of inherited disease. McGraw-Hill, New York, pp 2817–2834

37. Kuivenhoven JA, Pritchard H, Hill J, Frohlich J, Assmann G, Kastelein J (1997) The molecular pathology of lecithin:cholesterol acyltransferase (LCAT) deficiency syndromes. J Lipid Res 38:191–205

38. Rader DJ, Ikewaki K, Duverger N, Schmidt H, Pritchard H, Frohlich J, Clerc M, Dumon MF, Fairwell T, Zech L et al (1994) Markedly accelerated catabolism of apolipoprotein A-II (apoA-II) and high density lipoproteins containing apoA-II in classic lecithin:cholesterol acyltransferase deficiency and fish-eye disease. J Clin Invest 93:321–330

39. Kennedy MA, Venkateswaran A, Tarr PT, Xenarios I, Kudoh J, Shimizu N, Edwards PA (2001) Characterization of the human ABCG1 gene: liver X receptor activates an internal promoter that produces a novel transcript encoding an alternative form of the protein. J Biol Chem 276:39438–39447

40. Klucken J, Buchler C, Orso E, Kaminski WE, Porsch-Ozcurumez M, Liebisch G, Kapinsky M, Diederich W, Drobnik W, Dean M et al (2000) ABCG1 (ABC8), the human homolog of the Drosophila white gene, is a regulator of macrophage cholesterol and phospholipid transport. Proc Natl Acad Sci USA 97:817–822

41. Kobayashi A, Takanezawa Y, Hirata T, Shimizu Y, Misasa K, Kioka N, Arai H, Ueda K, Matsuo M (2006) Efflux of sphingomyelin, cholesterol, and phosphatidylcholine by ABCG1. J Lipid Res 47(8):1791–1802

42. Adorni MP, Zimetti F, Billheimer JT, Wang N, Rader DJ, Phillips MC, Rothblat GH (2007) The roles of different pathways in the release of cholesterol from macrophages. J Lipid Res 48(11):2453–2462

43. Wang N, Silver DL, Costet P, Tall AR (2000) Specific binding of apoA-I, enhanced cholesterol efflux, and altered plasma membrane morphology in cells expressing ABC1. J Biol Chem 275:33053–33058

44. Tall AR, Coster P, Wang N (2002) Regulation and mechanisms of macrophage cholesterol efflux. J Clin Invest 110:899–904

45. Wang N, Lan D, Chen W, Matsuura F, Tall AR (2004) ATP-binding cassette transporters G1 and G4 mediate cellular cholesterol efflux to high-density lipoprotein. Proc Natl Acad Sci USA 101:9774–9779

46. Hassan HH, Denis M, Lee DY, Iatan I, Nyholt D, Ruel I, Krimbou L, Genest J (2007) Identification of an ABCA1-dependent phospholipid-rich plasma membrane apolipoprotein A-I binding site for nascent HDL formation: implications for current models of HDL biogenesis. J Lipid Res 48(11):2428–2442

47. Van Eck M, Pennings M, Hoekstra M, Out R, Van Berkel TJ (2005) Scavenger receptor BI and ATP-binding cassette transporter A1 in reverse cholesterol transport and atherosclerosis. Curr Opin Lipidol 16(3):307–315

48. Sankaranarayanan S, Oram JF, Asztalos BF, Vaughan AM, Lund-Katz S, Adorni MP, Phillips MC, Rothblat GH (2009) Effects of acceptor composition and mechanism of ABCG1-mediated cellular free cholesterol efflux. J Lipid Res 50(2):275–284

49. Qiu X, Mistry A, Ammirati MJ, Chrunyk BA, Clark RW, Cong Y, Culp JS, Danley DE, Freeman TB, Geoghegan KF et al (2007) Crystal structure of cholesteryl ester transfer protein reveals a long tunnel and four bound lipid molecules. Nat Struct Mol Biol 14:106–113

50. Rye KA, Hime NJ, Barter PJ (1997) Evidence that cholesteryl ester transfer protein-mediated reductions in reconstituted high density lipoprotein size involve particle fusion. J Biol Chem 272:3953–3960

51. Zambon A, Deeb SS, Bensadoun A, Foster KE, Brunzell JD (2000) In vivo evidence of a role for hepatic lipase in human apoB-containing lipoprotein metabolism, independent of its lipolytic activity. J Lipid Res 41(12):2094–2099

52. Webb NR, de Beer MC, Asztalos BF, Whitaker N, van der Westhuyzen DR, de Beer FC (2004) Remodeling of HDL remnants generated by scavenger receptor class B type I. J Lipid Res 45(9):1666–1673

53. de la Llera-Moya M, Rothblat GH, Connelly MA, Kellner-Weibel G, Sakr SW, Phillips MC, Williams DL (1999) Scavenger receptor BI (SR-BI) mediates free cholesterol flux independently of HDL tethering to the cell surface. J Lipid Res 40(3):575–580

54. Gelissen IC, Harris M, Rye KA, Quinn C, Brown AJ, Kockx M, Cartland S, Packianathan M, Kritharides L, Jessup W (2006) ABCA1 and ABCG1 synergize to mediate cholesterol export to apoA-I. Arterioscler Thromb Vasc Biol 26(3):534–540

55. Vaughan AM, Oram JF (2006) ABCA1 and ABCG1 or ABCG4 act sequentially to remove cellular cholesterol and generate cholesterol-rich HDL. J Lipid Res 47(11):2433–2443

56. Jaye M, Lynch KJ, Krawiec J, Marchadier D, Maugeais C, Doan K, South V, Amin D, Perrone M, Rader DJ (1999) A novel endothelial-derived lipase that modulates HDL metabolism. Nat Genet 21:424–428

57. Jahangiri A, Rader DJ, Marchadier D, Curtiss LK, Bonnet DJ, Rye KA (2005) Evidence that endothelial lipase remodels high density lipoproteins without mediating the dissociation of apolipoprotein A-I. J Lipid Res 46:896–903

58. Settasatian N, Duong M, Curtiss LK, Ehnholm C, Jauhiainen M, Huuskonen J, Rye KA (2001) The mechanism of the remodeling of high density lipoproteins by phospholipid transfer protein. J Biol Chem 276:26898–26905

59. van Haperen R, Samyn H, Moerland M, van Gent T, Peeters M, Grosveld F, van Tol A, de Crom R (2008) Elevated expression of phospholipid transfer protein in bone marrow derived cells causes atherosclerosis. PLoS One 3:e2255

60. Valenta DT, Ogier N, Bradshaw G, Black AS, Bonnet DJ, Lagrost L, Curtiss LK, Desrumaux CM (2006) Atheroprotective potential of macrophage-derived phospholipid transfer protein in low-density lipoprotein receptor-deficient mice is overcome by apolipoprotein AI overexpression. Arterioscler Thromb Vasc Biol 26:1572–1578

61. Hammad SM, Stefansson S, Twal WO, Drake CJ, Fleming P, Remaley A, Brewer HBJr, Argraves WS (1999) Cubilin, the endo-cytic receptor for intrinsic factor-vitamin B(12) complex, mediates high-density lipoprotein holoparticle endocytosis. Proc Natl Acad Sci USA 96(18):10158–10163

62. Hammad SM, Barth JL, Knaak C, Argraves WS (2000) Megalin acts in concert with cubilin to mediate endocytosis of high density lipoproteins. J Biol Chem 275(16):12003–12008

63. Rye KA, Barter PJ (2004) Formation and metabolism of prebeta-migrating, lipid-poor apolipoprotein A-I. Arterioscler Thromb Vasc Biol 24:421–428

64. Rye KA, Wee K, Curtiss LK, Bonnet DJ, Barter PJ (2003) Apolipoprotein A-II inhibits high density lipoprotein remodeling and lipid-poor apolipoprotein A-I formation. J Biol Chem 278:22530–22536

65. Hime NJ, Barter PJ, Rye KA (1998) The influence of apolipoproteins on the hepatic lipase-mediated hydrolysis of high density lipoprotein phospholipid and triacylglycerol. J Biol Chem 273:27191–27198

66. Rye KA, Duong M, Psaltis MK, Curtiss LK, Bonnet DJ, Stocker R, Barter PJ (2002) Evidence that phospholipids play a key role in pre-beta apoA-I formation and high-density lipoprotein remodeling. Biochemistry 41:12538–12545

67. Caiazza D, Jahangiri A, Rader DJ, Marchadier D, Rye KA (2004) Apolipoproteins regulate the kinetics of endothelial lipase-mediated hydrolysis of phospholipids in reconstituted high-density lipoproteins. Biochemistry 43:11898–11905

68. Glass C, Pittman RC, Civen M, Steinberg D (1985) Uptake of high-density lipoprotein-associated apoprotein A-I and cholesterol esters by 16 tissues of the rat in vivo and by adrenal cells and hepatocytes in vitro. J Biol Chem 260(2):744–750

69. Le NA, Ginsberg HN (1988) Heterogeneity of apolipoprotein A-I turnover in subjects with reduced concentrations of plasma high density lipoprotein cholesterol. Metabolism 37(7):614–617

70. Jäckle S, Rinninger F, Lorenzen T, Greten H, Windler E (1993) Dissection of compartments in rat hepatocytes involved in the intra-cellular trafficking of high-density lipoprotein particles or their selectively internalized cholesteryl esters. Hepatology 17(3):455–465

71. Acton S, Rigotti A, Landschulz KT, Xu S, Hobbs HH, Krieger M (1996) Identification of scavenger receptor SR-BI as a high density lipoprotein receptor. Science 271(5248):518–520

72. Rigotti A, Trigatti BL, Penman M, Rayburn H, Herz J, Krieger M (1997) A targeted mutation in the murine gene encoding the high density lipoprotein (HDL) receptor scavenger receptor class B type I reveals its key role in HDL metabolism. Proc Natl Acad Sci USA 94(23):12610–12615

HDL Structure, Function, and Antiinflammatory Properties

Kerry-Anne Rye and Philip J. Barter

Introduction

High density lipoproteins (HDL) are the smallest and the densest of all plasma lipoproteins. They consist of several distinct subpopulations of particles of varying size, shape, density, surface charge, and composition. Large-scale epidemiological studies and studies in animals have identified an inverse relationship between HDL levels and the incidence of cardiovascular disease [1, 2]. In addition to preventing atherosclerotic lesion progression, the results of animal studies indicate that HDL also have the capacity to mediate lesion regression [3].

The cardioprotective properties of HDL have been attributed to several processes. The best understood of these involves their ability to accept cholesterol from peripheral cells, including macrophages in the artery wall, in the first step of the reverse cholesterol transport pathway [4]. HDL also inhibit LDL oxidation [5], enhance endothelial repair [6], and improve endothelial function [7]. In addition, HDL display antithrombotic and antiinflammatory properties [7, 8] and have recently been shown to inhibit the activation and binding of monocytes to the endothelium [9].

Origins and Structure of HDL

HDL originate as discoidal particles that are secreted from the liver or assembled in the plasma from the individual constituents (Fig. 1). Discoidal HDL consist of a phospholipid bilayer, the acyl chains of which are shielded from the aqueous environment by an annulus consisting of two or more

K.-A. Rye (✉)
Lipid Research Group, The Heart Research Institute,
Sydney, NSW, Australia

Faculty of Medicine, University of Sydney,
Sydney, NSW, Australia

Department of Medicine, University of Melbourne,
Melbourne, VIC, Australia
e-mail: ryek@hri.org.au

apolipoprotein molecules (Fig. 1). These particles also contain a small amount of unesterified cholesterol that is available for esterification by lecithin:cholesterol acyltransferase (LCAT), the enzyme responsible for most of the cholesteryl ester formation in plasma. The cholesteryl esters that are formed by LCAT are very hydrophobic and partition rapidly into the HDL core in a process that converts the discs into small spherical HDL and subsequently into the large, spherical HDL particles that predominate in normal human plasma (Fig. 1). Spherical HDL contain a central core of neutral lipids (cholesteryl esters and some triglyceride) surrounded by a surface monolayer of phospholipids, unesterified cholesterol and apolipoproteins (Fig. 2). The two main apolipoproteins associated with HDL are apoA-I and apoA-II. Approximately 5–10% of the apoA-I in human plasma exists in a lipid-free/lipid-poor form, which plays a key role in HDL metabolism.

Heterogeneity of HDL

HDL are heterogeneous in terms of density, size, composition, and surface charge. They can be separated in the ultracentrifuge on the basis of density into two main subfractions: HDL_2 and HDL_3. HDL_2 are larger and less dense than HDL_3 (Fig. 3a). HDL can also be resolved on the basis of particle size by nondenaturing gradient gel electrophoresis into five distinct subpopulations of particles HDL_{2b}, HDL_{2a}, HDL_{3a}, HDL_{3b}, and HDL_{3c} with mean diameters of 10.6, 9.2, 8.4, 8.0, and 7.6 nm, respectively (Fig. 3b) [10]. They have also been classified on the basis of their apolipoprotein composition into two populations of particles: those that contain apoA-I but not apoA-II, (A-I)HDL, and those that contain apoA-I and apoA-II, (A-I/A-II)HDL (Fig. 3c) [11]. In normal human plasma, apoA-I is distributed approximately equally between (A-I)HDL and (A-I/A-II)HDL, while apoA-II is mostly associated with (A-I/A-II)HDL.

When subjected to agarose gel electrophoresis, HDL migrate to a γ-, α- or preβ-position (Fig. 3d). Spherical (A-I)HDL and (A-I/A-II)HDL display α-migration, while

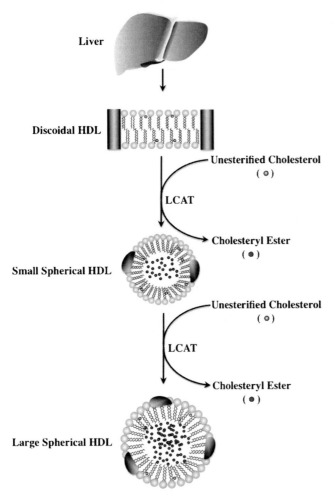

Fig. 1 Origins of HDL. Discoidal HDL are secreted from the liver and converted by LCAT into small spherical HDL and then into large spherical HDL. Vertical sections of discoidal HDL, small spherical HDL and large spherical HDL are shown

discoidal HDL and lipid-free apoA-I are preβ-migrating. A small population of large, spherical HDL that contain apoE, a minor HDL apolipoprotein with well characterized cardioprotective properties, migrate to a γ-position [12].

HDL Remodeling and Its Relationship to Atherogenesis

The above variations in HDL size, shape, surface charge, and composition are, to a large extent, a consequence of interactions with a range of plasma factors in processes that are collectively termed remodeling. Plasma factors that remodel HDL include LCAT, cholesteryl ester transfer protein (CETP), phospholipid transfer protein (PLTP), hepatic lipase (HL), and endothelial lipase (EL).

One of the key events in HDL remodeling is the dissociation of lipid-free or lipid-poor apoA-I from spherical HDL that are decreasing in size. Lipid-free/lipid-poor apoA-I is generated during the remodeling of HDL by CETP, PLTP, and HL but not by EL (Fig. 4) [13, 14]. ApoA-I that has dissociated from spherical HDL accepts the cholesterol and phospholipids that are exported from cell membranes via the ATP-binding cassette transporter ABCA1 in the first step of the reverse cholesterol transport pathway (Fig. 4). The progressive lipidation of apoA-I via this pathway generates discoidal HDL that interact with LCAT. As HDL acquire increasing amounts of cholesteryl esters in their core and are progressively converted from discoidal HDL into spherical particles, they must acquire additional surface constituents to prevent their structural integrity becoming compromised. This imbalance is rectified by the incorporation of lipid-free/lipid-poor apoA-I back into the HDL fraction, a process that has the

Fig. 2 Structure of spherical HDL. Spherical HDL contain a neutral lipid core (cholesteryl esters and triglycerides) surrounded by a monolayer of phospholipids, apolipoproteins and a small amount of unesterified cholesterol

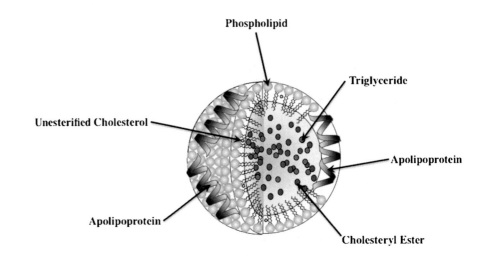

added advantage of decreasing the clearance of lipid-free/lipid-poor apoA-I from the circulation, thus helping to maintain circulating HDL levels.

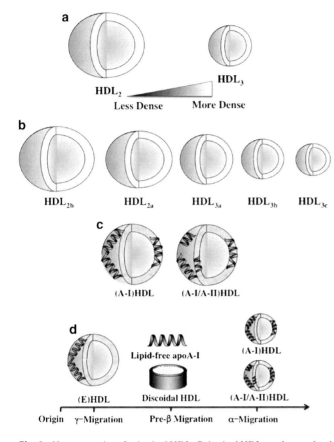

Fig. 3 Heterogeneity of spherical HDL. Spherical HDL can be resolved on the basis of density (**a**), particle size (**b**), apolipoprotein composition (**c**) and surface charge (**d**)

CETP is a member of the lipopolysaccharide-binding/lipid transfer protein family. CETP transfers cholesteryl esters and triglycerides between HDL, VLDL, and LDL. When VLDL levels are elevated, CETP-mediated transfers of core lipids from HDL to VLDL exceed the transfer of core lipids in the opposite direction, from VLDL to HDL (Fig. 5). This generates core lipid-depleted, triglyceride-enriched HDL with an excess of surface constituents relative to core lipids, an imbalance that is rectified by the dissociation of lipid-free/lipid-poor apoA-I and a reduction in HDL size [15]. CETP deficiency in humans is associated with increased HDL levels [16] and appears to be associated with cardioprotective benefit, although this has been disputed by some investigators [17].

PLTP is a member of the same gene family as CETP. It transfers phospholipids between HDL and VLDL, as well as between different HDL particles. PLTP remodels HDL into large and small particles by processes that involve particle fusion and the generation of lipid-free/lipid-poor apoA-I (Fig. 6) [18]. The role of PLTP in atherogenesis is unclear, with evidence that it both enhances and inhibits atherosclerosis in mice [19, 20]. On balance, PLTP appears to have an unfavorable effect on atherosclerosis.

EL and HL are members of the triglyceride lipase family. HDL that are enriched in triglycerides following interaction with CETP are excellent substrates for HL. HL rapidly hydrolyses triglycerides in triglyceride-enriched HDL, generating small HDL and mediating the dissociation of lipid-free/lipid-poor apoA-I (Fig. 7) [21]. In contrast to HL, EL has high phospholipase and low triglyceride lipase activity [22]. EL remodels HDL into small particles via a process that does not involve the dissociation of lipid-free/lipid-poor apoA-I [14, 22]. EL and HL both regulate plasma HDL levels, but their influence on atherosclerosis is not well understood.

Fig. 4 Formation of lipid-free/lipid-poor apoA-I. Lipid-free/lipid-poor apoA-I is generated during the remodelling of spherical HDL by CETP, PLTP and HL. The lipid-free/lipid-poor apoA-I either reassociates with spherical HDL that are increasing in size by interacting with LCAT, or acquire cholesterol and phospholipids from cell membranes that contain ABCA1. The progressive lipidation of apoA-I via the latter pathway generates discoidal rHDL that are converted into spherical HDL by LCAT

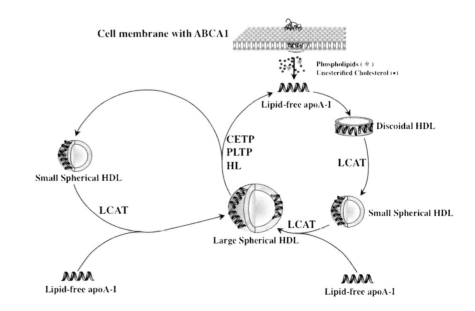

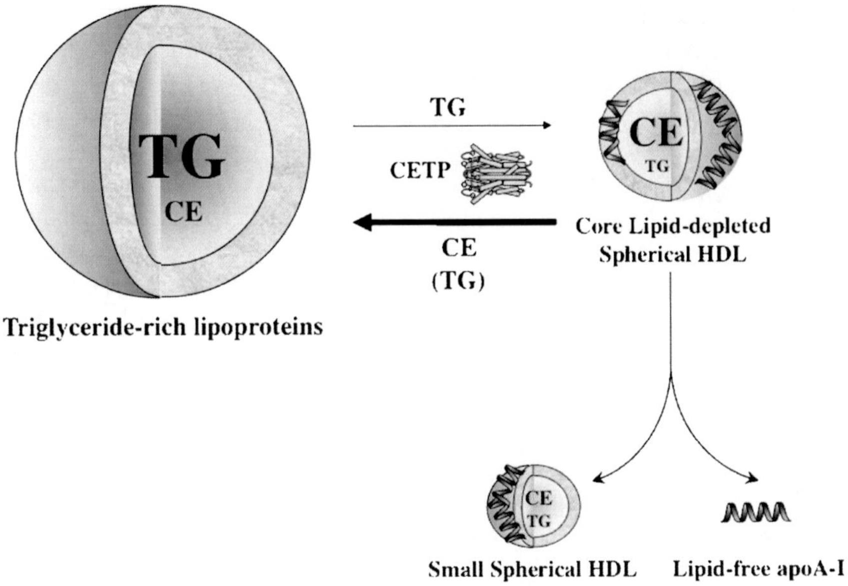

Fig. 5 Remodelling of HDL by CETP. CETP transfers cholesteryl esters and triglycerides between HDL and VLDL. When VLDL levels are high the transfers of core lipids from HDL to VLDL exceed the transfers from VLDL to HDL. The resulting core lipid-depleted HDL are remodelled into small particles by a process that is accompanied by the dissociation of lipid-free/lipid-poor apoA-I

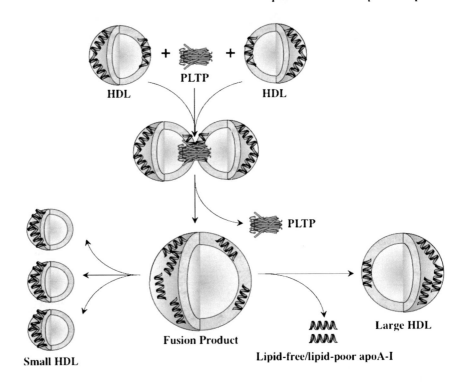

Fig. 6 Remodelling of HDL by PLTP. PLTP mediates the fusion of spherical HDL, generating an unstable product that is remodelled into large and small particles by a process that also generates lipid-free/lipid-poor apoA-I

Studies with reconstituted HDL (rHDL) assembled in the laboratory from the individual constituents have established that HDL composition has a significant impact on HDL remodelling. ApoA-II has been shown to inhibit remodeling and the dissociation of lipid-free/lipid-poor apoA-I from HDL [23]. The phospholipid composition of the particles can also affect CETP-mediated remodeling of HDL and the dissociation of apoA-I [24]. Enrichment with triglyceride enhances both HDL remodelling by PLTP and the dissociation of apoA-I [18]. ApoA-I and apoA-II also regulate the EL-mediated hydrolysis of HDL phospholipids, and the hydrolysis of HDL phospholipids and triglycerides by HL [25, 26].

Cardioprotective Properties of HDL Subpopulations

Human population and transgenic animal studies have suggested that HDL subpopulations do not all protect against atherosclerosis equally well. Information about the cardioprotective properties of specific HDL subpopulations is, however, conflicting. For example, the notion that preβ-migrating lipid-free/lipid-poor apoA-I is more cardioprotective than spherical, α-migrating HDL is based on in vitro observations, which show that lipid-free/lipid-poor apoA-I is superior to spherical HDL as an acceptor of cholesterol from cells in the

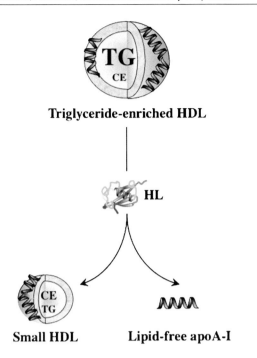

Fig. 7 Remodelling of HDL by HL. HL hydrolyses triglycerides in triglyceride-enriched HDL in a process that reduces the size of the particles and mediates the dissociation of lipid-free/lipid-poor apoA-I

first step of reverse cholesterol transport. However, this assumption is not supported by epidemiological evidence, with a recent analysis of the Veterans Affairs HDL Intervention Trial (VA-HIT), showing that subjects with new cardiovascular events have significantly lower levels of large, α-migrating spherical HDL than event-free subjects [27]. When apoA-I-containing HDL subpopulations from these individuals were quantified by 2-D gel electrophoresis, the cases had lower levels of large α-migrating HDL and significantly higher levels of small, poorly lipidated, preβ-migrating HDL compared to event-free subjects [27]. Large, α-migrating spherical HDL also appear to be the best negative predictors of recurrent cardiovascular events, while small, α-migrating spherical HDL are positive predictors of new events [27]. (A-I)HDL also seem to be superior to the smaller and more dense (A-I/A-II) HDL as predictors of coronary heart disease [28].

Increasing HDL Levels and Atherosclerosis

The possibility that HDL subpopulations are functionally distinct raises the important question as to which subpopulations should be targets for raising HDL levels. One intervention that is known to elevate HDL levels is pharmacological inhibition of CETP activity. This causes cholesteryl esters to accumulate in HDL and selectively increases HDL_2 levels [29]. The CETP inhibitor, torcetrapib, is markedly antiatherogenic in rabbits [2]. In humans, however, torcetrapib

does not reduce atherosclerosis [30, 31] and has caused an excess of deaths and cardiovascular events in a large-scale endpoint trial, probably as a consequence of off-target effects [32]. The impact of other CETP inhibitors, which do not appear to share the off-target effects of torcetrapib, on cardioprotection in humans is currently under investigation.

Another strategy for increasing HDL levels that is also being investigated is infusions of rHDL or mimetic peptides of apoA-I. Short-term administration of high doses of rHDL containing phosphatidylcholine and apoA-I$_{Milano}$, a naturally occurring dimeric form of apoA-I, (ETC-216), has recently been shown to reduce atherosclerotic plaque size in New Zealand White rabbits. In that study, two infusions of ETC-216 (75 mg/kg apoA-I$_{Milano}$) administered 4 days apart significantly decreased the size and increased the stability of abdominal aortic lesions [33]. In a further study, atheroma volume was significantly decreased in animals that received ETC-216 at doses of either 40 or 150 mg/kg apoA-I$_{Milano}$ once every 4 days for a total of 20 days. In that study, two 150 mg/kg infusions were sufficient to induce significant lesion regression [34]. In an earlier study, intravenous administration of ETC-216 at either 15 or 45 mg/kg at weekly intervals over 5 weeks to acute coronary syndrome subjects also reduced atherosclerotic lesion volume [35].

Increasing HDL levels by transgenic overexpression of apoA-I has also been reported to inhibit atherosclerotic lesion progression in the thoracic aortas of high fat fed apoE−/− mice [36].

Infusions of rHDL that contain full length, wild type apoA-I also appear to be beneficial in humans and animals. A single intravenous infusion of rHDL containing phosphatidylcholine and apoA-I (80 mg/kg apoA-I) normalized endothelium-dependent vasodilation in hypercholesterolemic men, presumably by increasing NO bioavailability [37], and improved glucose tolerance in subjects with type 2 diabetes [38]. Infusions of rHDL (40 or 80 mg/kg apoA-I) also improve plaque burden, although liver function may be adversely affected in some subjects at the higher dose [39]. Short term infusions of much smaller amounts of rHDL (8 mg/kg apoA-I) have also been shown to reduce atherosclerotic lesion size in cholesterol-fed New Zealand White rabbits [40].

ApoA-I mimetics are short peptides that have antiinflammatory properties and are structurally analogous to full length apoA-I. When administered orally to apoE−/− mice, the apoA-I mimetics D-4F and 5F inhibit atherosclerosis and LDL-induced monocyte chemotactic activity [41]. D-4F has also been reported to increase reverse cholesterol transport and decrease the lipid hydroperoxide content of VLDL, LDL, and HDL [41]. These beneficial effects have been attributed to the interaction of D-4F with HDL [41], although a recent report suggests that this may not be the case [42].

While these in vivo studies are consistent with interventions that raise HDL levels having a potential therapeutic benefit, it has yet to be established in large population studies that this approach reduces atherosclerotic lesion development, improves lesion composition, or promotes lesion regression. We also do not know if it is necessary to raise HDL levels, or whether the observed benefit reflects altered gene expression and signalling in the artery wall that can be achieved with much lower doses of HDL. If this does turn out to be the case, the possibility that administration of much smaller amounts of apoA-I or rHDL might reduce cardiovascular risk as effectively as large doses needs to be considered.

HDL and Inflammation

Atherosclerosis is a chronic inflammatory disorder that is characterized by the presence of macrophages and other inflammatory cells in the artery wall. HDL inhibit the inflammation that is associated with atherosclerotic plaque development, including the proinflammatory events that characterize the initial stages of the disease, such as the adherence of monocytes to the endothelium and their subsequent transmigration into the artery wall (Fig. 8). Under normal circumstances, the endothelium is quiescent and resistant to leukocyte adhesion. However, in the presence of inflammatory stimuli, the endothelium becomes activated and expresses adhesion molecules such as intercellular adhesion molecule 1 (ICAM-1), vascular adhesion molecule 1 (VCAM-1), P-selectin, and E-selectin to which

monocytes adhere and eventually become firmly tethered. The monocytes then migrate across the endothelium in a process that requires expression of the chemokine, monocyte chemotactic protein-1 (MCP-1) (Fig. 8). Low density lipoproteins (LDL) that are retained in the artery wall under conditions of hypercholesterolemia can become oxidized and exacerbate these events by releasing inflammatory lipids that increase endothelial adhesion molecule expression. Once in the vessel wall, monocytes differentiate into macrophages, the hallmark cells of atherosclerotic lesion development (Fig. 8). Macrophages also express scavenger receptors that take up oxidized LDL in an unregulated manner in a process that eventually culminates in the development of atherosclerotic plaques. In vitro and in vivo studies have established that HDL can inhibit these events by reducing endothelial adhesion molecule and MCP-1 expression, inhibiting monocyte recruitment into the artery wall and preventing LDL oxidation (Fig. 8) [8, 43].

Antiinflammatory Properties of HDL: In Vitro Studies

Cockerill et al. were the first to report that HDL inhibit inflammation in vitro [8]. In that study, HDL from human plasma and discoidal rHDL containing apoA-I and phosphatidylcholine inhibited VCAM-1, ICAM-1, and E-selectin protein and mRNA expression in tumour necrosis factor (TNF)-α-activated human umbilical vein endothelial cells

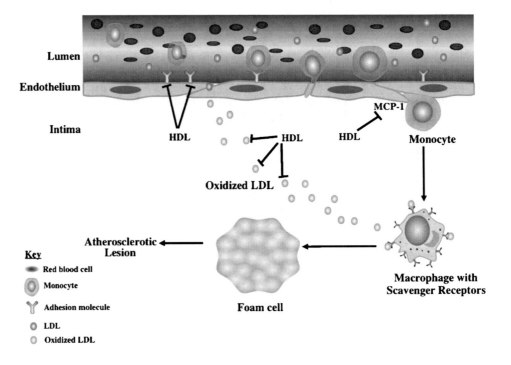

Fig. 8 Anti-inflammatory properties of HDL. HDL decrease endothelial adhesion molecule expression and inhibit monocyte adhesion to the endothelial surface. HDL prevent endothelial transmigration of monocytes by inhibiting monocyte chemoattractant protein 1 (MCP-1) expression. HDL also prevent the oxidation of LDL in the artery wall

(HUVECs) [8]. Discoidal rHDL containing apoA-II, or apoA-I$_{Milano}$, also inhibit VCAM-1 and ICAM-1 expression in cultured HUVECs [44]. The ability of HDL to inhibit sphingosine kinase and reduce nuclear translocation of NF-kB appears to be responsible, at least in part, for these effects [45, 46]. A more recent report showing that HDL increase the expression of 3β-hydroxysteroid-Δ24 reductase (DHCR24), the enzyme that catalyses the final step in cholesterol synthesis has shed further light on the mechanism of the antiinflammatory properties of HDL [47]. In addition to its role in cholesterol synthesis, DHCR24 has antioxidant and antiapoptotic properties, and the ability of HDL to increase its expression in cultured human coronary artery endothelial cells (HCAECs) appears to be related directly to a reduction in NF-kB activity and VCAM-1 expression [47].

HDL have also been reported to inhibit MCP-1 expression and monocyte transmigration in a co-culture system consisting of aortic endothelial cells and smooth muscle cells stimulated with oxidized LDL [48]. The observation that the ability of HDL isolated from different human subjects to inhibit VCAM-1 expression in cultured HUVECs varies widely, with the antiinflammatory capacity of HDL$_3$ being superior to that of HDL$_2$, serves to further highlight the functional heterogeneity of HDL subfractions [49].

Antiinflammatory Properties of HDL: In Vivo Studies

There is mounting evidence that HDL are antiinflammatory in vivo. Alternate daily intravenous infusions of rHDL containing apoA-I (40 mg/kg) complexed with phosphatidylcholine over 3 weeks into cholesterol-fed apoE−/− mice with periarterial carotid cuffs have been shown to reduce endothelial VCAM-1 expression, monocyte/macrophage infiltration into the artery wall, and oxidized LDL formation [50]. These beneficial effects were apparent in the absence of significant changes in plasma total and HDL cholesterol levels, as well as in arterial tissue cholesterol levels [50].

Infusions of small amounts of rHDL containing apoA-I (8 mg/kg) and phosphatidylcholine, or lipid-free apoA-I (8 mg/kg) alone, can also inhibit the acute inflammatory response that is associated with periarterial carotid collar insertion into normocholesterolemic New Zealand White rabbits [43]. These infusions markedly decreased collar-induced intima-media neutrophil infiltration and reduced endothelial expression of VCAM-1, ICAM-1, and MCP-1. When considered together, these results indicate that rHDL infusions may be of potential therapeutic value in acute coronary syndromes and stroke.

Concluding Remarks

While considerable progress in understanding the functionality of HDL subpopulations and their impact on cardiovascular disease has been made in recent years, much remains unknown. As new strategies for increasing HDL levels are identified, it will be important to ascertain how they affect HDL subpopulation distribution and function. This will enhance our understanding of HDL subpopulation functionality and identify specific populations of particles that are potential therapeutic targets for reducing cardiovascular risk.

Acknowledgments This work was funded by NHMRC Program Grant 482800.

References

1. Gordon DJ, Probstfield JL, Garrison RJ et al (1989) High-density lipoprotein cholesterol and cardiovascular disease. Four prospective American studies. Circulation 79:8–15
2. Morehouse LA, Sugarman ED, Bourassa PA et al (2007) Inhibition of CETP activity by torcetrapib reduces susceptibility to diet-induced atherosclerosis in New Zealand White rabbits. J Lipid Res 48:1263–1272
3. Tangirala RK, Tsukamoto K, Chun SH, Usher D, Pure E, Rader DJ (1999) Regression of atherosclerosis induced by liver-directed gene transfer of apolipoprotein A-I in mice. Circulation 100:1816–1822
4. Lewis GF, Rader DJ (2005) New insights into the regulation of HDL metabolism and reverse cholesterol transport. Circ Res 96:1221–1232
5. Negre-Salvayre A, Dousset N, Ferretti G, Bacchetti T, Curatola G, Salvayre R (2006) Antioxidant and cytoprotective properties of high-density lipoproteins in vascular cells. Free Radic Biol Med 41:1031–1040
6. Tso C, Martinic G, Fan WH, Rogers C, Rye KA, Barter PJ (2006) High-density lipoproteins enhance progenitor-mediated endothelium repair in mice. Arterioscler Thromb Vasc Biol 26:1144–1149
7. Mineo C, Deguchi H, Griffin JH, Shaul PW (2006) Endothelial and antithrombotic actions of HDL. Circ Res 98:1352–1364
8. Cockerill GW, Rye KA, Gamble JR, Vadas MA, Barter PJ (1995) High-density lipoproteins inhibit cytokine-induced expression of endothelial cell adhesion molecules. Arterioscler Thromb Vasc Biol 15:1987–1994
9. Murphy AJ, Woollard KJ, Hoang A et al (2008) High-density lipoprotein reduces the human monocyte inflammatory response. Arterioscler Thromb Vasc Biol 28:2071–2077
10. Blanche PJ, Gong EL, Forte TM, Nichols AV (1981) Characterization of human high-density lipoproteins by gradient gel electrophoresis. Biochim Biophys Acta 665:408–419
11. Cheung MC, Albers JJ (1984) Characterization of lipoprotein particles isolated by immunoaffinity chromatography. Particles containing A-I and A-II and particles containing A-I but no A-II. J Biol Chem 259:12201–12209
12. Huang Y, von Eckardstein A, Wu S, Maeda N, Assmann G (1994) A plasma lipoprotein containing only apolipoprotein E and with gamma mobility on electrophoresis releases cholesterol from cells. Proc Natl Acad Sci USA 91:1834–1838

13. Rye KA, Barter PJ (2004) Formation and metabolism of prebeta-migrating, lipid-poor apolipoprotein A-I. Arterioscler Thromb Vasc Biol 24:421–428

14. Jahangiri A, Rader DJ, Marchadier D, Curtiss LK, Bonnet DJ, Rye KA (2005) Evidence that endothelial lipase remodels high density lipoproteins without mediating the dissociation of apolipoprotein A-I. J Lipid Res 46:896–903

15. Rye KA, Hime NJ, Barter PJ (1995) The influence of cholesteryl ester transfer protein on the composition, size, and structure of spherical, reconstituted high density lipoproteins. J Biol Chem 270:189–196

16. Brown ML, Inazu A, Hesler CB et al (1989) Molecular basis of lipid transfer protein deficiency in a family with increased high-density lipoproteins. Nature 342:448–451

17. Ishigami M, Yamashita S, Sakai N et al (1994) Large and cholesteryl ester-rich high-density lipoproteins in cholesteryl ester transfer protein (CETP) deficiency can not protect macrophages from cholesterol accumulation induced by acetylated low-density lipoproteins. J Biochem 116:257–262

18. Settasatian N, Duong M, Curtiss LK et al (2001) The mechanism of the remodeling of high density lipoproteins by phospholipid transfer protein. J Biol Chem 276:26898–26905

19. van Haperen R, Samyn H, Moerland M et al (2008) Elevated expression of phospholipid transfer protein in bone marrow derived cells causes atherosclerosis. PLoS One 3:e2255

20. Valenta DT, Ogier N, Bradshaw G et al (2006) Atheroprotective potential of macrophage-derived phospholipid transfer protein in low-density lipoprotein receptor-deficient mice is overcome by apolipoprotein AI overexpression. Arterioscler Thromb Vasc Biol 26:1572–1578

21. Clay MA, Newnham HH, Barter PJ (1991) Hepatic lipase promotes a loss of apolipoprotein A-I from triglyceride-enriched human high density lipoproteins during incubation in vitro. Arterioscler Thromb 11:415–422

22. Jaye M, Lynch KJ, Krawiec J et al (1999) A novel endothelial-derived lipase that modulates HDL metabolism. Nat Genet 21:424–428

23. Rye KA, Wee K, Curtiss LK, Bonnet DJ, Barter PJ (2003) Apolipoprotein A-II inhibits high density lipoprotein remodeling and lipid-poor apolipoprotein A-I formation. J Biol Chem 278:22530–22536

24. Rye KA, Duong M, Psaltis MK et al (2002) Evidence that phospholipids play a key role in pre-beta apoA-I formation and high-density lipoprotein remodeling. Biochemistry 41:12538–12545

25. Caiazza D, Jahangiri A, Rader DJ, Marchadier D, Rye KA (2004) Apolipoproteins regulate the kinetics of endothelial lipase-mediated hydrolysis of phospholipids in reconstituted high-density lipoproteins. Biochemistry 43:11898–11905

26. Hime NJ, Barter PJ, Rye KA (1998) The influence of apolipoproteins on the hepatic lipase-mediated hydrolysis of high density lipoprotein phospholipid and triacylglycerol. J Biol Chem 273:27191–27198

27. Asztalos BF, Collins D, Horvath KV, Bloomfield HE, Robins SJ, Schaefer EJ (2008) Relation of gemfibrozil treatment and high-density lipoprotein subpopulation profile with cardiovascular events in the Veterans Affairs High-Density Lipoprotein Intervention Trial. Metabolism 57:77–83

28. Luc G, Bard JM, Ferrieres J et al (2002) Value of HDL cholesterol, apolipoprotein A-I, lipoprotein A-I, and lipoprotein A-I/A-II in prediction of coronary heart disease: the PRIME Study. Prospective Epidemiological Study of Myocardial Infarction. Arterioscler Thromb Vasc Biol 22:1155–1161

29. Brousseau ME, Schaefer EJ, Wolfe ML et al (2004) Effects of an inhibitor of cholesteryl ester transfer protein on HDL cholesterol. N Engl J Med 350:1505–1515

30. Nissen SE, Tardif JC, Nicholls SJ et al (2007) Effect of torcetrapib on the progression of coronary atherosclerosis. N Engl J Med 356:1304–1316

31. Bots ML, Visseren FL, Evans GW et al (2007) Torcetrapib and carotid intima-media thickness in mixed dyslipidaemia (RADIANCE 2 study): a randomised, double-blind trial. Lancet 370:153–160

32. Barter PJ, Caulfield M, Eriksson M et al (2007) Effects of torcetrapib in patients at high risk for coronary events. N Engl J Med 357:2109–2122

33. Ibanez B, Vilahur G, Cimmino G et al (2008) Rapid change in plaque size, composition, and molecular footprint after recombinant apolipoprotein A-I Milano (ETC-216) administration: magnetic resonance imaging study in an experimental model of atherosclerosis. J Am Coll Cardiol 51:1104–1109

34. Parolini C, Marchesi M, Lorenzon P et al (2008) Dose-related effects of repeated ETC-216 (recombinant apolipoprotein A-I Milano/1-palmitoyl-2-oleoyl phosphatidylcholine complexes) administrations on rabbit lipid-rich soft plaques: in vivo assessment by intravascular ultrasound and magnetic resonance imaging. J Am Coll Cardiol 51:1098–1103

35. Nissen SE, Tsunoda T, Tuzcu EM et al (2003) Effect of recombinant ApoA-I Milano on coronary atherosclerosis in patients with acute coronary syndromes: a randomized controlled trial. JAMA 290:2292–2300

36. Rong JX, Li J, Reis ED et al (2001) Elevating high-density lipoprotein cholesterol in apolipoprotein E-deficient mice remodels advanced atherosclerotic lesions by decreasing macrophage and increasing smooth muscle cell content. Circulation 104:2447–2452

37. Spieker LE, Sudano I, Hurlimann D et al (2002) High-density lipoprotein restores endothelial function in hypercholesterolemic men. Circulation 105:1399–1402

38. Drew BG, Duffy SJ, Formosa MF et al (2009) High-density lipoprotein modulates glucose metabolism in patients with type 2 diabetes mellitus. Circulation 119:2103–2111

39. Tardif JC, Gregoire J, L'Allier PL et al (2007) Effects of reconstituted high-density lipoprotein infusions on coronary atherosclerosis: a randomized controlled trial. JAMA 297:1675–1682

40. Nicholls SJ, Cutri B, Worthley SG et al (2005) Impact of short-term administration of high-density lipoproteins and atorvastatin on atherosclerosis in rabbits. Arterioscler Thromb Vasc Biol 25:2416–2421

41. Navab M, Anantharamaiah GM, Reddy ST et al (2004) Oral D-4F causes formation of pre-beta high-density lipoprotein and improves high-density lipoprotein-mediated cholesterol efflux and reverse cholesterol transport from macrophages in apolipoprotein E-null mice. Circulation 109:3215–3220

42. Wool GD, Vaisar T, Reardon CA, Getz GS (2009) An apoA-I mimetic peptide containing a proline residue has greater in vivo HDL binding and anti-inflammatory ability than the 4F peptide. J Lipid Res 50:1889–1900

43. Nicholls SJ, Dusting GJ, Cutri B et al (2005) Reconstituted high-density lipoproteins inhibit the acute pro-oxidant and proinflammatory vascular changes induced by a periarterial collar in normocholesterolemic rabbits. Circulation 111:1543–1550

44. Calabresi L, Franceschini G, Sirtori CR et al (1997) Inhibition of VCAM-1 expression in endothelial cells by reconstituted high density lipoproteins. Biochem Biophys Res Commun 238:61–65

45. Xia P, Vadas MA, Rye KA, Barter PJ, Gamble JR (1999) High density lipoproteins (HDL) interrupt the sphingosine kinase signaling pathway. A possible mechanism for protection against atherosclerosis by HDL. J Biol Chem 274:33143–33147

46. Park SH, Park JH, Kang JS, Kang YH (2003) Involvement of transcription factors in plasma HDL protection against TNF-alpha-induced vascular cell adhesion molecule-1 expression. Int J Biochem Cell Biol 35:168–182

47. McGrath KC, Li XH, Puranik R et al (2009) Role of 3beta-hydroxysteroid-delta 24 reductase in mediating antiinflammatory effects of high-density lipoproteins in endothelial cells. Arterioscler Thromb Vasc Biol 29:877–882

48. Navab M, Imes SS, Hama SY et al (1991) Monocyte transmigration induced by modification of low density lipoprotein in cocultures of human aortic wall cells is due to induction of monocyte chemotactic protein 1 synthesis and is abolished by high density lipoprotein. J Clin Invest 88:2039–2046

49. Ashby DT, Rye KA, Clay MA, Vadas MA, Gamble JR, Barter PJ (1998) Factors influencing the ability of HDL to inhibit expression of vascular cell adhesion molecule-1 in endothelial cells. Arterioscler Thromb Vasc Biol 18:1450–1455

50. Dimayuga P, Zhu J, Oguchi S et al (1999) Reconstituted HDL containing human apolipoprotein A-1 reduces VCAM-1 expression and neointima formation following periadventitial cuff-induced carotid injury in apoE null mice. Biochem Biophys Res Commun 264:465–468

Human Apolipoprotein A-I Deficiency

Ernst J. Schaefer and Raul D. Santos

Abbreviations

Apo   Apolipoprotein
HDL   High density lipoproteins
LDL   Low density lipoproteins
CHD   Coronary heart disease
LCAT   Lecithin:cholesterol acyltransferase

Introduction

Our purpose is to review the characteristics of probands described with familial apolipoprotein (apo) A-I deficiency. Decreased plasma high density lipoprotein (HDL) cholesterol levels (<40 mg/dl in men and <50 mg/dl in women) have been associated with an increased risk of coronary heart disease (CHD) [1]. Marked HDL deficiency states (HDL cholesterol <5 mg/dl) and undetectable plasma apolipoprotein (apo) A-I levels have been reported in humans due to mutations at the AI/CIII/AIV gene locus [2–27]. These patients have a lack of apoA-I-containing HDL in plasma, normal or decreased triglyceride levels, normal low density lipoprotein (LDL) cholesterol levels, and often strikingly premature CHD [2–27]. In this regard, they differ from patients with homozygous Tangier disease, due to mutations in the ATP binding cassette A1 gene, who have detectable plasma apoA-I levels in preβ-1 HDL, defective cellular cholesterol efflux, hypertriglyceridemia, and decreased LDL cholesterol [28–30]. They also differ from patients with homozygous lecithin:cholesterol acyltransferase (LCAT) deficiency who have plasma apoA-I levels in the 10–20 mg/dl range found in both preβ-1 HDL and α-4 HDL, elevations of both plasma cholesterol and triglycerides, increased plasma free cholesterol, low density lipoprotein of abnormal electrophoretic mobility, and marked corneal opacification [31].

E.J. Schaefer (✉)
Lipid Metabolism Laboratory, Tufts University,
Boston, MA 02111, USA
e-mail: ernst.schaefer@tufts.edu

Familial Apolipoprotein AI/CIII/AIV Deficiency

A kindred originally of English origin was described by Schaefer and colleagues in 1982 containing one homozygote and multiple heterozygotes, residing in northern Alabama, United States. The index case had no xanthomas, marked HDL deficiency, low triglyceride and normal LDL cholesterol levels, and severe premature coronary artery disease. She had no history of diabetes, smoking, or hypertension, and was premenopausal. She died at the time of coronary artery bypass grafting surgery at age 43 years [2–6]. At autopsy severe diffuse coronary atherosclerosis was documented [2–4]. The defect in this kindred was subsequently found be due to a large deletion of the entire apoAI/CIII/AIV gene complex [5]. Decreased plasma levels of the fat soluble vitamins A, D, and E (less than 50% of normal) were also noted, as was a moderately prolonged prothrombin time consistent with vitamin K deficiency in the homozygote [5]. Heterozygotes were found to have plasma HDL cholesterol, apoA-I, apoC-III, and apoA-IV levels that were about 50% of normal [5]. ApoA-I gene transfection studies indicated that apoA-I was essential for HDL formation, similar to what was noted in this initial kindred [6]. When the molecular defect was described, this kindred was denoted as familial apoAI/CIII/AIV deficiency.

Familial Apolipoprotein AI/CIII Deficiency

Approximately 6 months later, also in 1982, a second kindred with apoA-I deficiency was described by Norum and colleagues in two sisters with marked HDL deficiency and planar xanthomas. They had premature CHD and underwent successful coronary artery bypass grafting surgery at ages 29 and 30 years [7]. They had no history of smoking, hypertension, or diabetes, and no evidence of fat malabsorption was reported. Their triglyceride levels were reduced, and their LDL cholesterol levels were normal. The genetic defect was found to be a DNA rearrangement affecting the adjacent apoA-I and apoC-III genes, resulting in a lack of production of these two apolipoproteins and their absence from plasma [8, 9]. It was subsequently reported that these homozygotes had small amounts of apoA-II containing HDL, and also had enhanced clearance of very low density lipoprotein apoB, presumably because there was no apoC-III present in their plasma to inhibit lipolysis [10–14]. This kindred was described as familial AI/CIII deficiency. A second kindred with premature CHD, marked HDL deficiency, and absence of apoA-I and apoC-III in plasma has been described [15].

Familial Apolipoprotein AI Deficiency

Since 1991, at least ten kindreds with isolated apoA-I deficiency have been described [16–27]. All homozygous probands had a lack of plasma apoA-I and marked HDL deficiency, as well as normal levels of triglycerides and LDL cholesterol. Matsunaga and colleagues in 1991 described a subject with apolipoprotein A-I deficiency due to a codon 84 nonsense mutation of the apolipoprotein A-I gene, as well as evidence of coronary heart disease (CHD) [16]. Funke et al. described a kindred in which the proband had a frameshift mutation in the human apolipoprotein A-I gene, which caused high density lipoprotein deficiency, partial lecithin:cholesterol-acyl-transferase deficiency and corneal opacities but not premature coronary artery disease [17]. Roemling et al. described a nonsense mutation in the apolipoprotein A-I gene, which was associated with high density lipoprotein deficiency but not coronary artery disease [18]. Deeb et al. described a patient with undetectable apoA-I due to a mutation in the apolipoprotein A-I gene [19]. Takada et al. reported a case of apoA-I deficiency with a codon 8 nonsense mutation of the apoA-I gene without evidence of coronary artery disease [20]. Miccoli and colleagues have reported compound heterozygosity for a structural apolipoprotein A-I variant, apoA-I (L141R) Pisa and an apolipoprotein A-I null allele in patients with absence of HDL, corneal opacification, and the presence of coronary heart disease [21]. Matsunaga et al. have reported that compound heterozygosity for an apolipoprotein AI gene promoter mutation and a structural nonsense mutation can cause apolipoprotein A-I deficiency [22]. Pisciotta et al. have reported recurrent mutations of the apolipoprotein A-I gene in three kindreds with severe HDL deficiency [23]. Ikewaki et al. have reported that a novel two nucleotide deletion in the apolipoprotein A-I gene, apoA-I Shinbashi, is associated in the homozygous state with high density lipoprotein deficiency, corneal opacities, planar xanthomas, and premature coronary artery disease [24].

One of the best characterized kindreds was reported by Ng et al. with an apoA-I gene mutation at Q[-2]X resulting in undetectable apoA-I in homozygotes in a Portuguese kindred living in Toronto, Canada [25, 26]. The index case was a 34-year-old female who presented with marked HDL deficiency, mildly thickened Achilles tendons, xanthelasmas, mild midline cerebellar ataxia, and asymmetric bilateral neurosensory hearing loss. She also had bilateral cataracts, and bilateral subretinal lipid deposition with exudative proliferative retinopathy, with resultant bilateral retinal detachments requiring surgical repair. Her apoA-I levels were undetectable and her HDL cholesterol was 2 mg/dl, her triglycerides were elevated at 254 mg/dl, as was her LDL cholesterol at 222 mg/dl. Four other homozygotes in this pedigree were found, who also had marked HDL deficiency (mean 4 mg/dl), normal triglycerides of 123 mg/dl (mean), and mean LDL cholesterol of 175 mg/dl (elevated). One homozygous sister at age 38 years, had xanthelasma, Achilles tendon xanthomas, planar xanthomas in the web spaces of the hands, and the cubital and popliteal fossae. She had sustained a myocardial at age 34 years, and had coronary artery bypass grafting surgery at age 37 years. A second homozygous sister had angina and documented reversible myocardial ischemia on stress testing, as well as cerebellar ataxia. The two other homozygotes at ages 26 and 28, as well as four heterozygotes (ages 14–39 years) were asymptomatic and had no evidence of CHD, neuropathy, or visual impairment. In the discussion, the authors concluded that there was combined hyperlipidemia in this kindred, which was probably not related to the apoA-I gene mutation.

Case Study of Familial Apolipoprotein Deficiency

Most recently, we have described a kindred with the same mutation as that described by Ng et al. [27]. The common features of our kindred and that of Ng et al. are the Q[-2]X mutation in the apoA-I gene, the planar xanthomas, and the marked HDL deficiency. The index case presented to the Lipid Clinic at the Heart Institute (INCOR) of the University of Sao Paulo Hospital, Sao Paulo, Brazil. He was a 39-year-old male with striking tuboeruptive xanthomas on his buttocks and lower back (see Fig. 1a), and a biopsy confirmed lipid-laden macrophages (see Fig. 1b). He also had palmar and planar xanthomas (see Fig. 1c), as well as corneal arcus and corneal opacification observed by slit lamp examination (see Fig. 1d). Because of the presence of the xanthomas and palmar creases, we searched for apoE deficiency, apoE mutations, and apoE 2/2 homozygosity but have not observed any of these abnormalities in the proband.

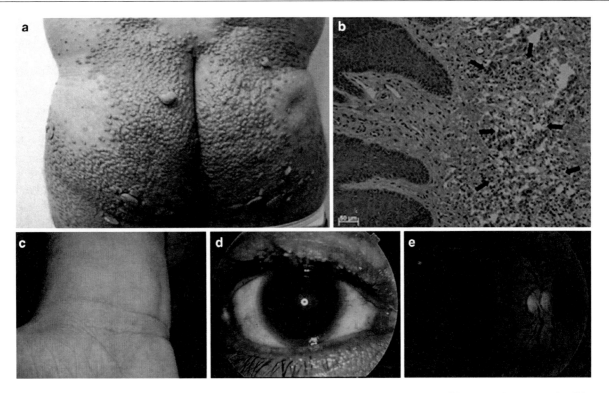

Fig. 1 Images of the index case's tuboeruptive xanthomas on the buttocks and lower back (**a**), a light micrograph showing lipid laden macrophages in a biopsy taken from these xanthomas (**b**), the *yellow palmar* creases on the palms of the hands and wrists (**c**), the planar xanthomas on the upper eyelids, corneal arcus, and mild corneal opacification in the index case (**d**), and an image of the retina of the index case, with no abnormalities

Examination of the proband's retina was normal (see Fig. 1e), as was his neurologic examination. On physical examination, he had a normal blood pressure, a body mass index of 29.0 kg/m², and no evidence of hepatosplenomegaly, or enlarged orange tonsils. On laboratory testing, he had normal liver, renal, and thyroid function, and a normal fasting glucose level and a normal complete blood count. He was noted to have an HDL cholesterol level of 4 mg/dl. He did not have any history of chest pain, heart disease, hypertension, diabetes, or cigarette smoking. He was asymptomatic but on coronary stress testing was noted to have significant ischemia. He was noted to have significant calcium deposition in his left coronary artery on computed tomography (see Fig. 2) and significant calcified and soft plaque on multidetector computed tomographic coronary angiography . He underwent standard coronary angiography, which revealed a complete obstruction of his right coronary artery, as well as an approximately 90% narrowing of his left anterior descending coronary artery (see Fig. 3). He then underwent successful coronary artery bypass grafting surgery, and since then has done well.

The proband had three children who were healthy at ages 3–8 years, and their HDL cholesterol levels were 14, 21, and 34 mg/dl, respectively. The proband's 41-year-old brother had previously sustained a myocardial infarction followed

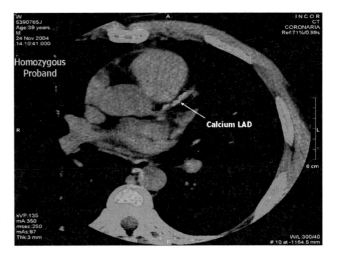

Fig. 2 Computed tomographic image of the index case's heart showing significant calcium deposition in the left anterior coronary artery

by coronary artery bypass grafting surgery at the age of 38 years. He was also noted to have tuboeruptive xanthomas, as well as corneal arcus. His HDL cholesterol was found to be 2 mg/dl. His daughter was in good health at age 12 years, and was presumably a heterozygote, but did not consent for to having her blood drawn. Two other siblings of the index case were examined and were found not to have xanthomas and to have HDL cholesterol values of 15 and 22 mg/dl, consistent with being heterozygotes. They were in good health at ages 33 and 35 years. Their children were in good health at ages 3–10 years with HDL cholesterol levels of 21, 45, and 42 mg/dl, respectively. The parents of the index case were alive and well at ages 65 and 66 years, respectively, with HDL cholesterol values that were both 24 mg/dl. They were first cousins, and their fathers were nonidentical twin brothers. Therefore, the index case, his homozygous brother, and his two heterozygous siblings were products of a consanguineous marriage. Control subjects matched for the age and gender of affected family members were also examined.

Data on plasma lipids, lipoprotein cholesterol, and apolipoproteins in controls ($n=10$), heterozygotes ($n=8$) and homozygotes ($n=2$) for this form of familial apoA-I deficiency are shown in Table 1. DNA sequencing of the apoA-I gene in the two homozygotes documented that they were homozygous for the Q[-2]X in the apoA-I gene, while the suspected heterozygotes were confirmed by DNA analysis. Homozygotes ($n=2$) had mean values of HDL-C, apoA-I, apoA-II, and apoE that were 6.7, 0, 28.9, and 55.9% of normal, respectively, and free cholesterol represented 30.2% of total cholesterol, and about the same percentage of HDL cholesterol as free cholesterol, ruling out the diagnosis of LCAT deficiency. Heterozygotes had HDL cholesterol, apoA-I, and apoA-II values that were 42.6, 46.4, and 68.4% of control values (all $p<0.05$), respectively, with relatively normal amounts of apoB, apoC-III, and apoE in plasma (see Table 1).

A schematic of normal apoA-I-containing HDL particles is shown in Fig. 4, and control values are provided in Table 2. These data are obtained by two-dimensional gel electrophoresis, followed by immunoblotting with specific apoA-I antibody, and then imaging with a phosphorimager. The data are expressed both in terms of the concentration of apoA-I in the different HDL subspecies, as well as in terms of percentages of total plasma apoA-I. In normals, about 12 mg/dl of apoA-I or 10% of the total is found in two small, discoidal preβ-1 HDL particles. About 22 mg/dl or about 20% of the total is found in either large, spherical α-1 HDL or in the adjacent large, spherical preα-1 HDL. All these HDL particles contain apoA-I without apoA-II. In contrast, intermediate sized spherical α-2 and α-3 HDL contain both apoA-I and apoA-II and have a combined apoA-I concentration of about 60 mg/dl or about 50% of the total plasma apoA-I and all of the plasma apoA-II in normal plasma. Adjacent to α-2 and α-3 HDL are the intermediate spherical preα-2 and preα-3 HDL, which contain apoA-I without apoA-II, and together have an apoA-I concentration of about 10 mg/dl or about 8% of total plasma apoA-I. The smallest α migrating HDL particles are α-4 HDL and the adjacent preα-4 HDL, which both contain apoA-I without apoA-II, and are discoidal particles, which together have an apoA-I concentration of about 2 mg/dl, and represent about 1.5% of total plasma apoA-I. Finally, there

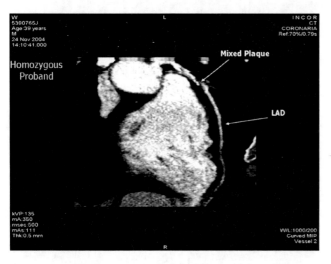

Fig. 3 Coronary angiogram showing a high grade narrowing of about 90% of the left anterior descending coronary artery of the index case

Table 1 Characteristics of study participants	Controls ($n=10$)	Heterozygotes ($n=8$)	Homozygotes ($n=2$)
Male/female	7/3	5/3	2/0
Total cholesterol (mg/dl)	200±38	181±37	157, 174
Triglyceride (mg/dl)	117±88	113±45	56, 94
HDL-C (mg/dl)	54±13	23±7*	4.0, 3.2
LDL-C (mg/dl)	126±33	140±33	126, 146
ApoA-I (mg/dl)	140±25	65±13*	Undetectable
ApoA-II (mg/dl)	38±4	26±5*	10, 12
ApoB (mg/dl)	96±16	97±17	90, 106
ApoC-III (mg/dl)	9.1±4.2	8.7±3.2	3.4, 4.0
ApoE (mg/dl)	7.6±3.6	4.1±1.2	4.7, 3.8

Data are mean±SD
*Significantly different ($p<0.05$) from controls; homozygotes ($n=2$) had mean values of HDL-C, apoA-I, apoA-II, apoC-III, and apoE that were 6.7%, 0%, 28.9%, and 55.9% of normal, respectively, and free cholesterol represented 30.2% of total cholesterol

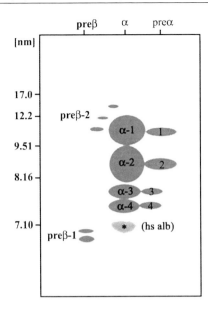

Fig. 4 Schematic representation of apoA-I-containing HDL subpopulations in human plasma separated by nondenaturing agarose–polyacrylamide gel electrophoresis. The nomenclature is based on HDL particle separation by electrophoretic charge relative to albumin (preβ, α, and preα) in the first dimension, and by size relative to the molecular weight standards in the second dimension

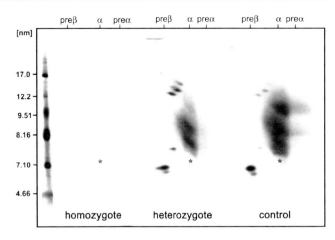

Fig. 5 Distribution of apoA-I containing HDL subpopulations of a homozygote (*left*), a heterozygote (*middle*) and a normal control subject (*right*) separated by two-dimensional, nondenaturing agarose-PAGE. Subpopulations were characterized by charge (preβ, α, preα) based on their relative mobility to albumin (first dimension); and size determined from molecular weight standards (Pharmacia high molecular weight standard proteins [7.1–17.0 nm] supplemented with LDH 4.66 nm) (second dimension). The *asterisk* indicates the endogenous human serum albumin marking the α-mobility front. The images indicate undetectable apoA-I containing HDL in the homozygote and decreases in large α-1 HDL in heterozygote

Table 2 Apo-A-I concentrations in HDL subpopulations (mg/dl)*

	Controls (*n* = 10)	Heterozygotes (*n* = 8)
Preβ-1	12.2 ± 3.2 (9.9%)	6.3 ± 2.0** (9.8%)
Preβ-2	1.7 ± 0.9 (1.4%)	3.8 ± 1.5** (6.0%)**
α-1	16.8 ± 8.9 (13.6%)	3.3 ± 2.4** (4.8%)**
α-2	39.3 ± 9.7 (31.8%)	24.3 ± 6.2** (37.1%)
α-3	24.0 ± 5.7 (19.4%)	17.1 ± 3.5** (26.5%)
α-4	13.5 ± 3.6 (10.9%)	4.1 ± 1.2**(6.4%)
Preα-1	5.3 ± 3.4 (4.3%)	0.3 ± 0.4** (0.5%)**
Preα-2	6.2 ± 2.4 (5.0%)	2.8 ± 0.6** (4.3%)
Preα-3	3.5 ± 1.4 (2.8%)	2.0 ± 0.7** (3.1%)
Preα-4	1.0 ± 0.4 (0.8%)	0.8 ± 0.3 (1.2%)

*Data are mean (mg/dl) ± standard deviations, with the percentage of the total value in parentheses
**Significantly different (*p* < 0.05) from controls

are three large preβ-2 HDL particles, which altogether have an apoA-I concentration of about 2 mg/dl or about 1.5% of the total. These particles do not contain apoA-II.

Table 2 also summarizes data on apoA-I-containing HDL subpopulations in heterozygous and control subjects. Homozygotes had undetectable levels of apoA-I containing HDL as shown in Fig. 5. They had HDL particles in the α-3 region containing apoA-II, but no apoA-I (Fig. 6), as well as relatively normal amounts of the separate apoA-IV and apoE containing HDL particles, which have slow α mobility (Figs. 7 and 8). ApoC-III in the homozygotes was entirely in the free form and not associated with other apolipoproteins (data not shown). Heterozygotes had a marked decrease in the mean apoA-I concentration in large α-1 HDL (19.6% of

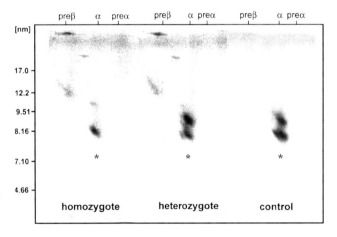

Fig. 6 ApoA-II-containing HDL subpopulations of a homozygote, a heterozygote, and a representative control subject, showing decreased amounts of apoA-II in the α-3 position only, whereas in the heterozygote and the control subjects, apoA-II is found in both the α-3 and the α-4 position

normal), some decrease in α-2 and α-3 HDL (61.8% and 71.3% of normal), and a more marked decrease in α-4 HDL (30.4% of normal). They also had preβ-1 HDL values that were 51.6% of normal, but their preβ-2 HDL levels were 2.24-fold higher than normal. With regard to gel photographs of apoA-I, apoA-II, apoA-IV, and apoE containing HDL in heterozygotes, please see Figs. 5–8. Heterozygotes had marked decreases in α-1 and α-4 HDL, and marked increases in preβ-2 HDL, with a relatively normal distribution and amount of apoA-II HDL, apoA-IV HDL, and apoE HDL.

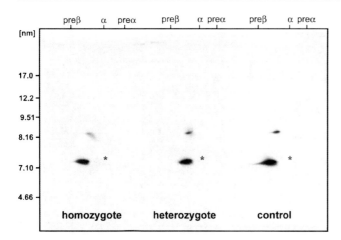

Fig. 7 ApoA-IV-containing HDL subpopulations of a homozygote, a heterozygote, and a control subject, showing normal amounts and distribution of apoA-IV HDL in the slowly migrating α position in all three subjects

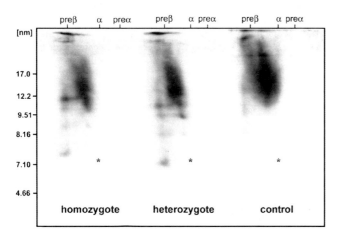

Fig. 8 ApoE-containing HDL subpopulations of a of a homozygote, a heterozygote, and a control subject, showing relatively normal amounts and distribution of apoE HDL in the slowly migrating α position in all three subjects. Please note that apoE HDL particles are larger than apoA-IV HDL particles

Levels of fat soluble vitamins were generally normal in this kindred in both homozygotes and heterozygotes with mean values (standard deviation) being in the normal range for retinol, 1,25 hydroxy vitamin D, and α-tocopherol.

The overall lesions from the apoA-I deficiency states are that apoA-I is essential for normal HDL formation, and its absence generally results in severe HDL deficiency, xanthomas, and premature CHD. The addition of apoC-III deficiency as observed in apoAI/CIII deficiency results in the same phenotype except very low triglyceride levels, consistent with the concept that apoC-III can impair lipolysis. ApoAI/CIII/AIV deficiency results in the same phenotype, except that there are no xanthomas, and there is evidence of fat malabsorption, consistent with the concept that apoA-IV

plays a role in the intestinal absorption of fat and fat-soluble vitamins. The overall data in the present kindred indicates that isolated familial apoA-I deficiency results in marked HDL deficiency, xanthomas, and premature CHD. Moreover, the evidence indicates that in the absence of apoA-I, apoA-II particles can be found in the α-migrating region of HDL at the α-3 position; although apoA-II levels are significantly decreased. Moreover, in familial apoA-I deficiency levels of apoA-IV and apoE containing HDL are relatively normal, and these HDL particles have normal electrophoretic mobility and particle size. These data suggest that there are at least three types of separate and distinct HDL particles: those containing apoA-I (the predominant HDL species), those containing apoA-IV (a relatively minor component), and those containing apoE (also a relatively minor component). Nevertheless these latter HDL particles may be of great functional significance. While not all reported kindreds with apoA-I deficiency have been reported to have premature CHD, those individuals in whom apoA-I is undetectable generally had evidence of premature CHD in the third and fourth decades of life. In contrast, homozygotes with Tangier disease due to defective cellular cholesterol efflux generally develop CHD in their fifth or sixth decade of life [28–30], while those subjects with mutations in apoA-I affecting LCAT activity or homozygotes with LCAT activity generally do not have any evidence of premature CHD [17, 18, 21, 31].

References

1. Expert Panel (2001) Executive summary of the third report of the National Cholesterol Education Program (NCEP) Expert Panel on Detection, Evaluation, and Treatment of High Blood Cholesterol in Adults (Adult Treatment Panel III). J Am Med Assoc 285: 2486–2497
2. Schaefer EJ, Heaton WH, Wetzel MG et al (1982) Plasma apolipoprotein A-I absence associated with marked reduction of high density lipoproteins and premature coronary artery disease. Arteriosclerosis 2:16–26
3. Schaefer EJ (1984) The clinical, biochemical, and genetic features in familial disorders of high density lipoprotein deficiency. Arteriosclerosis 4:303–322
4. Schaefer EJ, Ordovas JM, Law S et al (1985) Familial apolipoprotein A-I and C-III deficiency, variant II. J Lipid Res 26:1089–1101
5. Ordovas JM, Cassidy DK, Civeira F et al (1989) Familial apolipoprotein A-I, C-III, and A-IV deficiency with marked high density lipoprotein deficiency and premature atherosclerosis due to a deletion of the apolipoprotein A-I, C-III, and A-IV gene complex. J Biol Chem 264:16339–16342
6. Lamon-Fava S, Ordovas JM, Mandel G et al (1987) Secretion of apolipoprotein A-I in lipoprotein particles following transfection of the human apolipoprotein A-I gene into 3T3 cells. J Biol Chem 262:8944–8947
7. Norum RA, Lakier JB, Goldstein S et al (1982) Familial deficiency of apolipoproteins A-I and C-III and precocious coronary artery disease. N Engl J Med 306:1513–1519

8. Karathanasis SK, Norum RA, Zannis VI et al (1983) An inherited polymorphism in the human apolipoprotein A-I gene locus related to the development of atherosclerosis. Nature 301:718–720

9. Karathanasis SK, Ferris E, Haddad EA (1987) DNA inversion within the apolipoprotein AI/CIII/AIV-encoding gene cluster of certain patients with premature atherosclerosis. Proc Natl Acad Sci 84:7198–7202

10. Beher WT, Gabbard A, Norum RA et al (1983) Effect of blood high density lipoprotein cholesterol concentration on fecal steroid excretion in humans. Life Sci 32:2933–2937

11. Forte TM, Nichols AV, Krauss RM et al (1984) Familial apolipoprotein AI and apolipoprotein CIII deficiency. Subclass distribution, composition, and morphology of lipoproteins in a disorder associated with premature atherosclerosis. J Clin Invest 74:1601–1613

12. Ginsberg HN, Le NA, Goldberg IJ et al (1986) Apolipoprotein B metabolism in subjects with deficiency of apolipoproteins CIII and AI. Evidence that apoCIII inhibits catabolism of triglyceride-rich lipoproteins by lipoprotein lipase in vivo. J Clin Invest 78: 1287–1295

13. Subbaiah PV, Norum RA, Bagdade JD (1991) Effect of apolipoprotein activators on the specificity lecithin:cholesterol acyltransferase: determination of cholesteryl esters formed in A-I/C-III deficiency. J Lipid Res 32:1601–1609

14. Bekaert ED, Alaupovic P, Knight-Gibson CS et al (1991) Characterization of apoA-I and apoB containing lipoprotein particles in a variant of familial apolipoprotein A-I deficiency with planar xanthomas: the metabolic significance of LP-A-II particles. J Lipid Res 32:1587–1599

15. Hiasa Y, Maeda T, Mori H (1986) Deficiency of apolipoproteins A-I and C-III and severe coronary artery disease. Clin Cardiol 9:349–352

16. Matsunaga T, Hiasa Y, Yanagi H et al (1991) Apolipoprotein A-I deficiency due to a codon 84 nonsense mutation of the apolipoprotein A-I gene. Proc Natl Acad Sci 88:2793–2797

17. Funke HA, von Eckardstein A, Pritchard AH et al (1991) A frameshift mutation in the human apolipoprotein A-I gene causes high density lipoprotein deficiency, partial lecithin:cholesterol-acyl-transferase deficiency and corneal opacities. J Clin Invest 87:371–376

18. Roemling R, von Eckhardstein A, Funke H et al (1994) A nonsense mutation in the apolipoprotein A-I gene is associated with high density lipoprotein deficiency, but not coronary artery disease. Arterioscler Thromb 14:1915–1922

19. Deeb SS, Cheung MC, Peng R, Wolf AC, Stern R, Albers JJ, Knopp RH (1991) A mutation in the apolipoprotein A-I gene. J Biol Chem 266:13654–13660

20. Takada K, Saku K, Ohta T et al (1995) A new case of apoA-I deficiency showing codon 8 nonsense mutation of the apoA-I gene without evidence of coronary artery disease. Arterioscler Thromb Vasc Biol 15:1866–1874

21. Miccoli R, Bertolotto A, Navalesi R et al (1996) Compound heterozygosity for a structural apolipoprotein A-I variant, apoA-I (L141R) Pisa and an apolipoprotein A-I null allele in patients with absence of HDL, corneal opacification, and coronary heart disease. Circulation 94:1622–1628

22. Matsunaga A, Sasaki J, Han H et al (1999) Compound heterozygosity for an apolipoprotein AI gene promoter mutation and a structural nonsense mutation with apolipoprotein deficiency. Arterioscler Thromb Vasc Biol 19:348–355

23. Pisciotta L, Miccoli R, Cantafora A et al (2003) Recurrent mutations of the apolipoprotein A-I gene in three kindreds with severe HDL deficiency. Atherosclerosis 167(2):335–345

24. Ikewaki K, Matsunaga A, Han H et al (2004) A novel two nucleotide deletion in the apolipoprotein A-I gene, apoA-I Shinbashi, associated with high density lipoprotein deficiency, corneal opacities, planar xanthomas, and premature coronary artery disease. Atherosclerosis 172:39–45

25. Ng DS, Leiter LA, Vezina C et al (1994) Apolipoprotein A-I Q[-2] X causing isolated apolipoprotein deficiency in a family with analphalipoproteinemia. J Clin Invest 93:223–229

26. Ng DS, O'Connor PW, Mortimer CB et al (1996) Case report: retinopathy and neuropathy associated with complete apolipoprotein A-I deficiency. Am J Med Sci 312:30–33

27. Santos RD, Schaefer EJ, Asztalos BF et al (2008) Characterization of high density lipoprotein particles in familial apolipoprotein A-I deficiency with premature coronary atherosclerosis, corneal arcus and opacification, and tubo-eruptive and planar xanthomas. J Lipid Res 49:349–357

28. Asztalos BF, Brousseau ME, McNamara JR et al (2001) Subpopulations of high-density lipoproteins in homozygous and heterozygous Tangier disease. Atherosclerosis 156:217–225

29. Brousseau ME, Schaefer EJ, Dupuis J et al (2000) Novel mutations in the gene encoding ATP-binding cassette 1 in four Tangier disease kindreds. J Lipid Res 41:433–441

30. Brousseau ME, Eberhart GP, Dupuis J et al (2000) Cellular cholesterol efflux in heterozygotes for Tangier disease is markedly reduced and correlates with high density lipoprotein cholesterol concentration and particle size. J Lipid Res 41:1125–1135

31. Asztalos BF, Schaefer EJ, Horvath KV et al (2007) Role of LCAT in HDL remodeling: investigation of LCAT deficiency states. J Lipid Res 48:592–599

Human Apolipoprotein A-I Mutants

Guido Francheschini

Introduction

Apolipoprotein A-I (apoA-I) is the major protein constituent of the antiatherogenic high density lipoproteins (HDL), and functions as a critical mediator in reverse cholesterol transport (RCT), the process by which excess cholesterol in arterial macrophages is transported to the liver for excretion. ApoA-I is the preferential acceptor of cell cholesterol through the ABCA1 transporter, and acts as a cofactor for the lecithin:cholesterol acyltransferase (LCAT) enzyme. In addition, apoA-I displays unique properties, not directly related to its major activities in RCT but possibly involved in HDL protection against vascular disease, like inhibition of LDL oxidation, prevention of cytokine-induced cell adhesion molecules (CAMs) expression, and upregulation of endothelial nitric oxide synthase (eNOS).

Human apoA-I is a 243-residue polypeptide that contains characteristic 11- and 22-residue repeats of amphipathic α-helices [1] (Fig. 1). Structure–function relationships have been established for specific helical regions within apoA-I. The N- and C-terminal helices (1, 9, and 10) are essential for initial lipid binding [2]; the C-terminal helix 10 is involved in ABCA1 binding, ABCA1-mediated cholesterol efflux, and ABCA1-dependent HDL biogenesis [3]; a pair of central helices (6 and 7) is critical for maximal activation of LCAT [4].

Mutations in the *APOA1* gene may cause either a low-HDL phenotype or hereditary amyloidosis. Forty-six mutations in the human *APOA1* gene are listed in the Human Gene Mutation Database (HGMD, http://www.hgmd.cf.ac.uk/ac/index.php, interrogated May 2009). These mutations are spread from residue −2 to 178. There are five nonsense mutations, 19 missense mutations (five more missense mutations have been described which are not listed in the HGMD, Table 1), 14 deletions, 4 insertions, 1 splice site mutation, and 3 complex rearrangements. Only missense–nonsense mutations are discussed in this chapter.

G. Francheschini (✉)
Center E. Grossi Paoletti, Department of Pharmacological Sciences, Università degli Studi di Milano, via Balzaretti 9, Milano 20133, Italy
e-mail: guido.francheschini@unimi.it

Human ApoA-I Mutations Causing a Low-HDL Phenotype

Eighteen mutations in the *APOA1* gene have been shown to be associated with low plasma HDL concentrations (Table 1). These mutations are clustered at two different locations within the apoA-I sequence: the N-terminal region (residues −2 to 32) and the central region comprising helices 5–7 (Fig. 1). These two regions of apoA-I have been involved in lipid-binding and LCAT activation, respectively; indeed, many of the mutations in the central domain poorly activate LCAT [4].

The apoA-I$_{Milano}$ (A-I$_M$) has been the first apoA-I mutant described in humans. A 42-year-old man was referred to the E. Grossi Paoletti Lipid Clinic in Milano in 1975, because of a combined hyperlipidemia characterized by hypertriglyceridemia, ranging between 300 and 1,000 mg/dl, and mildly to markedly elevated cholesterolemia (range 240–412 mg/dl) [5]. On agarose gel electrophoresis, the α-band was barely visible. Evaluation of plasma HDL-cholesterol (HDL-C) levels by selective precipitation and later on by ultracentrifugation, gave findings ranging from 7 to 13 mg/dl. The clinical presentation was unremarkable; the man was generally healthy and presented only with a gerontoxon in both eyes. Interestingly, two of the three children of the man proved to have an essentially identical lipid profile; so did the father, at the time around 75 years of age, whereas the mother, clearly suffering from an atherosclerotic condition, had normal lipid levels [5]. Subsequent parallel work in Milano and at the Gladstone Foundation in San Francisco came to an identical conclusion: the proband's plasma contained two forms of apoA-I, one of which differed from wild-type apoA-I by the presence of a cysteine residue. Therefore, the subject was a heterozygous carrier of the first apoA-I mutant, which was called A-I$_M$ [5, 6]. Shortly thereafter, the mutation was established as a substitution of cysteine for arginine at position 173 in the apoA-I protein chain [7]. Disulfide-linked homodimers (A-I$_M$–A-I$_M$) and heterodimers with apoA-II (A-I$_M$–A-II), but very little A-I$_M$ monomer, were found in the plasma of the proband and of the two dyslipidemic children [8].

E.J. Schaefer (ed.), *High Density Lipoproteins, Dyslipidemia, and Coronary Heart Disease*,
DOI 10.1007/978-1-4419-1059-2_7, © Springer Science+Business Media, LLC 2010

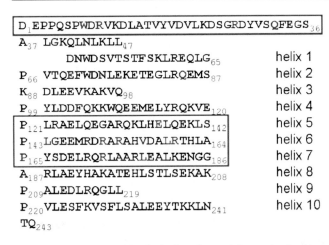

Fig. 1 Single amino acid substitutions in apoA-I associated with a low-HDL phenotype

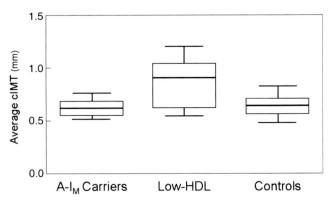

Fig. 2 cIMT values in A-I$_{Milano}$ carriers ($n=21$), age-sex matched low-HDL subjects not carrying the A-I$_{Milano}$ mutation ($n=21$), and matched nonaffected family members ($n=42$). The far wall of common carotid artery, bifurcation, and of the first proximal cm of the internal carotid artery were measured, and the values were averaged to calculate individual cIMT. The *box plot* displays median values with the 25th and 75th percentiles; capped bars indicate the 10th and 90th percentiles

Table 1 Missense-nonsense mutations in human apoA-I

Nucleotide change	Codon change	AA change	Codon	Phenotype	References
c.67C>T	CAG-TAG	Gln-Term	−2	Low-HDL	[22]
c.95G>A	TGG-TAG	Trp-Term	8	Low-HDL	[23]
c.101G>T	CGA-CTA	Arg-Leu	10	Low-HDL	[24]
c.148G>C	GGC-CGC	Gly-Arg	26	Amyloidosis	[25]
c.152G>C	AGA-ACA	Arg-Thr	27	Low-HDL?	[26]
c.166C>T	CAG-TAG	Gln-Term	32	Low-HDL	[27]
c.220T>C	TGG-CGG	Trp-Arg	50	Amyloidosis	[28]
c.251T>G	CTG-CGG	Leu-Arg	60	Amyloidosis	[29]
c.263T>C	CTC-CCC	Leu-Pro	64	Amyloidosis	[30]
c.296T>C	CTG-CCG	Leu-Pro	75	Amyloidosis	[31]
c.322C>T	CAG-TAG	Gln-Term	84	Low-HDL	[32]
c.341T>C	CTG-CCG	Leu-Pro	90	Amyloidosis	[33]
c.478G>T	GAG-TAG	Glu-Term	136	Low-HDL	[34]
c.494T>G	CTG-CGC	Leu-Arg	141	Low-HDL	[35]
c503T>G	CTG-CGG	Leu-Arg	144	Low-HDL	[36]
c.524G>A	CGC-CAC	Arg-Cys	151	Low-HDL	[37]
c.530G>C	GCC-CCC	Arg-Pro	153	Low-HDL	[38]
c.539T>A	GTG-GAG	Val-Glu	156	Low-HDL	[39]
c.548T>G	CTG-CGC	Leu-Arg	159	Low-HDL	[40]
c.548T>C	CTG-CCG	Leu-Pro	159	Low-HDL	[41]
c.551G>T	CGC-CTC	Arg-Leu	160	Low-HDL	[42]
c.566C>G	CCC-CGC	Pro-Arg	165	Low-HDL	[43]
c.581T>C	CTG-CCG	Leu-Pro	170	Amyloidosis	[20]
c.589C>T	CGC-TGC	Arg-Cys	173	Low-HDL	[7]
c.590G>C	CGC-CCC	Arg-Pro	173	Amyloidosis	[44]
c.593T>C	TTG-TCG	Leu-Ser	174	Amyloidosis	[45]
c.595G>C	GCC-CCC	Ala-Pro	175	Amyloidosis	[46]
c.605T>A	CTT-CAT	Leu-His	178	Amyloidosis	[47]
c.605T>C	CTT-CCT	Leu-Pro	178	Low-HDL	[17]

A survey of the population of Limone sul Garda, where the A-I$_M$ proband was born, led to the identification of another 40 carriers [9]. Interestingly, obligate carriers in the past centuries seemed to be relatively long-lived and the only early death, presumably due to an acute vascular condition, in this century occurred in a 53-year-old man, a heavy smoker with arterial hypertension. All carriers are heterozygous for the A-I$_M$ mutation, and have low plasma HDL-C levels, a partial LCAT deficiency, and variable expression of hypertriglyceridemia; in a small number of carriers significant hypercholesterolemia could also be detected. In the past 15 years, none of the carriers had suffered from any ischemic vascular condition.

The paradoxical observation of a high-risk dyslipidemic phenotype associated with the apparent lack of premature atherosclerotic vascular disease prompted a series of studies aimed at comparing vascular structure and function in A-I$_M$ carriers, unaffected relatives, and low-HDL subjects not carrying the A-I$_M$ mutation. Carotid intima-media thickness (cIMT) has been established as a surrogate marker for human atherosclerosis, and applied to the assessment of preclinical atherosclerosis in low-HDL patients carrying mutations in the *LCAT* and *ABCA1* genes [10–12]. cIMT was measured in 21 carriers of the A-I$_M$ mutation, 42 age-gender matched unaffected relatives (controls) and 21 age-gender matched low-HDL subjects not carrying the A-I$_M$ mutation [13]. The average cIMT values were remarkably similar in A-I$_M$ carriers and controls, and significantly lower than those of low-HDL subjects (Fig. 2). In a subsequent study, endothelial function was assessed by measuring vascular response to reactive hyperemia by a plethysmographic method [14]. The increase in forearm blood flow during the early phases of reactive hyperemia is believed to enhance shear stress, which induces the release of nitric oxide (NO), with consequent vasodilation and increased arterial compliance. The postischemic increase of arterial compliance in the apoA-I$_M$ carriers was twofold greater than in low-HDL subjects, and remarkably similar to that of controls (Fig. 3). Endothelial function was also assessed by measuring circulating CAMs levels [14].

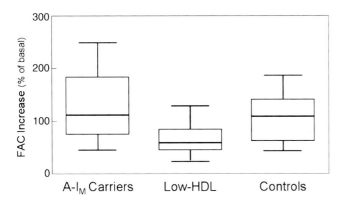

Fig. 3 Arterial compliance in A-I_{Milano} carriers, age-sex matched low-HDL subjects not carrying the A-I_{Milano} mutation, and matched nonaffected family members. Forearm arterial compliance (FAC) of the nondominant arm was measured at rest and during reactive hyperemia; postischemic change in FAC was calculated as the difference between preischemic and peak values, and expressed as percentage of the preischemic value. The *box plot* displays median values with the 25th and 75th percentiles; *capped bars* indicate the 10th and 90th percentiles

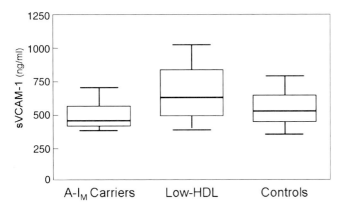

Fig. 4 Plasma levels of soluble VCAM-1 (sVCAM-1) in A-I_{Milano} carriers, age-sex matched Low-HDL subjects not carrying the A-I_{Milano} mutation, and matched nonaffected family members. The *box plot* displays median values with the 25th and 75th percentiles; *capped bars* indicate the 10th and 90th percentiles

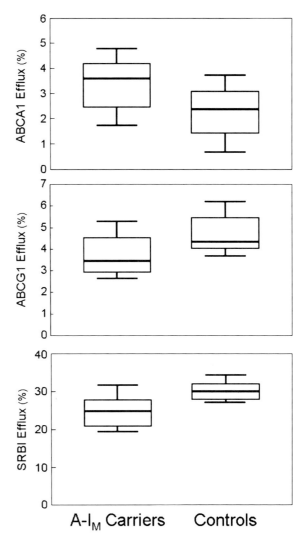

Fig. 5 Cell cholesterol efflux to sera from A-I_{Milano} carriers ($n = 14$) and age-sex matched nonaffected family members ($n = 14$). ABCA1-mediated efflux was essayed in cAMP-stimulated J774 macrophages (*top panel*), ABCG1-mediated efflux in CHO cells stably expressing hABCG1 (*middle panel*), and SRBI-mediated efflux in Fu5AH hepatoma cells (*bottom panel*). Cells were labeled with [3H]cholesterol and then incubated with 2% serum for 4–6 h. The *box plots* display median values with the 25th and 75th percentiles; *capped bars* indicate the 10th and 90th percentiles

As expected, the low-HDL subjects showed significantly higher plasma levels of sVCAM-1, sICAM-1, and sE-Selectin than controls; by contrast, no significant difference was found between A-I_M carriers and controls (Fig. 4). Therefore, despite the moderate to severe low-HDL phenotype, the A-I_M carriers do not present with structural and functional arterial changes indicative of enhanced atherosclerosis.

Considerable effort has been expended to understand the mechanism(s), whereby the A-I_M mutation might be linked to enhanced cardiovascular protection. Studies evaluating the ability of serum from carriers and controls to remove cell cholesterol through the three major protein-mediated pathways (ABCA1, ABCG1, and SR-B1) revealed a high capacity of A-I_M serum to extract cell cholesterol via ABCA1 (Fig. 5), likely because of the accumulation of an abnormal

HDL particle, containing a single molecule of the A-I_M–A-I_M dimer, and migrating in preβ-position on agarose gel [15]. The ABCG1- and SR-B1-mediated cholesterol effluxes were instead reduced (Fig. 5), reflecting the overall reduction in the serum HDL content. In a second set of experiments, HDL isolated from A-I_M carriers were compared with HDL from controls for their capacity to modulate endothelial function in cultured human umbilical vein endothelial cells [14]. A-I_M HDL were more effective than control HDL in stimulating eNOS expression and activation, and in downregulating TNFα-induced VCAM-1 expression (Fig. 6). These findings indicate that the A-I_M mutation exerts a gain-of-function

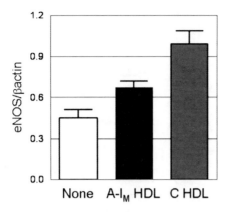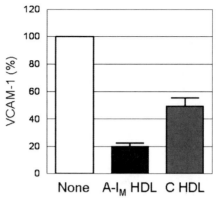

Fig. 6 Effect of HDL isolated from A-I$_{Milano}$ carriers (A-I$_M$ HDL) and controls (C HDL) in enhancing eNOS expression (*left panel*) and down-regulating TNFα-induced VCAM-1 release (*right panel*) in cultured human umbilical vein endothelial cells. Cells were incubated overnight with HDL (1.4 mmol/l cholesterol). eNOS protein levels were assessed by Western blotting and normalized by β-actin values. VCAM-1 concentrations were measured by ELISA and expressed as percentage of concentration in media of untreated, TNFα-stimulated cells

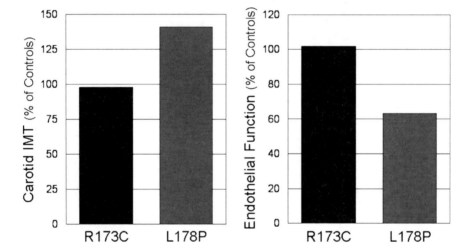

Fig. 7 cIMT and endothelial function in low-HDL subjects heterozygous for the A-I$_{Milano}$ (R173C) and the L178P mutations. Endothelial function was assessed by measuring arterial compliance in A-I$_{Milano}$ carriers, and flow-mediated vasodilation in L178P carriers

effect against the development of cardiovascular disease through at least two distinct mechanisms: promotion of ABCA1-mediated cell cholesterol removal from the arterial wall and prevention of endothelial dysfunction.

The combination of strong clinical and mechanistic data supporting a role for the mutant protein in atherosclerosis protection led to the idea of developing a biotechnological product to be used in conditions of HDL deficiency or even as a "drug" in the prevention/treatment of vascular disorders. The A-I$_M$–A-I$_M$ dimer was expressed in *E. coli* and used to produce synthetic HDL particles [16]. When injected into rabbits, such synthetic HDL were shown to be able to penetrate into the atherosclerotic plaque, remove cholesterol from macrophages and cause a rapid regression of the atherosclerotic lesion; even more strikingly, a short-term treatment with the same synthetic HDL caused a regression of atherosclerotic lesions in coronary patients [16].

A low-HDL phenotype is quite common among carriers of *APOA1* gene mutations, but it can be associated with an extremely variable atherosclerosis burden and coronary risk. While the complete apoA-I deficiency due to chromosomal aberration is definitely associated with premature coronary heart disease (this book), even marked reductions of plasma HDL-C caused by missense/nonsense mutations in the same gene do not necessarily lead to enhanced coronary risk. The carriers of the A-I$_M$ mutation behave clearly distinct from carriers of other missense apoA-I mutations associated with a low-HDL phenotype, like the apoA-I (L178P) mutation, who instead present with enhanced cIMT and endothelial dysfunction (Fig. 7), associated with a severe cardiovascular risk [17]. This dramatic difference in the clinical phenotype of carriers of two missense mutations in the *APOA1* gene, both leading to remarkably similar plasma HDL-C and apoA-I reductions [13, 17], illustrates that the plasma HDL-C level per se does not necessarily reflect the atheroprotective potential of HDL, and highlights the need for novel tools for cardiovascular risk prediction in individuals with low-HDL. Genetic testing aimed at the identification of the molecular defect causing the low-HDL state does not seem to have predictive properties, except for mutations already known to be associated with either low or high risk. Assessing HDL in terms of functions rather than just levels of cholesterol or apoA-I may provide relevant insight into the atheroprotective capacity of each individual HDL, but simple, reliable, and reproducible assays of HDL function are less likely to be applicable on a large scale or validated against clinical outcomes. Surrogate markers to assess atherosclerotic burden, such as cIMT, or endothelial function, although influenced by a variety of factors other than HDL, have already shown to be strong predictors of future cardiovascular events, and appear to be the best tools for screening of low-HDL individuals and for prioritizing antiatherogenic therapies aimed at increasing plasma HDL levels and function, when these will be made available.

Human ApoA-I Mutations Causing Hereditary Amyloidosis

Amyloidosis is a heterogeneous group of diseases characterized by the pathological aggregation of proteins (or protein fragments) that accumulate predominantly extracellularly in tissues and organs, causing damage and eventually death. Mutations in the *APOA1* gene may cause rare forms of hereditary amyloidosis that are inherited in an autosomal dominant manner, with the heterozygous carriers developing a "late onset" disease [18]. The carriers have a mild to moderate reduction of plasma HDL-C and apoA-I levels, but these are never below 50% of normal value. The clinical manifestations of apoA-I amyloidosis frequently involve liver, kidney, heart, larynx, skin, testis, and adrenal glands [18]. The predominant component of amyloid fibrils is a truncated form of apoA-I corresponding to its 90–100 N-terminal residues [18], which illustrates the propensity of this region to fibrillogenesis. The molecular mechanisms underlying the amyloidogenic properties of apoA-I mutants have not been widely investigated. However, it is likely that well-recognized, general mechanisms of in vivo amyloidogenesis, like misfolding of the native protein structure and generation of a critical concentration of the amyloidogenic precursor, may apply also to apoA-I amyloidosis. Indeed, amyloid deposits consisting mainly of N-terminal fragments of the precursor protein are also common in other types of amyloidosis [19].

Eleven amyloidogenic missense/nonsense apoA-I mutations have been identified since the molecular description of

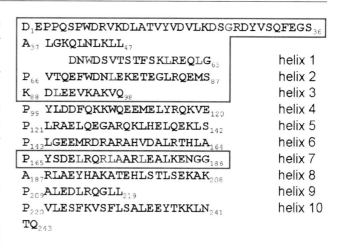

D₁EPPQSPWDRVKDLATVYVDVLKDSGRDYVSQFEGS₃₆	
A₃₇LGKQLNLKLL₄₇	
DNWDSVTSTFSKLREQLG₆₅	helix 1
P₆₆VTQEFWDNLEKETEGLRQEMS₈₇	helix 2
K₈₈DLEEVKAKVQ₉₈	helix 3
P₉₉YLDDFQKKWQEEMELYRQKVE₁₂₀	helix 4
P₁₂₁LRAELQEGARQKLHELQEKLS₁₄₂	helix 5
P₁₄₃LGEEMRDRARAHVDALRTHLA₁₆₄	helix 6
P₁₆₅YSDELRQRLAARLEALKENGG₁₈₆	helix 7
A₁₈₇RLAEYHAKATEHLSTLSEKAK₂₀₈	helix 8
P₂₀₉ALEDLRQGLL₂₁₉	helix 9
P₂₂₀VLESFKVSFLSALEEYTKKLN₂₄₁	helix 10
TQ₂₄₃	

Fig. 8 Single amino acid substitutions in apoA-I leading to hereditary amyloidosis

the first amyloidogenic mutant in the late 1980s (Table 1, Fig. 8). Six of these mutations cause single amino acid replacements within the first 90 apoA-I residues, with the loss of a hydrophobic residue, which is substituted by either a polar and positively charged amino acid, or a Pro residue. Five more mutations cluster in the middle of helix 7. Patients with mutations in the N-terminal region mainly suffer from hepatic and renal amyloidosis, while mutations within helix 7 mainly cause amyloidosis of the heart, larynx and skin [20]. Amyloidogenic mutations in the N-terminal region and those within helix 7 both cause the formation of amyloid fibrils that contain a ~10 kDa N-terminal apoA-I peptide as the major protein component [18], suggesting a common mechanism for apoA-I fibrillogenesis. In patients, who are invariably heterozygous for the mutation, the N-terminal fragment is not detectable in plasma, but it is highly concentrated in amyloid deposits. It is tempting to speculate that the fate of the proteolytic fragments of apoA-I mutants is a key pathogenic event in apoA-I amyloidogenesis. The absence of the peptide in carriers' plasma could be ascribed to a fast renal clearance in the preclinical phase, when deposits are not yet produced, but to a very fast absorption on the fibrils once the deposits are present. Additionally, differences in the compartment in which the proteolytic event takes place (either in the plasma and/or in the extracellular milieu around cell membranes) might account for the different fate of the N-terminal peptide, resulting in either degradation or deposition.

The wild-type apoA-I has been reported to be reproducibly overrepresented when compared with the mutant apoA-I in plasma of carriers of the two Italian amyloidogenic apoA-I mutations, one occurring in the N-terminal region, the other within helix 7 (L75P and L174S): in the L174S apoA-I carriers, the mutant represents 25% of total apoA-I, whereas in carriers of the L75P apoA-I mutant the unbalance is even more pronounced, with the mutant accounting for less than

10% of total apoA-I [18]. Either decreased secretion or enhanced catabolism of the mutant compared to wild-type apoA-I, or a combination of the two, may cause this unbalance. Preliminary data in eukaryotic cell cultures transiently expressing the two Italian amyloidogenic mutants suggest that the intracellular folding pathway is significantly impaired [18]. Nevertheless, an enhanced plasma clearance has been reported for the G26R mutant [21]. Altogether, these findings suggest that an accelerated catabolism and possibly an impaired secretion are intrinsic properties of amyloidogenic apoA-I mutants. However, how this altered metabolism is linked to the susceptibility of the protein to proteolytic remodeling and to its progressive deposition in tissues as amyloid fibrils remains a largely unknown feature of the disease.

Acknowledgments The author is indebted to Elda Favari and Franco Bernini of the University of Parma for the efflux studies.

References

1. Segrest JP, Jones MK, De Loof H, Brouillette CG, Venkatachalapathi YV, Anantharamaiah GM (1992) The amphipathic helix in the exchangeable apolipoproteins: a review of secondary structure and function. J Lipid Res 33:141–166
2. Tanaka M, Dhanasekaran P, Nguyen D et al (2006) Contributions of the N- and C-terminal helical segments to the lipid-free structure and lipid interaction of apolipoprotein a-I. Biochemistry 45:10351–10358
3. Chroni A, Koukos G, Duka A, Zannis VI (2007) The carboxy-terminal region of apoA-I Is required for the ABCA1-dependent formation of alpha-HDL but not prebeta-HDL particles in vivo. Biochemistry 46:5697–5708
4. Sorci-Thomas MG, Thomas MJ (2002) The effects of altered apolipoprotein A-I structure on plasma HDL concentration. Trends Cardiovasc Med 12:121–128
5. Franceschini G, Sirtori CR, Capurso A, Weisgraber KH, Mahley RW (1980) A-I$_{Milano}$ apoprotein. Decreased high density lipoprotein cholesterol levels with significant lipoprotein modifications and without clinical atherosclerosis in an italian family. J Clin Invest 66:892–900
6. Weisgraber KH, Bersot TP, Mahley RW, Franceschini G, Sirtori CR (1980) A-Imilano apoprotein. Isolation and characterization of a cysteine-containing variant of the A-I apoprotein from human high density lipoproteins. J Clin Invest 66:901–907
7. Weisgraber KH, Rall SC Jr, Bersot TP, Mahley RW, Franceschini G, Sirtori CR (1983) Apolipoprotein AI$_{Milano}$. Detection of normal AI in affected subjects and evidence for a cysteine for arginine substitution in the variant AI. J Biol Chem 258:2508–2513
8. Franceschini G, Sirtori M, Gianfranceschi G, Sirtori CR (1981) Relation between the HDL apoproteins and AI isoproteins in subjects with the AIMilano abnormality. Metabolism 30:502–509
9. Gualandri V, Franceschini G, Sirtori CR et al (1985) A-I$_{Milano}$ apoprotein. Identification of the complete kindred and evidence of a dominant genetic transmission. Am J Hum Genet 37:1083–1097
10. Hovingh GK, Hutten BA, Holleboom AG et al (2005) Compromised LCAT function is associated with increased atherosclerosis. Circulation 112:879–884
11. van Dam MJ, de Groot E, Clee SM et al (2002) Association between increased arterial-wall thickness and impairment in ABCA1-driven cholesterol efflux: an observational study. Lancet 359:37–42
12. Calabresi L, Baldassarre D, Castelnuovo S et al (2009) Functional LCAT is not required for efficient atheroprotection in humans. Circulation 120:628–635
13. Sirtori CR, Calabresi L, Franceschini G et al (2001) Cardiovascular status of carriers of the apolipoprotein A-I$_{Milano}$ mutant. The Limone sul Garda Study. Circulation 103:1949–1954
14. Gomaraschi M, Baldassarre D, Amato M et al (2007) Normal vascular function despite low levels of high-density lipoprotein cholesterol in carriers of the apolipoprotein A-I(Milano) mutant. Circulation 116:2165–2172
15. Favari E, Gomaraschi M, Zanotti I et al (2007) A unique protease-sensitive high density lipoprotein particle containing the apolipoprotein A-IMilano dimer effectively promotes ATP-binding cassette A1-mediated cell cholesterol efflux. J Biol Chem 282:5125–5132
16. Calabresi L, Sirtori CR, Paoletti R, Franceschini G (2006) Recombinant apolipoprotein A-I$_{Milano}$ for the treatment of cardiovascular diseases. Curr Atheroscler Rep 8:163–167
17. Hovingh GK, Brownlie A, Bisoendial RJ et al (2004) A novel apoA-I mutation (L178P) leads to endothelial dysfunction, increased arterial wall thickness, and premature coronary artery disease. J Am Coll Cardiol 44:1429–1435
18. Obici L, Franceschini G, Calabresi L et al (2006) Structure, function and amyloidogenic propensity of apolipoprotein A-I. Amyloid 13:191–205
19. Bohne S, Sletten K, Menard R et al (2004) Cleavage of AL amyloid proteins and AL amyloid deposits by cathepsins B, K, and L. J Pathol 203:528–537
20. Eriksson M, Schonland S, Yumlu S et al (2009) Hereditary apolipoprotein AI-associated amyloidosis in surgical pathology specimens: identification of three novel mutations in the APOA1 gene. J Mol Diagn 11:257–262
21. Rader DJ, Gregg RE, Meng MS et al (1992) In vivo metabolism of a mutant apolipoprotein, apoA-I$_{Iowa}$, associated with hypoalphalipoproteinemia and hereditary systemic amyloidosis. J Lipid Res 33:755–763
22. Ng DS, Leiter LA, Vezina C, Connelly PW, Hegele RA (1994) Apolipoprotein A-I Q[-2]X causing isolated apolipoprotein A-I deficiency in a family with analphalipoproteinemia. J Clin Invest 93:223–229
23. Takata K, Saku K, Ohta T et al (1995) A new case of apoA-I deficiency showing codon 8 nonsense mutation of the apoA-I gene without evidence of coronary heart disease. Arterioscler Thromb Vasc Biol 15:1866–1874
24. Ladias JA, Kwiterovich PO Jr, Smith HH, Karathanasis SK, Antonarakis SE (1990) Apolipoprotein A1 Baltimore (Arg10—Leu), a new ApoA1 variant. Hum Genet 84:439–445
25. Nichols WC, Gregg RE, HBJr B, Benson MD (1990) A mutation in apolipoprotein A-I in the Iowa type of familial amyloidotic polyneuropathy. Genomics 8:318–323
26. Cohen JC, Kiss RS, Pertsemlidis A, Marcel YL, McPherson R, Hobbs HH (2004) Multiple rare alleles contribute to low plasma levels of HDL cholesterol. Science 305:869–872
27. Romling R, von Eckardstein A, Funke H et al (1994) A nonsense mutation in the apolipoprotein A-I gene is associated with high-density lipoprotein deficiency and periorbital xanthelasmas. Arterioscler Thromb 14:1915–1922
28. Booth DR, Tan SY, Booth SE et al (1995) A new apolipoprotein AI variant, Trp50Arg, causes hereditary amyloidosis. Q J Med 88:695–702
29. Soutar AK, Hawkins PN, Vigushin DM et al (1992) Apolipoprotein AI mutation Arg-60 causes autosomal dominant amyloidosis. Proc Natl Acad Sci USA 89:7389–7393
30. Murphy CL, Wang S, Weaver K, Gertz MA, Weiss DT, Solomon A (2004) Renal apolipoprotein A-I amyloidosis associated with a novel mutant Leu64Pro. Am J Kidney Dis 44:1103–1109
31. Coriu D, Dispenzieri A, Stevens FJ et al (2003) Hepatic amyloidosis resulting from deposition of the apolipoprotein A-I variant Leu75Pro. Amyloid 10:215–223

32. Matsunaga T, Hiasa Y, Yanagi H et al (1991) Apolipoprotein A-I deficiency due to a codon 84 nonsense mutation of the apolipoprotein A-I gene. Proc Natl Acad Sci USA 88:2793–2797

33. Hamidi Asl L, Liepnieks JJ, Hamidi Asl K et al (1999) Hereditary amyloid cardiomyopathy caused by a variant apolipoprotein A1 [see comments]. Am J Pathol 154:221–227

34. Dastani Z, Dangoisse C, Boucher B et al (2006) A novel nonsense apolipoprotein A-I mutation (apoA-I(E136X)) causes low HDL cholesterol in French Canadians. Atherosclerosis 185:127–136

35. Miccoli R, Bertolotto A, Navalesi R et al (1996) Compound heterozygosity for a structural apolipoprotein A-I variant, apo A-I(L141R)Pisa, and an apolipoprotein A-I null allele in patients with absence of HDL cholesterol, corneal opacifications, and coronary heart disease. Circulation 94:1622–1628

36. Recalde D, Cenarro A, Civeira F, Pocovi M (1998) ApoA-IZaragoza(L144R): a novel mutation in the apolipoprotein A-I gene associated with familial hypoalphalipoproteinemia. Hum Mutat 11:416

37. Bruckert E, von Eckardstein A, Funke H et al (1997) The replacement of arginine by cysteine at residue 151 in apolipoprotein A-I produces a phenotype similar to that of apolipoprotein A-I$_{Milano}$. Atherosclerosis 128:121–128

38. Esperon P, Vital M, Raggio V, Alallon W, Stoll M (2008) A new APOA1 mutation with severe HDL-cholesterol deficiency and premature coronary artery disease. Clin Chim Acta 388:222–224

39. Huang W, Sasaki J, Matsunaga A et al (1998) A novel homozygous missense mutation in the apo A-I gene with apo A-I deficiency. Arterioscler Thromb Vasc Biol 18:389–396

40. Miettinen HE, Gylling H, Miettinen TA, Viikari J, Paulin L, Kontula K (1997) Apolipoprotein A-I$_{Fin}$. Dominantly inherited hypoalphali-poproteinemia due to a single base substitution in the apolipoprotein A-I gene. Arterioscler Thromb Vasc Biol 17:83–90

41. Miller M, Aiello D, Pritchard H, Friel G, Zeller K (1998) Apolipoprotein A-I(Zavalla) (Leu159→Pro): HDL cholesterol deficiency in a kindred associated with premature coronary artery disease. Arterioscler Thromb Vasc Biol 18:1242–1247

42. Leren TP, Bakken KS, Daum U et al (1997) Heterozygosity for apolipoprotein A-I(R160L)Oslo is associated with low levels of high density lipoprotein cholesterol and HDL- subclass LpA-I/A-II but normal levels of HDL-subclass LpA-I. J Lipid Res 38:121–131

43. von Eckardstein A, Funke H, Henke A, Altland K, Benninghoven A, Assmann G (1989) Apolipoprotein A-I Variants. Naturally occurring substitutions of proline residues affect plasma concentration of apolipoprotein A-I. J Clin Invest 84:1722–1730

44. Hamidi Asl K, Liepnieks JJ, Nakamura M, Parker F, Benson MD (1999) A novel apolipoprotein A-1 variant, Arg173Pro, associated with cardiac and cutaneous amyloidosis. Biochem Biophys Res Commun 257:584–588

45. Obici L, Bellotti V, Mangione P et al (1999) The new apolipoprotein A-I variant leu(174) → ser causes hereditary cardiac amyloidosis, and the amyloid fibrils are constituted by the 93- residue N-terminal polypeptide. Am J Pathol 155:695–702

46. Lachmann HJ, Booth DR, Booth SE et al (2002) Misdiagnosis of hereditary amyloidosis as AL (primary) amyloidosis. N Engl J Med 346:1786–1791

47. de Sousa MM, Vital C, Ostler D et al (2000) Apolipoprotein AI and transthyretin as components of amyloid fibrils in a kindred with apoAI Leu178His amyloidosis. Am J Pathol 156:1911–1917

ATP Binding Cassette A1 Transporter Function and Tangier Disease

Ernst J. Schaefer and H. Bryan Brewer

Introduction

Fredrickson and colleagues described two homozygous probands with Tangier disease with marked deficiency of plasma high density lipoproteins (HDL) and enlarged orange tonsils in 1961 [1]. Tangier Island is a small island in the Chesapeake Bay, which was originally discovered by Captain John Smith (see Fig. 1), and named as such by him because of its similarity to the harbor of Tangier in Morocco. The island was settled by families from Wales in the early 1600s, and the early and current inhabitants make their living by fishing and harvesting crabs from their traps (see Fig. 2).

The initial proband had his tonsils removed at age 5 on the eastern shore of Maryland. The surgeon removing the tonsils noted their unusual orange color and consistency, and sent tissue for pathologic analysis. The pathologist noted lipid laden macrophages, and referred the tissue on to the Armed Forces Institute of Pathology in Washington DC, where they were referred on to the National Institutes of Health (NIH). Dr. Donald Fredrickson of the Molecular Disease Branch of the National Heart Institute was consulted, and he asked the family to come to the Clinical Center at NIH in Bethesda, MD. It was noted that both the male proband and his 6-year-old sister had marked deficiency of alpha lipoproteins or HDL, and hepatosplenomegaly. The sister was also noted to have enlarged orange tonsils (see Fig. 3) [1–3]. Both parents were found to have HDL cholesterol levels that were about 50% of normal. Sampling of inhabitants (approximately 900 at the time) of the island revealed no more homozygotes. These original observations by Fredrickson and colleagues led to the discovery of much subsequent work on HDL deficiency and the finding of the ABCA1 transporter [1–46].

E.J. Schaefer (✉)
Tufts University, 711 Washington Street,
Boston, MA 02111, USA
e-mail: ernst.schaefer@tufts.edu

Pathologic Findings

Ferrans, working with Fredrickson, documented the presence of cholesterol laden macrophages in the tonsils, liver, and Schwann cells of these patients by both light and electron microscopy (see Fig. 4) [4]. Subsequently, Schaefer and colleagues at NIH documented the presence of orange omental mass filled with cholesterol laden macrophages in a homozygote, which had previously undergone a splenectomy (see Fig. 5) [5]. These data indicated an important role for the spleen in removing abnormal lipoproteins from plasma in these patients, and the emergence of omental masses to fulfill such a function when the spleen had been removed [5]. In addition, this patient presented with intestinal obstruction, but instead of removing a large portion of the patient's small intestine, Schaefer and colleagues elected to unobstruct this patient with a mercury filled bag attached to an naso-gastric tube. This approach worked along with frequent soft meals, and the patient passed away 15 years later in his sleep at home [5]. Chu and colleagues at NIH noted the presence of mild corneal opacification in patients with homozygous Tangier disease (see Fig. 6) [6].

Clinical Features of Tangier Disease

Engel and colleagues at NIH and Kocen and colleagues in the United Kingdom noted that patients with homozygous Tangier disease could have peripheral neuropathy, found to be present in about 1/3 of cases [7–9]. The neuropathy generally is not severe in these cases, and can be transient in nature [7–9]. The presence of premature coronary artery disease was reported by Schaefer and colleagues, who have extensively reviewed the literature in this regard [9–11] (see Fig. 7). They have estimated that Tangier homozygotes have about a threefold increased risk of coronary heart disease (CHD), while in heterozygotes it is estimated that CHD risk is about 1.5-fold increased [11]. Most patients have evidence

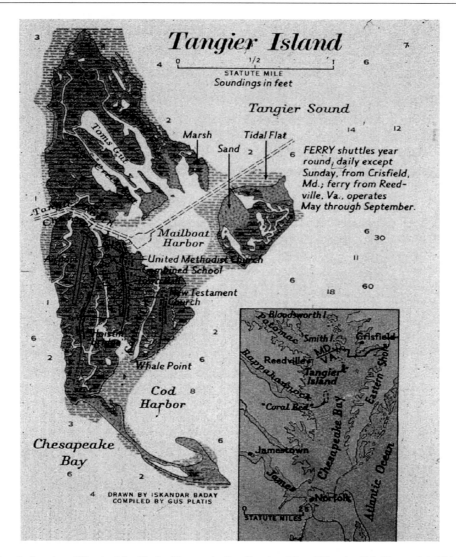

Fig. 1 A map showing the location of Tangier Island in the Chesapeake Bay. Reprinted from Wheatley HG, Harvey DA. This is my Island Tangier. National Geographic Magazine 1973;144(5): 700

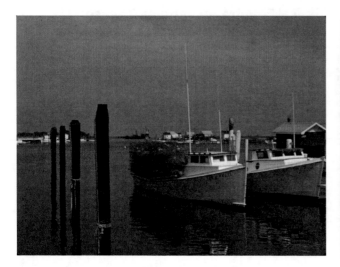

Fig. 2 A photograph of fishing and crabbing boats in the harbor of Tangier Island in the Chesapeake Bay

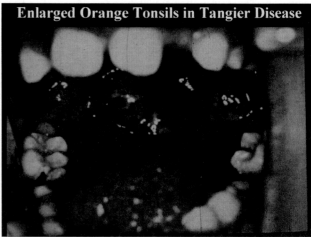

Fig. 3 A photograph of the enlarged orange tonsils of one of the original homozygotes from Tangier Island

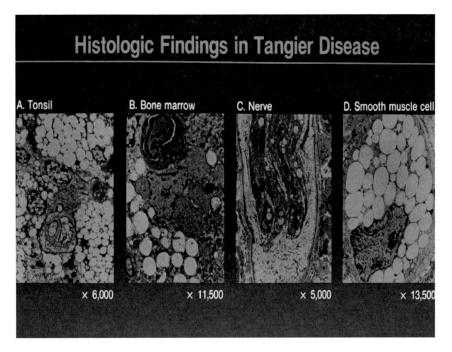

Fig. 4 Electron microscopy studies by Ferrans and Fredrickson documenting lipid deposition in the tonsils, bone marrow, nervous tissue, and smooth muscle cells of a homozygote with Tangier disease. Courtesy of Dr. Donald Fredrickson. Reprinted from Ferrans VJ, Fredrickson DS. The pathology of Tangier disease. A light and electron microscopic study. Am J Pathol 1975; 78:101–158

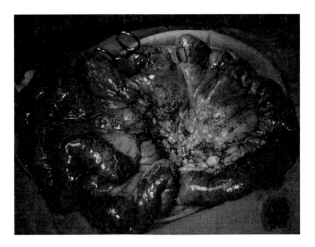

Fig. 5 A photograph of the omental masses that developed in a Tangier homozygote after splenectomy. Reprinted from Schaefer EJ, Triche TJ, Zech LA, Stein E, Kemeny MM, Brennan MF, Brewer HB Jr. Massive omental reticuloendothelial cell lipid uptake in Tangier disease following splenectomy. Am J Med 1983;75:521–526

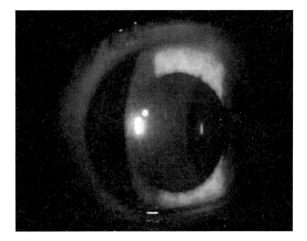

Fig. 6 Corneal opacification documented by slit lamp examination is shown in a Tangier homozygote. Reprinted from Chu FC, Kuwabara T, Cogan PG, Schaefer EJ, Brewer HB Jr. Ocular manifestations of familial high density lipoprotein deficiency (Tangier disease). Arch Opthalmol 1979;97:1926–1928

of hepatosplenomegaly. However it has been suggested by these authors that Tangier homozygotes may be somewhat protected from premature CHD because their LDL cholesterol are about 50% of normal [9–11].

Lipoprotein Metabolism

Work by Assmann, Fredrickson, and colleagues documented that patients with homozygous Tangier disease have mild hypertriglyceridemia, and low density lipoprotein (LDL)

cholesterol levels that are about 50% of normal, along with marked HDL deficiency, with very small HDL particles [12]. Moreover, the LDL in these patients was found to be triglyceride enriched [12]. The basis for these lipoprotein abnormalities have been examined by carrying radioiodinated HDL studies, HDL infusion studies, and more recently stable isotope lipoprotein metabolic studies [13–16]. In these studies, we documented that Tangier homozygotes had HDL apoA-I residence times of 0.18 days or 4.3 h, versus 4.79 days in controls [13], while heterozygotes had residence times of 2.41 days, indicating hypercatabolism of HDL

Fig. 7 Coronary angiography in a 58 year old Tangier homozygote showing significant stenosis in the left anterior descending coronary artery is shown. Reprinted from Schaefer EJ, Zech LA, Schwartz DS, Brewer HB Jr. Coronary heart disease prevalence and other clinical features in familial high density lipoprotein deficiency (Tangier disease). Ann Int Med 1980;93:261–266

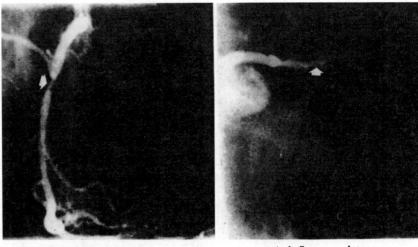

Right Coronary Artery   Left Coronary Artery

Right Anterior Oblique Projections

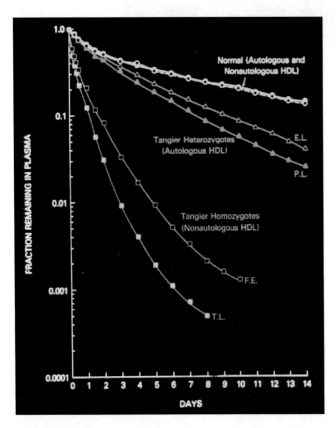

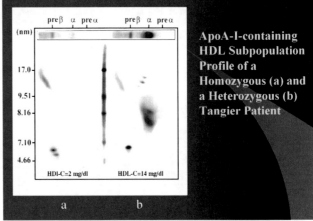

ApoA-I-containing HDL Subpopulation Profile of a Homozygous (a) and a Heterozygous (b) Tangier Patient

Fig. 9 Two dimensional gel electrophoresis of plasma HDL using anti-apoA-I immunoblotting documenting the presence of only pre-beta 1 HDL in a Tangier homozygote (*left*), and lack of large alpha 1 and alpha 2 in a Tangier heterozygote. Reprinted from Asztalos BF, Brousseau ME, McNamara JR, Horvath KV, Roheim PS, Schaefer EJ. Subpopulations of high-density lipoproteins in homozygous and heterozygous Tangier disease. Atherosclerosis 2001;156:217–225

Fig. 8 Plasma decay curves for radioiodinated HDL protein are shown for a homozygote, a heterozygote, and the normal subject, consistent with hypercatabolism of HDL particles in patients with Tangier disease. Reprinted from Schaefer EJ, Blum CB, Levy RI, Jenkins LL, Alaupovic P, Foster DM, Brewer HB Jr. Metabolism of high density lipoprotein apolipoproteins in Tangier disease. N Eng J Med 1978;299:905–910. © 1978 Massachusetts Medical Society. All rights reserved

apoA-I in homozygous and heterozygous Tangier patients (see Fig. 8) [13]. Moreover, HDL apoA-I was more rapidly catabolized than HDL apoA-II, especially in homozygotes,

and homozygotes have very small prebeta 1 migrating HDL only (see Fig. 9). These data have been confirmed by HDL infusion studies [14, 15].

In addition, Schaefer and colleagues documented that Tangier homozygotes have normal cholesterol synthesis and absorption, but their LDL apoB fractional catabolism is about twofold enhanced, accounting for the low LDL cholesterol levels of about 50% [16]. Moreover, the LDL in Tangier homozygotes is cholesterol poor and triglyceride-enriched, and very small [16]. In addition, their LDL particles are enriched in beta carotene to make up for the lack of cholesteryl ester in the core of their LDL particles [16]. Tangier homozygotes with HDL cholesterol <5 mg/dl can be distinguished from those lacking apoA-I because of their elevated triglycerides and decreased LDL cholesterol, whereas apoA-I deficient patients have normal values for these two parameters [17, 18]. In addition, having well standardized immunoassays for apoA-I is also valuable because Tangier homozygotes have detectable apoA-I levels (about 2–6 mg/dl), while apoA-I deficient patients have undetectable levels of apoA-I [17–19]. Tangier homozygotes do not have significant abnormalities in other apolipoproteins [17].

Defective ABCA1 Transporter Function in Tangier Disease

Oram and Bierman first reported that existence of a putative cellular HDL receptor or transporter important for reverse cholesterol [20]. Chimini and colleagues in Marseilles characterized a variety of ABC transporters, involved in active transport of specific molecules out of cells, including ABCA1 [21]. Subsequently, it was recognized by Francis, Oram, and colleagues in Seattle as well as Rogler, Schmitz, and colleagues in Regensburg that fibroblasts obtained from Tangier patients were defective in their ability to efflux free cholesterol and phospholipids onto apoA-I or HDL particles in vitro [22, 23]. Then, Rust, Assmann, and colleagues in Muenster documented that the disease locus for Tangier disease was at the chromosomal location 9q31 [24]. Subsequently, Langmann, Schmitz, Chimini, and colleagues cloned and sequenced ABCA1 in humans and documented that the gene is involved in cellular sterol transport [25]. Shortly thereafter, six different research groups reported that specific mutations in ABCA1 were causative for Tangier disease [26–31]. The first three research groups to make these observations were groups headed by Hayden in Vancouver, Schmitz in Regensburg, and Assmann in Muenster [26–28]. Moreover, heterozygotes were also shown to have decreased cellular cholesterol efflux (see Fig. 10) [32]. A model for the ABCA1 transporter process is shown in Fig. 11 [33].

Subsequently, population studies have indicated that specific ABCA1 genetic variants are linked to an increased risk of CHD in the general population [34–39]. In addition, over-expression of human ABCA1 in animal models resulted in elevated HDL levels and increased biliary cholesterol excretion [40]. In addition, ABCA1 overexpression was shown to decrease atherosclerosis in apoE or LDL receptor knockout mice [41]. It has also been shown by Remaley and colleagues that a variety of peptides containing amphipathic helices similar to apoA-I can promote ABCA1 mediated cholesterol efflux [42]. In addition, elegant studies by Neufeld, Brewer, and colleagues have documented that ABCA1 is involved in late endocytic cellular cholesterol trafficking [43]. In addition, von Eckhardstein and colleagues have shown that

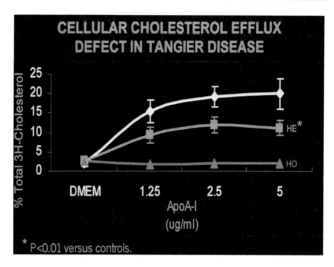

Fig. 10 Cellular cholesterol efflux studies using labeled cholesterol and apolipoprotein A-I are shown documenting almost no cholesterol efflux from skin fibroblasts obtained from homozygotes, and about half normal cholesterol efflux from skin fibroblasts obtained from obligate heterozygotes as compared to control fibroblasts. Reprinted from Brousseau ME, Eberhart GP, Dupuis J et al. Cellular cholesterol efflux in heterozygotes for Tangier disease is markedly reduced and correlates with high density lipoprotein cholesterol concentration and particle size. J Lipid Res 2000;41:1125–1135

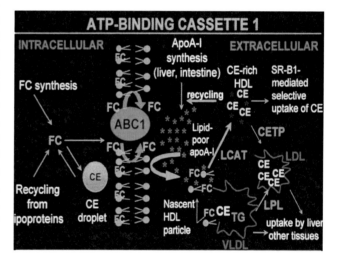

Fig. 11 Schematic representation of the ATP binding cassette protein A1 (ABCA1) transporter is shown. Reprinted from Young SJ. Fielding CJ. The ABCs of cholesterol efflux. Nat Genet 1999;22:316–318

ABCA1 gene expression modulates macrophage secretion of apoE [44]. In addition, it has been reported that the activation of peroxosomal proliferation activator receptor alpha and peroxosomal proliferation activator receptor gamma activation includes cholesterol removal from human macrophage foam cells through stimulation of the ABCA1 transporter [45]. Upregulation of ABCA1 gene expression may be an excellent strategy for CHD risk reduction [46].

We have recently documented that niacin not only increases the synthesis of apoA-I in humans significantly, but also significantly upregulates the liver gene expression of ABCA1 in animal studies [47, 48].

Conclusions

The lessons from Tangier disease are that ABCA1 is critical for cellular cholesterol efflux. In the absence of ABCA1 function, patients develop marked deposition of cholesteryl esters in macrophages in the tonsils, liver, spleen, arteries, and other tissues in the body. Clinically this results in enlarged orange tonsils, hepatosplenomegaly, peripheral neuropathy, premature CHD, and on endoscopy orange colored mucosa [1–11]. The cause of the low HDL is the lack of cellular cholesterol efflux onto pre-beta 1 HDL particles [11, 22, 23, 32]. Without cholesterol and phospholipids coming onto prebeta 1 HDL, the particles are rapidly cleared from the plasma, mainly by the kidney [13–15]. This lack of cholesterol on HDL results in no cholesterol esterification on HDL, and no cholesteryl ester transfer to apoB containing lipoproteins. This in turn results in very low density lipoproteins (VLDL) and LDL that are enriched in triglyceride and poor in cholesterol. In our view, this lack of cholesteryl ester in the core of LDL, results in the replacement of cholesteryl ester in the core of LDL with either triglyceride or beta carotene [16]. This excess beta carotene in LDL particles that are removed at twice the normal fractional catabolic rate, in our view results in excess tissue beta carotene, and the orange color observed in various tissues in Tangier homozygotes [1–10]. The treatment of this disease requires the aggressive treatment of CHD risk factors other than HDL in our view. Both peroxosomal proliferation activator receptor alpha and gamma agonists and niacin appear to upregulate ABCA1 gene expression. In niacin, this effect is particularly prominent and adds information about the mechanism of action of this agent, and its beneficial effects on CHD risk reduction [45, 48].

References

1. Fredrickson DS, Altrocchi PH, Avioli LC, Goodman DS, Goodman HC (1961) Tangier disease: combined clinical staff conference at the National Institute of Health. Ann Intern Med 55:1016–1122
2. Fredrickson DS (1964) The inheritance of high density lipoprotein deficiency (Tangier disease). J Clin Invest 43:228–243
3. Lux SE, Levy RI, Gotto AM, Fredrickson DS (1972) Studies on the protein defect in Tangier disease: isolation and Characterization of an abnormal high density lipoprotein. J Clin Invest 51:2505–2514
4. Ferrans VJ, Fredrickson DS (1975) The pathology of Tangier disease. A light and electron microscopic study. Am J Pathol 78:101–158
5. Schaefer EJ, Triche TJ, Zech LA, Stein E, Kemeny MM, Brennan MF, Brewer HB Jr (1983) Massive omental reticuloendothelial cell lipid uptake in Tangier disease following splenectomy. Am J Med 75:521–526

6. Chu FC, Kuwabara T, Cogan PG, Schaefer EJ, Brewer HB Jr (1979) Ocular manifestations of familial high density lipoprotein deficiency (Tangier disease). Arch Opthalmol 97:1926–1928
7. Engel WK, Dorman JD, Levy RI, Fredrickson DS (1967) Neuropathy in Tangier disease: alpha lipoprotein deficiency manifesting as familial recurrent neuropathy and intestinal lipid storage. Arch Neurol 17:1–10
8. Kocen RS, Lloyd JK, Lascelles PT, Fosbrooke AS, Williams D (1967) Familial alpha lipoprotein deficiency (Tangier disease) with neurologic abnormalities. Lancet 1:1341–1344
9. Schaefer EJ, Zech LA, Schwartz DS, Brewer HB Jr (1980) Coronary heart disease prevalence and other clinical features in familial high density lipoprotein deficiency (Tangier disease). Ann Int Med 93:261–266
10. Serfaty-Lacrosniere C, Lanzberg A, Civeira F, Isaia P, Berg J, Janus ED, Smith MP, Pritchard PH, Frohlich J, Lees RS, Ordovas JM, Schaefer EJ (1994) Homozygous Tangier disease and cardiovascular disease. Atherosclerosis 107:85–98
11. Asztalos BF, Brousseau ME, McNamara JR, Horvath KV, Roheim PS, Schaefer EJ (2001) Subpopulations of high-density lipoproteins in homozygous and heterozygous Tangier disease. Atherosclerosis 156:217–225
12. Assmann G, Herbert PN, Fredrickson DS, Forte T (1977) Isolation and characterization of an abnormal high density lipoprotein in Tangier disease. J Clin Invest 60:242–251
13. Schaefer EJ, Blum CB, Levy RI, Jenkins LL, Alaupovic P, Foster DM, Brewer HB Jr (1978) Metabolism of high density lipoprotein apolipoproteins in Tangier disease. N Eng J Med 299:905–910
14. Assmann G, Smootz E (1978) High density lipoprotein infusion and partial plasma exchange in Tangier disease. Eur J Clin Invest 8:131–140
15. Schaefer EJ, Anderson DW, Zech LA, Lindgren FT, Bronzert TJ, Rubalcaba EA, Brewer HB Jr (1981) Metabolism of high density lipoprotein subfractions and constituents in Tangier disease following the infusion of high density lipoproteins. J Lipid Res 22:217–226
16. Schaefer EJ, Brousseau ME, Diffenderfer MR, Cohn JS, Welty FK, O'Connor J, Dolnikowski GG, Wang J, Hegele RA, Jones PJ (2001) Cholesterol and apolipoprotein B metabolism in Tangier disease. Atherosclerosis 159:231–236
17. Alaupovic P, Schaefer EJ, McConathy WJ, Fesmire JD, Brewer HB Jr (1981) Plasma apolipoprotein concentrations in familial apolipoprotein A-I and A-II deficiency (Tangier disease). Metabolism 30:805–809
18. Schaefer EJ (1984) The clinical, biochemical, and genetic features in familial disorders of high density lipoprotein deficiency. Arteriosclerosis 4:303–322
19. Schaefer EJ, Lamon-Fava S, Ordovas JM, Cohn SD, Schaefer MM, Castelli WP, Wilson PWF (1994) Factors associated with low and elevated plasma high density lipoprotein cholesterol and apolipoprotein A-1 levels in the Framingham Offspring Study. J Lipid Res 35:871–882
20. Oram JF, Brinton EA, Bierman EL (1983) Regulation of high density lipoprotein receptor activity in cultured human skin fibroblasts and human arterial smooth muscle cells. J Clin Invest 72:1611–1621
21. Luciani MF, Denizot F, Savary S, Mattei MG, Chimini G (1994) Cloning of two novel ABC transporters mapping on human chromosome 9. Genomics 21:150–159
22. Francis GA, Knopp RH, Oram JF (1995) Defective removal of cellular cholesterol and phospholipids by apolipoprotein A-I in Tangier disease. J Clin Invest 96:78–87
23. Rogler G, Trumbach B, Klima B, Lackner KJ, Schmitz G (1995) HDL-mediated efflux of intracellular cholesterol is impaired in fibroblasts from Tangier disease patients. Arterioscler Thromb Vasc Biol 15:683–689

24. Rust S, Walter M, Funke H, von Eckhardstein A et al (1998) Assignment of Tangier disease To chromosome 9q31 by a graphical linkage exclusion strategy. Nat Genet 20:96–98

25. Langmann T, Klucken J, Reil M, Liebisch U et al (1999) Molecular cloning of the human ATP binding cassette transporter 1 (hABC1): evidence for sterol dependent regulation. Biochem Biohys Res Comm 257:29–33

26. Brooks-Wilson A, Marcil M, Clee SM et al (1999) Mutations in ABC1 in Tangier disease and familial high-density lipoprotein deficiency. Nat Genet 22:336–346

27. Bodzioch M, Orso E, Klucken J et al (1999) The gene encoding ATP-binding cassette transporter 1 is mutated in Tangier disease. Nat Gen 22:347–351

28. Rust S, Rosier M, Funke H et al (1999) Tangier disease is caused by mutations in the gene encoding ATP-binding cassette transporter 1. Nat Genet 22:352–355

29. Remaley AT, Rust S, Rosier M et al (1999) Human ATP-binding cassette transporter 1 (ABC1): genomic organization and identification of the genetic defect in the original Tangier disease kindred. Proc Natl Acad Sci USA 96:12685–126890

30. Lawn RM, Wade DP, Garvin J (1999) The Tangier disease gene product ABC1 controls the cellular apolipoprotein mediated lipid removal pathway. J Clin Invest 104:25–31

31. Brousseau ME, Schaefer EJ, Dupuis J et al (2000) Novel mutations in the gene encoding ATP-binding cassette 1 in four Tangier disease kindreds. J Lipid Res 41:433–441

32. Brousseau ME, Eberhart GP, Dupuis J et al (2000) Cellular cholesterol efflux in heterozygotes for Tangier disease is markedly reduced and correlates with high density lipoprotein cholesterol concentration and particle size. J Lipid Res 41:1125–1135

33. Young SJ (1999) Fielding CJ The ABCs of cholesterol efflux. Nat Genet 22:316–318

34. Brousseau ME, Bodzioch M, Schaefer EJ et al (2001) Common variants in the gene encoding ATP-binding cassette transporter 1 in men with low HDL cholesterol levels and coronary heart disease. Atherosclerosis 154:607–611

35. Probst MC, Thumann H, Aslanidas C et al (2004) Screening for functional sequence variants and mutations in ABCA1. Atherosclerosis 175:269–279

36. Frikke-Schmidt R, Nordestgaard BG, Schnohr P et al (2005) Mutations in ABCA1 predict risk of ischemic heart disease in the Copenhagen City Heart Study population. J Am Coll Cardiol 46:1516–1520

37. Soro-Paavonen A, Naukkarinen J, Lee-Ruechert M et al (2007) Common ABCA1 variants, HDL levels, and cellular cholesterol efflux in subjects with low HDL. J Lipid Res 48:1409–1416

38. Kyriakou T, Rontrefrant DE, Viturro E et al (2007) Functional polymorphisms in ABCA1 influence age of onset in coronary artery disease patients. Hum Mol Genet 16:1412–1422

39. Iatan I, Alrasadi K, Ruel I et al (2008) Effects of ABCA1 mutations on risk of myocardial infarction. Curr Atheroscler Rep 10:413–426

40. Vaisman BL, Lambert G, Amar MJ et al (2001) ABCA1 overexpression leads to hyperalphalipoproteinemia and increased biliary cholesterol excretion. J Clin Invest 108:303–309

41. Joyce CV, Amar MJ, Lambert G et al (2002) The ATP binding cassette transporter A1 (ABCA1) modulates the development of atherosclerosis in C57BL/6 and apoE-knockout mice. Proc Natl Acad Sci USA 99:407–412

42. Remaley AT, Thomas F, Stonik J et al (2003) Synthetic amphipathic helical peptides promote lipid efflux from cells by an ABCA1 dependent and an ABCA1 independent pathway. J Lipid Res 44:829–836

43. Neufeld EB, Stonik JA, Demosky SJ Jr et al (2004) The ABCA1 transporter mediates late endocytic trafficking: insights from the correction of the genetic defect in Tangier disease. J Biol Chem 279:15571–15578

44. Eckardstein A, Langer C, Engel T et al (2001) ATP binding cassette transporter ABCA1 modulates the secretion of apolipoprotein E from human monocyte derived macrophages. FASEB J 15:1555–1561

45. Chinetti G, Lestavel S, Bocher V et al (2001) Peroxisomal proliferation activator receptor alpha and peroxisomal proliferation activator receptor gamma activation includes cholesterol removal from human macrophage foam cells through stimulation of the ABCA1 transporter. Nat Med 7:53–58

46. Brewer HB Jr, Remaley AT, Neufeld EB et al (2004) Regulation of plasma HDL levels by the ABCA1 transporter and the emerging role of HDL in the treatment of cardiovascular disease. Arterioscler Thromb Vasc Biol 24:1755–1760

47. Lamon-Fava S, Diffenderfer MR, Barrett PHR, Buchsbaum A, Nyaku M, Horvath K, Asztalos BF, Otokozawa S, Ai M, Matthan NR, Lichtenstein AH, Dolnikowski GG, Schaefer EJ (2008) Extended-release niacin alters the metabolism of plasma apolipoprotein (apo) A-I and apoB-containing lipoproteins. Arterioscler Thromb Vasc Biol 28:1672–1678

48. Lamon-Fava S, Asztalos BF, Schaefer EJ (unpublished observations)

The Role ABCG1 in Cellular Cholesterol Efflux: Relevance to Atherosclerosis and Endothelial Function

Alan R. Tall

Introduction: ABC Transporters and Cholesterol Efflux Pathways

While HDL levels are known to have a strong inverse relationship to atherosclerotic CVD, the underlying mechanisms responsible for this association remain incompletely understood. Considerable cell culture and animal data support the idea that the atheroprotective properties of HDL are related to its ability to stimulate reverse cholesterol transport, i.e., efflux of cholesterol from macrophage foam cells in atheromata, followed by transport to the liver for excretion [1]. A variety of different anti-inflammatory, antithrombotic, and antioxidant effects of HDL have been described, but in vivo relevance to atherosclerosis remains uncertain [2, 3]. Several mechanisms of cellular cholesterol efflux have been identified, including passive cholesterol efflux, scavenger receptor B1 (SR-BI) mediated cholesterol efflux, and active cholesterol efflux by the ATP binding cassette transporters ABCA1 and ABCG1 [1, 4]. The latter transporters are highly induced in cholesterol loaded macrophages as a result of transcriptional induction by the transcription factors LXR/RXR [5, 6]. ABCA1 promotes cholesterol efflux to lipid-poor apoA-1, while ABCG1 promotes cholesterol efflux to HDL particles [7]. The activity of ABCA1 gives rise to a nascent HDL particle which may then interact with ABCG1.

ABC Transporters and Atherosclerosis

Although $Abcg1^{-/-}$ mice accumulate macrophage foam cells in lung and spleen on chow or high cholesterol diets [8], bone marrow transplantation from $Abcg1^{-/-}$ mice into $Apoe^{-/-}$ or $Ldlr^{-/-}$ mice resulted in either unchanged or reduced atherosclerosis [9, 10]. This unexpected outcome has been attributed to the upregulation of $ABCA1$ and ApoE secretion in ABCG1 deficient macrophages [10] as well as to increased apoptosis of $Abcg1^{-/-}$ macrophages in response to challenge with oxidized LDL or 7-oxysterols [9]. Bone marrow transplantation using donors deficient in ABCA1 and ABCG1 resulted in additive defects in macrophage reverse cholesterol transport in wild type mice [11], and dramatically accelerated atherosclerosis in LDL receptor deficient mice [12].

HDL and Endothelial Functions

Endothelial dysfunction, involving reduced bioavailability of NO and increased expression of cell adhesion molecules, is a key feature of early atherosclerotic lesions [13–16]. A part of the protective effect of HDL in atherosclerosis appears to be mediated by its ability to improve endothelial functions both in humans and in animal models [17–22]. This may involve both increases in the activity of endothelial nitric oxide synthase (eNOS) [20, 21, 23–27] as well as reduced expression of cell adhesion molecules [28, 29]. Infusions of reconstituted phospholipid/apoA-1 complexes were reported to improve the impaired endothelial function of patients with Tangier Disease, who have mutations in ABCA1 and very low HDL levels [30]. The beneficial effects of HDL on ECs may include stimulation of proliferation, cell survival, migration, and increased endothelial progenitor cell formation [31]. HDL may increase NO bioavailability and suppress increased expression of VCAM-1, E-selectin, and ICAM-1 following the treatment of ECs with TNF [29], and reduce LDL-induced endothelial MCP-1 expression [32]. The mechanisms of these effects are poorly understood, and relevance to chronic atherosclerosis remains uncertain [33], and worthy of further investigation. In a coculture system of endothelial cells and smooth muscle cells, HDL-2 and phospholipid liposomes but not apoA-1 suppressed the LDL-induced, MCP-1-dependent transmigration of monocytes to the subendothelial space. HDL has been shown to reverse

A.R. Tall (✉)
Department of Medicine, Columbia University,
630 W 168th St, New York, NY 10032, USA
e-mail: art1@columbia.edu

E.J. Schaefer (ed.), *High Density Lipoproteins, Dyslipidemia, and Coronary Heart Disease,*
DOI 10.1007/978-1-4419-1059-2_9, © Springer Science+Business Media, LLC 2010

decreased eNOS activity in cultured human ECs treated with oxidized LDL [24], and to reverse the decreased eNOS dependent arterial relaxation induced by a high cholesterol diet [34]. After feeding a high cholesterol diet, $Apoe^{-/-}$ mice expressing the human apoA-1 transgene showed improved arterial eNOS activity when compared to $Apoe^{-/-}$ control mice [34]. Interestingly, decreased Ach-induced vasorelaxation was observed in nonatherosclerotic cerebral arterioles of $Apoe^{-/-}$ mice on both chow and high fat diets, and the defect was reversed by apocynin (an inhibitor of NADPH oxidase) and Luminol (a scavenger of superoxide), implicating increased NADPH oxidase activity and ROS formation in the decreased bioavailability of NO [35]. Arterial rings from SR-BI knock-out mice have been reported to have impaired eNOS dependent relaxation [26], and SR-BI mediated cholesterol efflux can increase eNOS activity in transfected cells [36]. However, relaxation of arterial rings was very rapid (mins), occurred at very low HDL concentrations and showed different dose relationships in different preparations [26]. It remains uncertain whether reported in vivo effects are directly mediated by SR-BI in endothelial cells, or are secondary to hypercholesterolemia and altered composition of HDL and other lipoproteins in SR-BI knock-out mice. While minor components of HDL, such as estrogen [27] or sphingosine-1-phosphate [21], could have a role in improving eNOS activity, it has been suggested that concentrations are not high enough to be physiologically relevant [37]. Notably, while a variety of mechanisms responsible for antiatherogenic effects of HDL have been proposed, the contribution of endothelial effects of HDL (such as increases in NO bioavailability, or suppression of cell adhesion molecule or inflammatory chemokine responses) to its overall antiatherogenic role has never been directly evaluated.

ABC Transporters and Endothelial Function

The ABC transporters ABCA1 and ABCG1 are expressed in endothelial cells, and appear to have important effects on endothelial function [25, 38]. $Abca1$ and $Abcg1$ are induced in cholesterol loaded-cells including endothelium as a result of oxysterol mediated activation of LXR/RXR transcription factors [5, 6]. Laminar shear stress also induces expression of these transporters in endothelium, in part by induction and activation of LXR gene expression [38]. Recently, we have shown impaired eNOS-mediated arterial relaxation in $Abcg1^{-/-}$ or $Abca1^{-/-}$ mice after feeding a high cholesterol diet [25]. The defect was more severe in $Abcg1^{-/-}$ mice than in $Abca1^{-/-}$ mice, and similar to that of $Abca1^{-/-}Abcg1^{-/-}$ mice, suggesting a major role of ABCG1 in preserving arterial eNOS activity in mice fed high cholesterol diets. In part, these findings may be related to a specific role of ABCG1 in

promoting the efflux of 7-oxysterols accumulating in endothelial cells in mice fed high cholesterol diets [39]. Accumulation of 7-oxysterols in endothelium likely causes increased ROS formation, combining with NO to produce peroxynitrite and causing reduction of the active, dimeric form of eNOS.

$Abcg1^{-/-}$ Mice Show a Severe Defect in Endothelial-Dependent Vasorelaxation When Challenged with a Western-Type Diet or a High Cholesterol/Bile Salt Diet

We studied the Ach-induced relaxation of phenylephrine-preconstricted femoral artery rings in mice with knock-outs of $Abca1$ or $Abcg1$ fed the Western type diet (WTD) for 11 weeks [25]. This showed a similar severe defect in $Abcg1^{-/-}$ mice and in $Abca1^{-/-}Abcg1^{-/-}$ mice, and a milder defect in $Abca1^{-/-}$ mice. In contrast, there was no difference in relaxation in response to the endothelium-independent vasorelaxant, sodium nitroprusside (SNP). The EC50 values for vasorelaxation induced by Ach were determined for $Abcg1^{-/-}$ mice on chow, Western or high cholesterol diets (HCD). While there was no difference in response of WT and $Abcg1^{-/-}$ mice on the chow diet, there was a progressive increase in the EC50 value as the cholesterol content of the diet was increased from about fourfold control on the WTD to about tenfold control on the HCD. We also showed decreased eNOS activity, measured by the conversion of ^{3}H-arginine into ^{3}H-citrulline, in aortic homogenates of $Abcg1^{-/-}$ mice [25]. The decreased eNOS activities paralleled a decrease in the active, dimeric form of eNOS without significant change in the level of eNOS monomer. The $Abcg1^{-/-}$ mice were created by knock-in of LacZ into the ABCG1 locus, and thus we were able to monitor the expression of ABCG1 in nonatherosclerotic aortas. This showed a prominent signal over the endothelial layer; staining with PECAM-1 indicated an intact endothelium [39].

Measurements of sterol levels in nonatherosclerotic thoracic and abdominal aortas by gas–liquid chromatography showed increased contents of 7-ketocholesterol in $Abcg1^{-/-}$ mice fed either WTD or Paigen diets, while the increase in cholesterol content was not significant. In $Abca1^{-/-}Abcg1^{-/-}$ mice both cholesterol and 7-KC levels were significantly increased when compared to controls [25]. However, these measurements of overall cholesterol levels would not be sufficiently precise to detect subtle differences in specific membrane compartments. We also showed increased 7-ketocholesterol levels in isolated aortic endothelial cells from $Abcg1^{-/-}$ mice. These findings are consistent with our earlier work showing a specific role of ABCG1 in mediating cellular efflux of 7-oxysterols [39].

Together, these findings suggested that lack of ABCG1 led to accumulation of 7-KC in aortic endothelial cells, and this in turn might be responsible for a lower level of the active eNOS dimer. To assess this hypothesis further, we conducted experiments in isolated human aortic endothelial cells (HAECs). We showed that 7-KC reduced levels of eNOS dimer, paralleling a reduction in eNOS activity [25]; these effects were reversed by addition of HDL, in an ABCG1-dependent fashion. The reduction of eNOS dimer occurred at low concentration of 7-KC, comparable to those we observed in endothelial cells in vivo [25]. Only at higher concentrations of 7-KC, in the range of 20–40 μg/ml 7-KC, were there effects on ER stress and apoptosis of HAECs, suggesting that such effects were irrelevant to in vivo responses in $Abcg1^{-/-}$ mice.

In studies of the efflux of cholesterol and 7-KC from HAECs to HDL, we found that ABCG1 mediated the major pathway involved, while efflux to lipid-poor apoA-1 was very low, and knock-down of ABCA1 or SR-BI had little effect on cholesterol or 7-KC efflux. Using an ROS sensitive dye, we showed that 7-KC induced formation of ROS in HAECs, with reversal by HDL in an ABCG1-dependent fashion. The ability of 7-KC to generate ROS and reduce eNOS dimer was abolished by N-acetylcysteine and by Glutathione-SH [25]. Also, inhibition of eNOS activity with L-NAME abolished ability of 7-KC to reduce eNOS dimer formation [25]. These observations suggested that 7-KC induced formation of ROS, combining with NO to produce peroxynitrite, followed by reduction of eNOS dimers. Although mitochondrial poisons reduced the production of ROS, the source of increased ROS was not elucidated and will be investigated further in this proposal. In these studies, we also showed that the human apoA-1 transgene was able to increase eNOS activity in Ldlr+/− mice fed the Paigen diet, in association with reduced cholesterol and 7-KC accumulation in aorta and increased eNOS dimer formation [25].

Clinical Relevance and the Gap in Understanding of HDL Biology

The most effective treatments for raising HDL levels in humans have involved the use of CETP inhibitors or niacin. Both approaches raise HDL at least in part by reducing catabolism, and lead to the accumulation of large, HDL-2 particles. Particularly after high level CETP inhibition, these particles have a high content of ApoE. There is a theoretical concern that inhibition of CETP will lead to a reduced exchange of HDL CE for TG in triglyceride-rich lipoproteins, with decreased subsequent remodeling by hepatic lipase that leads to diminished release of lipid-poor apoA-1 and thus reduced cholesterol efflux via the ABCA1 pathway [40].

However, ApoE-enriched HDL isolated from subjects with complete deficiency of CETP, or treated with CETP inhibitors, appears to have superior ability to control HDL in promoting cholesterol efflux from macrophage foam cells, in part via the ABCG1 pathway [41, 42]. Since the ABCG1 pathway of cholesterol efflux appears to be predominant in endothelial cells [25], HDL from subjects treated with CETP inhibitors or niacin could lead to improvements in endothelial functions by promoting efflux of cholesterol and 7-oxysterols via the ABCG1 pathway, leading to an increased eNOS activity and reduced cell adhesion molecule expression. Niacin treatment has been shown to improve NO-mediated vascular relaxation in humans [22]. Interestingly, posthoc analyses of clinical outcomes and coronary atheroma burden as assessed by IVUS suggested benefit in subjects who achieved HDL cholesterol >70 mg/dl on treatment [43]. Subjects with higher baseline HDL levels are more likely to acquire large, apoE-rich HDL when treated with CETP inhibitors than subjects with low HDL levels at baseline. Such large, apoE-rich HDL may exert beneficial effects on endothelial functions. Whether or not clinical benefit accrues from adding a CETP inhibitor to statins may ultimately be resolved by ongoing clinical trials with other CETP inhibitors that lack the off-target toxicity of torcetrapib [44]. It is nonetheless clear that a deeper understanding of the functions of HDL and their relationship to CVD is badly needed. Clinical trial data is unlikely to provide further insight into relevant mechanisms, which may be better elucidated by cell culture and animal studies.

References

1. Tall AR, Yvan-Charvet L, Terasaka N, Pagler T, Wang N (2008) HDL, ABC transporters, and cholesterol efflux: implications for the treatment of atherosclerosis. Cell Metab 7(5):365–375
2. Tall AR (2008) Cholesterol efflux pathways and other potential mechanisms involved in the athero-protective effect of high density lipoproteins. J Intern Med 263(3):256–273
3. Duffy D, Rader DJ (2009) Update on strategies to increase HDL quantity and function. Nat Rev Cardiol 6(7):455–463
4. Adorni MP, Zimetti F, Billheimer JT et al (2007) The roles of different pathways in the release of cholesterol from macrophages. J Lipid Res 48(11):2453–2462
5. Costet P, Luo Y, Wang N, Tall AR (2000) Sterol-dependent transactivation of the ABC1 promoter by the liver X receptor/retinoid X receptor. J Biol Chem 275(36):28240–28245
6. Kennedy MA, Venkateswaran A, Tarr PT et al (2001) Characterization of the human ABCG1 gene: liver X receptor activates an internal promoter that produces a novel transcript encoding an alternative form of the protein. J Biol Chem 276(42):39438–39447
7. Wang N, Lan D, Chen W, Matsuura F, Tall AR (2004) ATP-binding cassette transporters G1 and G4 mediate cellular cholesterol efflux to high-density lipoproteins. Proc Natl Acad Sci USA 101(26):9774–9779

8. Kennedy MA, Barrera GC, Nakamura K et al (2005) ABCG1 has a critical role in mediating cholesterol efflux to HDL and preventing cellular lipid accumulation. Cell Metab 1(2):121–131

9. Baldan A, Pei L, Lee R et al (2006) Impaired development of atherosclerosis in hyperlipidemic Ldlr-/- and ApoE-/- mice transplanted with Abcg1-/- bone marrow. Arterioscler Thromb Vasc Biol 26(10):2301–2307

10. Ranalletta M, Wang N, Han S, Yvan-Charvet L, Welch C, Tall AR (2006) Decreased atherosclerosis in low-density lipoprotein receptor knockout mice transplanted with Abcg1-/- bone marrow. Arterioscler Thromb Vasc Biol 26(10):2308–2315

11. Wang X, Collins HL, Ranalletta M et al (2007) Macrophage ABCA1 and ABCG1, but not SR-BI, promote macrophage reverse cholesterol transport in vivo. J Clin Invest 117(8):2216–2224

12. Yvan-Charvet L, Ranalletta M, Wang N et al (2007) Combined deficiency of ABCA1 and ABCG1 promotes foam cell accumulation and accelerates atherosclerosis in mice. J Clin Invest 117(12):3900–3908

13. Hink U, Li H, Mollnau H et al (2001) Mechanisms underlying endothelial dysfunction in diabetes mellitus. Circ Res 88(2):E14–E22

14. Gimbrone MA Jr, Topper JN, Nagel T, Anderson KR, Garcia-Cardena G (2000) Endothelial dysfunction, hemodynamic forces, and atherogenesis. Ann N Y Acad Sci 902:230–239, discussion 239–240

15. Ashfaq S, Abramson JL, Jones DP et al (2008) Endothelial function and aminothiol biomarkers of oxidative stress in healthy adults. Hypertension 52(1):80–85

16. Cai H, Harrison DG (2000) Endothelial dysfunction in cardiovascular diseases: the role of oxidant stress. Circ Res 87(10):840–844

17. Kuvin JT, Patel AR, Sidhu M et al (2003) Relation between high-density lipoprotein cholesterol and peripheral vasomotor function. Am J Cardiol 92(3):275–279

18. O'Connell BJ, Genest J Jr (2001) High-density lipoproteins and endothelial function. Circulation 104(16):1978–1983

19. Drew BG, Fidge NH, Gallon-Beaumier G, Kemp BE, Kingwell BA (2004) High-density lipoprotein and apolipoprotein AI increase endothelial NO synthase activity by protein association and multisite phosphorylation. Proc Natl Acad Sci USA 101(18):6999–7004

20. Mineo C, Shaul PW (2003) HDL stimulation of endothelial nitric oxide synthase: a novel mechanism of HDL action. Trends Cardiovasc Med 13(6):226–231

21. Nofer JR, van der Giet M, Tolle M et al (2004) HDL induces NO-dependent vasorelaxation via the lysophospholipid receptor S1P3. J Clin Invest 113(4):569–581

22. Kuvin JT, Ramet ME, Patel AR, Pandian NG, Mendelsohn ME, Karas RH (2002) A novel mechanism for the beneficial vascular effects of high-density lipoprotein cholesterol: enhanced vasorelaxation and increased endothelial nitric oxide synthase expression. Am Heart J 144(1):165–172

23. Matsuda Y, Hirata K, Inoue N et al (1993) High density lipoprotein reverses inhibitory effect of oxidized low density lipoprotein on endothelium-dependent arterial relaxation. Circ Res 72(5):1103–1109

24. Uittenbogaard A, Shaul PW, Yuhanna IS, Blair A, Smart EJ (2000) High density lipoprotein prevents oxidized low density lipoprotein-induced inhibition of endothelial nitric-oxide synthase localization and activation in caveolae. J Biol Chem 275(15):11278–11283

25. Terasaka N, Yu S, Yvan-Charvet L et al (2008) ABCG1 and HDL protect against endothelial dysfunction in mice fed a high-cholesterol diet. J Clin Invest 118(11):3701–3713

26. Yuhanna IS, Zhu Y, Cox BE et al (2001) High-density lipoprotein binding to scavenger receptor-BI activates endothelial nitric oxide synthase. Nat Med 7(7):853–857

27. Gong M, Wilson M, Kelly T et al (2003) HDL-associated estradiol stimulates endothelial NO synthase and vasodilation in an SR-BI-dependent manner. J Clin Invest 111(10):1579–1587

28. Nicholls SJ, Lundman P, Harmer JA et al (2006) Consumption of saturated fat impairs the anti-inflammatory properties of high-density lipoproteins and endothelial function. J Am Coll Cardiol 48(4):715–720

29. Cockerill GW, Rye KA, Gamble JR, Vadas MA, Barter PJ (1995) High-density lipoproteins inhibit cytokine-induced expression of endothelial cell adhesion molecules. Arterioscler Thromb Vasc Biol 15(11):1987–1994

30. Bisoendial RJ, Hovingh GK, Levels JH et al (2003) Restoration of endothelial function by increasing high-density lipoprotein in subjects with isolated low high-density lipoprotein. Circulation 107(23):2944–2948

31. Tso C, Martinic G, Fan WH, Rogers C, Rye KA, Barter PJ (2006) High-density lipoproteins enhance progenitor-mediated endothelium repair in mice. Arterioscler Thromb Vasc Biol 26(5):1144–1149

32. Navab M, Hama SY, Van Lenten BJ, Drinkwater DC, Laks H, Fogelman AM (1993) A new antiinflammatory compound, leumedin, inhibits modification of low density lipoprotein and the resulting monocyte transmigration into the subendothelial space of cocultures of human aortic wall cells. J Clin Invest 91(3):1225–1230

33. Dansky HM, Barlow CB, Lominska C et al (2001) Adhesion of monocytes to arterial endothelium and initiation of atherosclerosis are critically dependent on vascular cell adhesion molecule-1 gene dosage. Arterioscler Thromb Vasc Biol 21(10):1662–1667

34. Deckert V, Lizard G, Duverger N et al (1999) Impairment of endothelium-dependent arterial relaxation by high-fat feeding in ApoE-deficient mice: toward normalization by human ApoA-I expression. Circulation 100(11):1230–1235

35. Kitayama J, Faraci FM, Lentz SR, Heistad DD (2007) Cerebral vascular dysfunction during hypercholesterolemia. Stroke 38(7):2136–2141

36. Assanasen C, Mineo C, Seetharam D et al (2005) Cholesterol binding, efflux, and a PDZ-interacting domain of scavenger receptor-BI mediate HDL-initiated signaling. J Clin Invest 115(4):969–977

37. Shaul PW, Mineo C (2004) HDL action on the vascular wall: is the answer NO? J Clin Invest 113(4):509–513

38. Zhu M, Fu Y, Hou Y et al (2008) Laminar shear stress regulates liver X receptor in vascular endothelial cells. Arterioscler Thromb Vasc Biol 28(3):527–533

39. Terasaka N, Wang N, Yvan-Charvet L, Tall AR (2007) High-density lipoprotein protects macrophages from oxidized low-density lipoprotein-induced apoptosis by promoting efflux of 7-ketocholesterol via ABCG1. Proc Natl Acad Sci USA 104(38):15093–15098

40. Tall AR, Yvan-Charvet L, Wang N (2007) The failure of torcetrapib: was it the molecule or the mechanism? Arterioscler Thromb Vasc Biol 27(2):257–260

41. Yvan-Charvet L, Matsuura F, Wang N et al (2007) Inhibition of cholesteryl ester transfer protein by torcetrapib modestly increases macrophage cholesterol efflux to HDL. Arterioscler Thromb Vasc Biol 27(5):1132–1138

42. Matsuura F, Wang N, Chen W, Jiang XC, Tall AR (2006) HDL from CETP-deficient subjects shows enhanced ability to promote cholesterol efflux from macrophages in an apoE- and ABCG1-dependent pathway. J Clin Invest 116(5):1435–1442

43. Nicholls SJ, Tuzcu EM, Brennan DM, Tardif JC, Nissen SE (2008) Cholesteryl ester transfer protein inhibition, high-density lipoprotein raising, and progression of coronary atherosclerosis: insights from ILLUSTRATE (Investigation of Lipid Level Management Using Coronary Ultrasound to Assess Reduction of Atherosclerosis by CETP Inhibition and HDL Elevation). Circulation 118(24):2506–2514

44. Krishna R, Anderson MS, Bergman AJ et al (2007) Effect of the cholesteryl ester transfer protein inhibitor, anacetrapib, on lipoproteins in patients with dyslipidaemia and on 24-h ambulatory blood pressure in healthy individuals: two double-blind, randomised placebo-controlled phase I studies. Lancet 370(9603):1907–1914

In Vitro Studies and Mass Flux of Cholesterol Between Serum and Macrophages

Ginny Kellner-Weibel, Margarita de la Llera-Moya, Sandhya Sankaranarayanan, and George H. Rothblat

Introduction

The concept of reverse cholesterol transport (RCT) as first formulated by Glomset [3] is that excess cholesterol in peripheral tissues is transported by HDL, or subfractions of HDL, to the liver for excretion. We now know that RCT is a complex process. Several steps, utilizing enzymes and transfer proteins, occur within the plasma compartment before the cholesterol molecules are delivered from peripheral cells to hepatocytes [1, 2, 4] and both intracellular and extracellular factors affect the direction of cholesterol transport at the tissue level [5].

When cells are incubated with serum in vitro there is flux of free cholesterol (FC) out of the cell (*efflux*) while simultaneously there is movement of lipoprotein FC and cholesteryl ester (CE) into the cell (*influx*). Net cholesterol flux is the difference between influx and efflux, and this difference may result in net accumulation, net depletion, or no change in cell cholesterol content. The net flux of cholesterol plays a major role in maintaining cell cholesterol homeostasis, and this is particularly important for macrophages in the vessel wall where net influx results in the deposition of excess cholesterol with the subsequent formation of foam cells, the hallmark of atherosclerosis. It is clear from both epidemiological and animal studies that elevated HDL-C is a negative risk factor for atherosclerosis. However, HDL is a complex mixture of particles, which differ in their ability to stimulate cell CE hydrolysis, efflux, as well as the influx of both CE and FC. Moreover, both the interaction of various HDL particles with serum transfer proteins and enzymes and their ability to deliver cholesterol to the liver has not been established. Therefore, the efflux efficiency of serum is influenced not just by HDL-C level but also by the distribution and composition of the HDL particles or HDL "quality." However, since efflux is the only one component of net flux, the expression of cholesterol transporters on the cell surface and the content of cell cholesterol which affects influx of lipoprotein cholesterol, will also determine net cholesterol flux. Most investigators have measured the efflux of labeled cholesterol from cells, rather than attempt to measure the flux of cholesterol mass.

Although much has been learned about the mechanisms underlying cell cholesterol flux many questions remain unresolved. Among these are: (1) what cholesterol transport proteins are present and how does expression vary among cell types? (2) what are the relationships between intracellular cholesterol content, intracellular cholesterol transport, and FC efflux pathways? (3) how does cell cholesterol content influence flux of cholesterol mass?

Cholesterol Efflux to Serum

Most efflux studies have been done with purified apolipoproteins and lipoproteins and have measured the movement of radioactive cholesterol between cells and these extracellular acceptors[6]. These studies cannot provide accurate estimates of net FC movement particularly when either serum or lipoprotein mixtures are used as the extracellular acceptors [6], but can be very useful for establishing underlying mechanisms. However, in vivo, cells are exposed to the complex mixture of lipoprotein acceptors, enzymes, and transfer proteins present both in plasma and interstitial fluid. Since the concentration and composition of lipoproteins can be modified by enzymes and lipid transfer proteins in serum, the activity of these serum components will play a critical, but as yet unknown role, in the regulation of lipid flux between cells and lipoproteins.

The discoveries of SR-B1 [7–11], ABCA1, and ABCG1 [12], cellular proteins that mediate cholesterol transport, further highlight the complexity of cholesterol movement between cells and extracellular acceptors. Additionally ABCA1, SR-B1, and ABCG1 have been shown to reorganize intracellular pools of cholesterol and thereby impact cholesterol mobilization [13–15]. The importance of ABCA1

G. Kellner-Weibel (✉)
Department of Pediatrics, Children's Hospital of Philadelphia, Philadelphia, PA 10104, USA
e-mail: weibel@email.chop.edu

in lipoprotein metabolism is demonstrated by the fact that defects in ABCA1 lead to very low HDL levels in Tangier patients [16–20] and in ABCA1-KO mice [21]. The role of SR-BI has been demonstrated by the fact that genetic manipulation of SR-BI in mouse models has a major impact on HDL levels, lipoprotein turnover, and atherosclerosis [9, 22–26]. The role of ABCG1 has not been as well elucidated, yet it is clear that this transporter does play an important role in cell cholesterol metabolism as demonstrated by a number of observations such as: ABCG1 KO mice accumulate lipids in hepatocytes and macrophages when on a high fat diet and that the expression of ABCG1 in cells stimulates the efflux of cholesterol in some cell systems [27–30]. An additional pathway that has been overshadowed by the discovery of cell protein-mediated cholesterol flux is aqueous diffusion, the process that occurs with all cells when FC molecules are desorbed from the cell membrane, and once in the aqueous phase can be incorporated into extracellular acceptors that contain phospholipid[31]. Increased cholesterol efflux in cells expressing SR-BI and ABCG1 likely has a component of aqueous diffusion as expression of these receptors leads to FC enrichment of the plasma membrane thus promoting the passive desorption of FC.

Impact of Cell Cholesterol Content on Cholesterol Flux

Cell cholesterol flux to serum depends on both the type and concentration of lipoproteins in serum and the array of transport proteins expressed by the cells. The expression level of these transport proteins is greatly influenced by cell cholesterol content. The data in Fig. 1 demonstrates that the cholesterol content of J774 cells modulates the relative contribution of each efflux pathway. Cholesterol loading modulates the expression of transport proteins and increases the contribution of ABCA1, and ABCGI, while decreasing the contribution of SRBI to total fractional efflux. These changes in transporter expression ultimately result in changes in fractional cholesterol efflux (Fig. 1). In addition to these receptor-dependent pathways, the aqueous transfer pathway plays a large role in cholesterol efflux from cholesterol-normal J774 cells and, to a lesser extent, in cholesterol-enriched macrophages (Fig. 1).

Net Flux of Cholesterol Mass

The measurement of the efficiency of serum or isolated lipoproteins to mediate cell cholesterol efflux has been a valuable tool in elucidating the pathways and mechanisms involved in the removal of cell cholesterol. In addition, recent

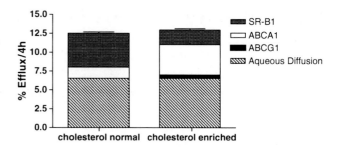

Fig. 1 Comparison of the contribution of cholesterol efflux pathways in cholesterol-normal and -enriched J774 macrophage cells. J774 cells were incubated with [^{3}H]cholesterol ± acLDL for 24 h. Efflux of [^{3}H] cholesterol to a pool of human serum (2.5%) was then measured in untreated cells to measure total efflux or from cells pretreated 2 h with Probucol to block ABCA1 or BLT-1 to block SR-B1. Aqueous diffusion was measured as residual efflux in cells treated with both inhibitors. ABCG1 was the difference in total efflux in the cholesterol-enriched and -normal cells. See ref. [36] for details of the assay

studies have demonstrated a relationship between efflux from macrophages and the deposition of lipids in vessels, as measured by IMT [32]. However, of prime importance with respect to understanding the process of RCT is measuring the net flux of cholesterol mass that occurs when cells are incubated with serum or isolated lipoproteins. In the present study, we have quantitated the net flux of cholesterol mass by directly measuring the change in cell cholesterol mass upon incubation of J774 macrophages with human sera. This is demonstrated in Fig. 2a, which shows the net cholesterol flux measured in cholesterol-normal and -enriched J774 cells exposed to: a pool of human serum (2.5%), the same pool after removal of apo B-lipoproteins (3.5% equivalent to 2.5% serum), human HDL$_3$ (50 µg/ml), and human apolipoprotein A-1 (25 µg/ml). Incubation with serum produced a net increase in cell cholesterol mass in cholesterol-normal cells and a substantial reduction in cholesterol-enriched cells. In contrast, incubation with the same serum after removal of the apo B lipoproteins resulted in little or no accumulation in cholesterol-normal cells but reduced cholesterol mass in cholesterol-enriched cells to almost the same extent as serum. Thus, as expected, apo B-containing lipoproteins contribute significantly to uptake but have a marginal effect on net cholesterol release. We can also see in Fig. 2a that, at the concentrations used in these experiments, both HDL and apo A-1 produced net mass efflux from enriched cells and had little or no impact on the cell cholesterol content of cholesterol-normal cells. Thus, the ability of serum HDL to remove cell cholesterol depends on cell cholesterol content and significant net release occurs only in cholesterol-enriched cells. In agreement with these results, Fig. 2b shows that exposure of cholesterol-enriched J774 to 23 normolipemic human sera for 8 h produced net depletion of cell cholesterol mass but, in contrast, exposure of cholesterol-normal J774 to the same sera produced net cholesterol mass accumulation. These data are

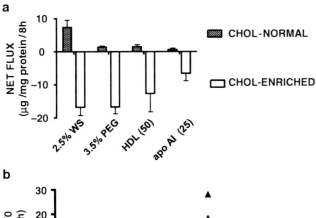

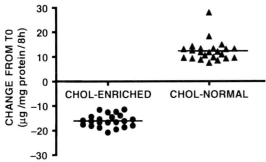

Fig. 2 Cellular cholesterol concentration impacts on net flux. Net flux of cell cholesterol upon incubation of cholesterol-normal (6.0 µg/mg protein) and FC-enriched (56 µg/mg protein) J774 cells with human sera or serum components. (**a**) Net cholesterol flux when J774 cells were incubated for 8 h with 2.5% serum pool, 3.5% apo B depleted serum, 50 µg/ml human HDL or 25 µg/ml human apo A-1. Each value is the average of triplicate determinations. (**b**) Net cholesterol flux when FC-enriched or cholesterol-normal cells were incubated with 23 individual human serum specimens (2.5%)

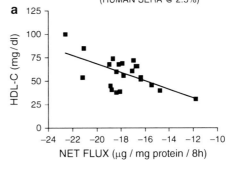

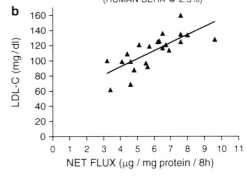

Fig. 3 Net flux of cholesterol correlates to HDL-C and LDL-C. (**a**) Relationship between the net efflux of cholesterol mass from cholesterol-enriched J774 and the HDL-C concentration of human sera. (**b**) Relationship between net increase in cell cholesterol mass in cholesterol-normal cells and the LDL-C concentration of human sera. Values for **a** are the average of four independent experiments, each run in triplicate. Values for **b** are the average from a single experiment run in triplicate

consistent with the significant association obtained between net efflux from cholesterol-loaded J774 cells and serum HDL-C levels (Fig. 3a) and net influx into cholesterol-normal cells and serum LDL-C (Fig. 3b).

Relationship Between Efflux of Labeled Cholesterol and Reduction of Cell Cholesterol Mass

As discussed earlier, the great majority of studies on cell cholesterol flux have followed the release of radiolabeled cho-lesterol from the cells since the protocols for this type of experiment are straightforward and readily adapted to high throughput assays. Using the data collected in the present study it is possible to establish the relationship between the fractional efflux of labeled cholesterol to the net reduction of cholesterol mass in J774 macrophages enriched with FC. As illustrated in Fig. 4a, when the cells are enriched in FC, and incubated with serum, there is a statistically significant positive correlation between the fraction of labeled cholesterol

that was released and the reduction in cell cholesterol mass ($r^2 = 0.43$, $p = 0.001$). The significant relationship between the release of radioactive cholesterol from cholesterol-enriched J774 macrophages and the actual decrease in cell cholesterol content was confirmed in studies using cholesterol-enriched mouse peritoneal macrophages (Fig. 4b).

Relationship Between Transporter Expression and Mobilization of Cell Cholesterol Mass

It is well documented that LDL receptor expression is down-regulated by increasing cell cholesterol content. As cells accumulate cholesterol, saturation of the plasma membrane also occurs, promoting cholesterol movement via concentra-tion gradients (aqueous diffusion). Both of these cellular

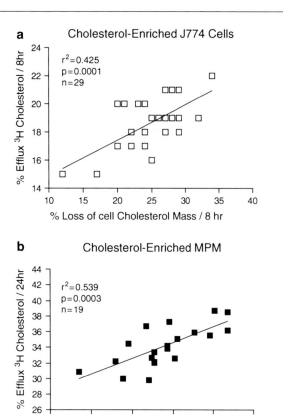

a Cholesterol-Enriched J774 Cells

$r^2 = 0.425$
$p = 0.0001$
$n = 29$

y-axis: % Efflux ^{3}H Cholesterol / 8hr
x-axis: % Loss of cell Cholesterol Mass / 8 hr

b Cholesterol-Enriched MPM

$r^2 = 0.539$
$p = 0.0003$
$n = 19$

y-axis: % Efflux ^{3}H Cholesterol / 24hr
x-axis: % Loss of Cell Cholesterol Mass / 24hr

Fig. 4 Relationship between reduction of cell cholesterol mass and fractional release of radiolabeled cholesterol from cholesterol-enriched J774 cells or primary mouse peritoneal macrophages. Cells were cholesterol-enriched by incubation with acLDL plus [^{3}H]cholesterol for 24 h. Cholesterol mass and [^{3}H]cholesterol efflux to 10% serum was measured at 8 or 24 h. These values were compared to the mass and [^{3}H]cholesterol levels before the efflux period. Values for **a** are the average of four independent experiments, each run in triplicate ($r^2 = 0.43$, $p = 0.001$). Values for **b** are from a single experiment run in triplicate ($r^2 = 0.539$, $p = 0.0003$)

mechanisms are evidence of the cell's ability to counteract an over accumulation of intracellular cholesterol which, if left unchecked, will become toxic [33, 34]. It is now known that cells modulate cholesterol transporter expression to promote net efflux of cholesterol [35, 36]. As discussed earlier with J774 macrophages, when primary mouse peritoneal macrophages (MPM) are cholesterol-enriched, there is an increase in ABCAI and ABCGI expression with a concurrent decrease in SR-B1 expression (Figs. 1 and 5). Since SRBI promotes the bi-directional flux of cholesterol and ABCAI and ABCGI promote the unidirectional flow of cholesterol out of the cell, modulating the transporter expression favors cholesterol efflux and reduces cell cholesterol mass. The data in Table 1 indicate that cholesterol transporters other than SRBI drive cholesterol mass reduction in MPM. When cholesterol-enriched MPM are exposed to HDL$_3$ for 18 h, 44% of the cell cholesterol mass is released (Table 1) and

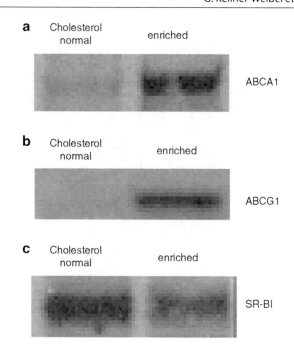

a Cholesterol normal   enriched — ABCA1

b Cholesterol normal   enriched — ABCG1

c Cholesterol normal   enriched — SR-BI

Fig. 5 Effect of cholesterol enrichment on transporter protein levels in primary mouse peritoneal macrophages. MPM were incubated for 24 h in the presence or absence of acLDL. 30 µg of cell protein was applied to each lane. ABCA1 (**a**), ABCGI (**b**), and SRBI (**c**) protein levels were determined as previously described [37]

27% of this occurs via ABCA1, as shown by the substantial reduction in mass efflux seen in cells treated with Probucol to block ABCA1. Treatment with BLT-1 to block SRBI, reduced cholesterol mass release by 12%, suggesting that ABCA1 plays a major role in removing excess cholesterol mass from macrophages. The important role of ABCA1 in promoting efflux of cholesterol mass in MPM documented in Table 1 agrees with the increase in ABCA1 mediated release of labeled cholesterol obtained with cholesterol-enriched J774 macrophage cells (Fig. 1).

Conclusion

In vivo, net movement of cholesterol in and out of cells, particularly aortic macrophages, will, in part, determine progression or regression of atherosclerotic lesions and modulate RCT. Various aspects of the movement of cholesterol between cells in culture and serum or isolated serum lipoproteins have been investigated for many years. The majority of these investigations have focused on the movement of FC, with the emphasis being on the efflux of radiolabeled cholesterol previously incorporated into the cells. The measurement of the release of labeled cholesterol is relatively simple since only FC undergoes efflux. Data generated by this approach have been valuable in identifying a number of pathways that participate in the release of cell cholesterol to maintain homeostasis, but fail to

Table 1 Contribution of SR-B1 and ABCAl to cholesterol mass reduction in mouse peritoneal macrophages. Mouse peritoneal macrophage (C57Bl/6 strain) cells were plated in growth medium, allowed to attach for 24 h and thereafter incubated with acLDL for 24 h to enrich with cholesterol. After 2 h equilibration, the cells were incubated with HDL_3 with or without inhibitors for 18 h. Cholesterol mass was determined by GLC. The experiment was done in quadruplicate ($n=4$). Cell cholesterol mass at $t=0$ (before the efflux phase) was 53.3 ± 0.95 μg cholesterol/mg protein

Acceptor	Treatment	Net efflux/18 h (μg cholesterol/mg protein)	% mass efflux/18 h	% inhibition	% contribution (to total efflux)
HDL3	–	23.8 ± 1.1	44.6 ± 1.4	–	–
HDL3	Probucol	9.5 ± 1.4	17.7 ± 1.7	$60.3 \pm 2.2\%$ (ABCA1)	$26.9 \pm 1.9\%$ (ABCA1)
HDL3	BLT-1	20.9 ± 1.3	39.2 ± 1.6	$12.3 \pm 2.1\%$ (SRB-1)	$7.44 \pm 20.9\%$ (SRB-1)

address the intricacies of the interplay of cell cholesterol, cholesterol transporters, and HDL. Measurement of the fractional release of labeled cell cholesterol is a functional assay that can be used to assess the efficiency of serum or lipoproteins in stimulating efflux and can be applied to the evaluation of drugs or diets for their ability to modulate cholesterol efflux, a process that is the first step in RCT. Indeed the significant relationship between net cholesterol removal and the fractional efflux of tracer cholesterol seen in cholesterol-enriched cells (Fig. 4) suggests that in vitro isotopic measures of serum efflux efficiency may be valid surrogate measure of the capacity of serum to remove excess tissue cholesterol in vivo. However, more rigorous experimental systems must be employed to measure net cholesterol flux. Clearly, we do not fully understand the roles of ABCA1, ABCG1, SR-BI and aqueous transfer in this process. Neither do we know the relative role of these pathways in RCT, or the role of each of the many subclasses of HDL. What is clear is that elevated levels of HDL-C are atheroprotective and that knowledge has prompted numerous attempts to develop agents that will raise the level of HDL in humans. More research is needed to not only provide fundamental information on the metabolism of lipoproteins, cell cholesterol and CE clearance, but more importantly, on the roles of HDL, ABCA1, ABCG1, and SR-BI in RCT and in the development of atherosclerosis.

References

1. Franceschini G, Maderna P, Sirtori CR (1991) Reverse cholesterol transport: physiology and pharmacology. Atherosclerosis 88:99–107
2. Von Eckardstein A, Nofer J-R, Assmann G (2001) High density lipoproteins and arteriosclerosis: role of cholesterol efflux and reverse cholesterol transport. Arterioscler Thromb Vasc Biol 21:13–27
3. Glomset JA (1968) The plasma lecithin:cholesterol acyltransferase reaction. J Lipid Res 9:155–167
4. Fielding CJ (1991) Reverse cholesterol transport. Curr Opin Lipidol 2:376–378
5. Rothblat GH, de la Llera-Moya M, Atger V, Kellner-Weibel G, Williams DL, Phillips MC (1999) Cell cholesterol efflux: integration of old and new observations provides new insights. J Lipid Res 40:781–796
6. Rothblat GH, de la Llera-Moya M, Favari E, Yancey PG, Kellner-Weibel G (2002) Cellular cholesterol flux studies: methodological considerations. Atherosclerosis 163:1–8
7. Acton S, Rigotti A, Landschulz KT, Xu S, Hobbs HH, Krieger M (1996) Identification of scavenger receptor SR-BI as a high density lipoprotein receptor. Science 271:518–520
8. Rigotti A, Trigatti B, Babitt J, Penman M, Xu S, Krieger M (1997) Scavenger receptor BI – a cell surface receptor for high density lipoprotein. Curr Opin Lipidol 8:181–188
9. Ji Y, Wang N, Ramakrishnan R, Sehayek E, Huszar D, Breslow JL et al (1999) Hepatic scavenger receptor BI promotes rapid clearance of high density lipoprotein free cholesterol and its transport into bile. J Biol Chem 274:33398–33402
10. Trigatti BL, Rigotti A, Braun A (2001) Cellular and physiological roles of SR-BI, a lipoprotein receptor which mediates selective lipid uptake. Biochim Biophys Acta 1529:276–286
11. Williams DL, Connelly MA, Temel RE, Swanakar S, Phillips MC, de la Llera-Moya M et al (1999) Scavenger receptor BI and cholesterol trafficking. Curr Opin Lipidol 10:329–339
12. Bodzioch M, Orsó E, Klucken T, Langmann T, Böttcher L, Diederich W et al (1999) The gene encoding ATP-binding cassette transporter 1 is mutated in Tangier disease. Nat Genet 22(4):347–351
13. Chen W, Sun Y, Welch C, Gorelik A, Leventhal AR, Tabas I et al (2001) Preferential ATP-binding cassette transporter A1-mediated cholesterol efflux from late endosomes/lysosomes. J Biol Chem 276:43564–43569
14. Neufeld EB, Remaley AT, Demosky SJ, Stonik JA, Cooney AM, Comly M et al (2001) Cellular localization and trafficking of the human ABCA1 transporter. J Biol Chem 276:27584–27590
15. Wang N, Ranalletta M, Matsuura F, Peng F, Tall AR (2006) LXR induced redistribution of ABCG1 to plasma membrane in macrophages enhances cholesterol mass efflux to HDL. Arterioscler Thromb Vasc Biol 26:1310–1316
16. Brooks-Wilson A, Marcil M, Clee SM, Zhang LH, Roomp K, Van Dam M et al (1999) Mutations in *ABC1* in Tangier disease and familial high-density lipoprotein deficiency. Nat Genet 22(4): 336–345
17. Hayden MR, Clee SM, Brooks-Wilson A, Genest JJr, Attie A, Kastelein JJP (2000) Cholesterol efflux regulatory protein, Tangier disease and familial high-density lipoprotein deficiency. Curr Opin Lipidol 11:117–122
18. Lawn RM, Wade DP, Garvin MR, Wang X, Schwartz K, Porter JG et al (1999) The Tangier disease gene product ABC1 controls the cellular apolipoprotein-mediated lipid removal pathway. J Clin Invest 104:R25–R31
19. Oram JF (2001) Tangier disease and ABCA1. Biochim Biophys Acta 1529:321–330
20. Remaley AT, Schumacher UK, Stonik JA, Farsi BD, Nazih H, Brewer HB (1997) Decreased reverse cholesterol transport from Tangier Disease Fibroblasts: acceptor specificity and effect of brefeldin on lipid efflux. Arterioscler Thromb Vasc Biol 17:1813–1821
21. McNeish J, Aiello RJ, Guyot D, Turley SD, Gaben-Cogneville A-M, Aldinger C et al (2000) High density lipoprotein deficiency and foam cell accumulation in mice with targeted disruption of ATP-binding cassette transporter-1. Proc Natl Acad Sci USA 97:4245–4250

22. Arai T, Wang N, Bezouevski M, Welch C, Tall AR (1999) Decreased atherosclerosis in heterozygous low density lipoprotein receptor-deficient mice expressing the scavenger receptor BI transgene. J Biol Chem 274:2366–2371

23. Krieger M, Kozarsky K (1999) Influence of the HDL receptor SR-BI on atherosclerosis. Curr Opin Lipidol 10:491–497

24. Tall AR, Jiang X, Luo Y, Silver D (1999) Lipid transfer proteins, HDL metabolism, and atherogenesis. Arterioscler Thromb Vasc Biol 20:1185–1188

25. Huszar D, Varban ML, Rinninger F, Feeley R, Arai T, Fairchild-Huntress V et al (2000) Increased LDL cholesterol and atherosclerosis in LDL receptor-deficient mice with attenuated expression of scavenger receptor B1. Arterioscler Thromb Vasc Biol 20(4):1068–1073

26. Kozarsky KF, Donahee MH, Glick JM, Krieger M, Rader DJ (2000) Gene transfer and hepatic overexpression of the HDL receptor SR-BI reduces atherosclerosis in the cholesterol-fed LDL receptor-deficient mouse. Arterioscler Thromb Vasc Biol 20:721–727

27. Wang N, Lan D, Chen W, Matsuura F, Tall AR (2004) ATP-binding cassette transporters G1 and G4 mediate cellular cholesterol efflux to high-density lipoprotein. Proc Natl Acad Sci USA 101:9774–9779

28. Kennedy MA, Barrera GC, Nakamura K, Baldan A, Tarr PT, Fishbein MC et al (2005) ABCG1 has a critical role in mediating cholesterol efflux to HDL and preventing cellular lipid accumulation. Cell Metab 1:121–129

29. Vaughan AM, Oram JF (2005) ABCG1 redistributes cell cholesterol to domains removable by high density lipoprotein but not by lipid-depleted apolipoproteins. J Biol Chem 280(34):30150–30157

30. Gelissen IC, Harris M, Rye KA, Quinn C, Brown AJ, Kockx M et al (2006) ABCA1 and ABCG1 synergize to mediate cholesterol export to apoA-I. Arterioscler Throm Vasc Biol 26:534–540

31. Johnson WJ, Mahlberg FH, Rothblat GH, Phillips MC (1991) Cholesterol transport between cells and high density lipoproteins. Biochim Biophys Acta 1085:273–298

32. Cuchel M, de la Llera-Moya M, Phillips JA, Wolfe ML, Rothblat GH, Rader DJ (2008) Cholesterol efflux capacity of serum predicts carotid internal-medial thickness independently of HDL-C and apo A-I levels. Circulation 118(Suppl):371, Abstract

33. Kellner-Weibel G, Jerome WG, Small DM, Warner GJ, Stoltenborg JK, Kearney MA et al (1998) Effects of intracellular free cholesterol accumulation on macrophage viability: a model for foam cell death. Arterioscler Thromb Vasc Biol 18:423–431

34. Shiratori Y, Okwu AK, Tabas I (1994) Free cholesterol loading of macrophages stimulates phosphatidylcholine biosynthesis and up-regulation of CTP:phosphocholine cytidylyltransferase. J Biol Chem 269:11337–11348

35. Tall AR, Yvan-Charvet L, Terasaka N, Pagler T, Wang N (2008) HDL, ABC transporters, and cholesterol efflux: implications for the treatment of atherosclerosis. Cell Metab 7(5):365–375

36. Adorni MP, Zimetti F, Billheimer JT, Wang N, Rader DJ, Phillips MC et al (2007) The role of different pathways in the release of cholesterol from macrophages. J Lipid Res 48:2453–2462

37. Duong M-N, Jin W, Zanotti I, Favari E, Rothblat GH (2006) The relative contributions of ABCA1 and SR-BI to cholesterol efflux to serum from fibroblasts and macrophages. Arterioscler Thromb Vasc Biol 26:541–547

Genetic LCAT Deficiency: Molecular Diagnosis, Plasma Lipids, and Atherosclerosis

Laura Calabresi and Guido Francheschini

Introduction

Lecithin:cholesterol acyltransferase (LCAT, phosphatidylcholine:sterol-O-acyltransferase; EC 2.3.1.43) is a glycoprotein of 416 residues [1]. A single copy of the human *LCAT* gene, which contains six exons, is present on chromosome 16 (region 16q 22). LCAT is synthesized mainly by the liver and secreted into the plasma compartment, where it circulates bound to small and large high density lipoprotein (HDL) particles, with a minor portion bound to apoB-containing lipoproteins. LCAT has both a phospholipase A$_2$ and an acyltransferase activity, as it catalyzes the transacylation of the *sn*-2 fatty acid of lecithin to the free 3-β hydroxyl group of cholesterol, generating cholesteryl ester (CE) and lysolecithin [1]. By this way, the LCAT reaction accounts for the synthesis of most of the plasma CE. Cholesterol esterification occurs mainly on HDL, via α-LCAT activity, but also on apoB-containing lipoproteins, via β-LCAT activity [1]. The preferred HDL substrate for LCAT is a newly assembled small, discoidal HDL migrating in the preβ position on agarose gel, thus called preβ-HDL [2]. The formation and accumulation of CE within these particles leads to conversion into spherical, α-migrating HDL, which comprise most of the plasma HDL. Preβ-HDL have a short plasma half-life, being rapidly cleared through the kidney [3], while mature α-HDL have a much slower turnover. LCAT thus plays a central role in intravascular HDL metabolism and in the determination of plasma HDL levels. LCAT is also believed to contribute to macrophage cholesterol efflux and reverse cholesterol transport, by keeping the cholesterol gradient between the cell membrane and the HDL acceptor surfaces [1].

Mutations in the LCAT gene cause two LCAT deficiency syndromes, classical familial LCAT deficiency (FLD, OMIM# 245900) and fish-eye disease (FED, OMIM# 136120). The differential diagnosis of FLD and FED is restricted to homozygotes or compound heterozygotes and requires measurement of cholesterol esterification rate (CER) in whole plasma (α-LCAT activity + β-LCAT activity) and of the ability of plasma to esterify cholesterol incorporated into a synthetic HDL substrate (α-LCAT activity). FLD cases have a completely defective cholesterol esterification; in FED cases, the mutant enzyme lacks α-LCAT activity but maintains β-LCAT activity. FLD cases reportedly present with corneal opacity and anemia, and many of them unpredictably develop renal disease; FED cases seem to have a milder clinical phenotype [4].

Most LCAT mutations have been identified through the investigation of single cases, or small nuclear families in which a defect in the *LCAT* gene was predicted from the biochemical or clinical presentation. General conclusions on the impact of such mutations on LCAT function in human health and disease have been attempted through a systematic review of the data published in these scattered reports [4, 5]. We have recently identified 16 Italian families carrying mutations in the *LCAT* gene, the largest series reported to date [6]. The investigation of these families may provide some new insights on the role of LCAT gene on lipid/lipoprotein metabolism and atherosclerosis.

LCAT Gene Mutations and Lipid/Lipoprotein Phenotype

Seventy-five mutations in the human *LCAT* gene are listed in the Human Gene Mutation Database (HGMD, http://www.hgmd.cf.ac.uk/ac/index.php, interrogated May 2009). These mutations are spread from residue −13 to 399. There are 3 nonsense mutations, 56 missense mutations, 9 deletions, 5 insertions, 1 indel, and 1 splice site mutation.

Sequence analysis of the Italian probands' DNA identified 22 different mutations [6]. All mutations are private mutations. Overall, 18 out of the 79 examined individuals carry two mutant *LCAT* alleles (nine homozygotes and nine compound heterozygotes), 41 carry one mutant *LCAT* allele, and 20 have a normal genotype.

L. Calabresi (✉)
Center E. Grossi Paoletti, Department of Pharmacological Sciences, Università degli Studi di Milano, via Balzaretti 9, Milano 20133, Italy
e-mail: laura.calabresi@unimi.it

E.J. Schaefer (ed.), *High Density Lipoproteins, Dyslipidemia, and Coronary Heart Disease*,
DOI 10.1007/978-1-4419-1059-2_11, © Springer Science+Business Media, LLC 2010

Eleven out of the 18 carriers of two mutant *LCAT* alleles had undetectable α-LCAT and β-LCAT activities, and were diagnosed as FLD cases; seven had detectable β-LCAT but no α-LCAT activity, and were classified as FED cases. Since carriers of one mutant *LCAT* allele cannot be classified as FLD or FED based on neither biochemical nor clinical criteria [4], differential genetic diagnosis in heterozygotes was performed by expressing LCAT mutants, as well as the wild-type LCAT protein, in COS-1 cells, and measuring LCAT concentration and α-LCAT and β-LCAT activities in the cell medium [7] (Table 1). Thirty heterozygotes were found to carry either a truncated LCAT mutant (*n* = 8), or an LCAT mutant displaying undetectable α-LCAT and β-LCAT activities (*n* = 22), and were thus classified as FLD. Eleven heterozygotes were found to carry an LCAT mutant displaying no α-LCAT activity but detectable β-LCAT activity, and were classified as FED.

The study of the Italian families confirms earlier findings from single family reports that inheritance of 2 mutant *LCAT* alleles causes remarkably low plasma HDL-cholesterol, apoA-I, and apoA-II levels [6]. However, the severity of the hypoalphalipoproteinemia (HA) varies widely among cases with different LCAT genotypes, as exemplified by the sixfold variation in plasma HDL-cholesterol levels among the 19 Italian cases. The HA in the carriers of 2 mutant *LCAT* alleles is associated with multiple alterations in HDL structure and particle distribution, with a selective depletion of LpA-I:A-II particles, a predominance of small, preβ-migrating HDL3, and a complete lack of HDL2 [6, 8]. Such changes likely reflect the accumulation in plasma of CE-poor, apoA-I-containing, discoidal HDL [9], which cannot mature into spherical HDL due to the lack of LCAT activity, and are rapidly cleared from the circulation [3]. All Italian cases had remarkably low plasma LCAT protein concentrations [6], which can be either due to impaired expression and secretion, or increased

catabolism of the mutant LCAT. The striking positive correlation between plasma LCAT and HDL-cholesterol levels suggests that HDL may function as a vehicle for LCAT in plasma, stabilizing the enzyme and preventing its catabolism. Elevated plasma triglycerides and VLDL-cholesterol were a frequent finding among Italian cases, consistent with previous reports in isolated families [4]; similarly, hypertriglyceridemia has been reported in mouse models of human LCAT deficiency generated through gene targeting [10, 11]. A decreased postheparin lipoprotein lipase activity has been detected in LCAT-deficient mice [10] and in some FLD cases [12], suggesting that defective lipolysis may contribute to the elevated plasma triglycerides. More intriguing is the observation of enhanced hepatic triglyceride synthesis in LCAT-deficient mice [10, 11]. As a partial LCAT deficiency is found in monogenic forms of HA due to mutations in HDL-related genes other than *LCAT* [13, 14], hepatic triglyceride overproduction may represent a general mechanism for the rise of plasma triglycerides in genetic HA.

Scattered reports of heterozygous carriers of LCAT mutations indicate that they may have either low or normal plasma HDL-cholesterol levels. The Italian heterozygotes had lower average plasma HDL-cholesterol and apoA-I levels than controls, and half of them classify as low-HDL individuals, according to current guidelines [15]. The availability of a relatively large number of carriers of 2 and 1 mutant *LCAT* alleles allowed us to identify a significant *LCAT* gene-dose-dependent effect on plasma lipid and apolipoprotein levels, cholesterol esterification measurements, and HDL-related parameters [6]. These findings underline the importance of proper LCAT function for efficient lipid and lipoprotein metabolism. No significant difference in plasma HDL lipid, apolipoprotein, and subfraction levels was found between FLD and FED individuals carrying either two [6] or one (Table 2) mutant *LCAT* alleles.

Table 1 Concentration and activity of missense LCAT mutants expressed in COS-1 cells

Mutant	LCAT mass (μg/ml)	LCAT activity (nmol/ml/h)		Mutant phenotype
		α activity	β activity	
WT	0.28 ± 0.05	12.7 ± 1.8	76.2 ± 10.7	
T-13M	0.28 ± 0.10	0	45.1	FED
V46E	0.24 ± 0.08	0	45.1	FED
S91P	0.40 ± 0.14	0	0	FLD
R140C	0.30 ± 0.08	0	0	FLD
A141T	0.27 ± 0.08	0	117.3	FED
R147W	0.16 ± 0.02	0	0	FLD
S181N	0.45 ± 0.02	0	0	FLD
K218N	0.22 ± 0.05	0	0	FLD
R244H	0.39 ± 0.02	0	110.2	FED
T274A	0.15 ± 0.02	0	18.3	FED
T274I	0.27 ± 0.06	0	0	FLD
V309M	0.32 ± 0.03	0	0	FLD
L372R	0.16 ± 0.07	0	0	FLD

Data are expressed as mean ± SD

Table 2 Lipid/lipoprotein levels, lipoprotein subpopulations, and cholesterol esterification in FLD and FED carriers of one mutant *LCAT* allele

	FLD	FED	P
n	30	11	
Gender (M/F)	16/14	7/4	
Age (years)	48.9±22.0	44.5±23.7	0.58
BMI (kg/m²)	24.8±4.8	24.5±3.9	0.86
Total cholesterol (mg/dl)	162.4±39.1	162.6±63.1	0.99
Unesterified cholesterol (mg/dl)	48.7±12.9	51.2±18.4	0.63
Unesterified/total cholesterol	0.31±0.07	0.33±0.07	0.42
LDL cholesterol (mg/dl)	97.2±33.4	97.4±62.9	0.99
HDL cholesterol (mg/dl)	39.3±11.7	41.8±15.4	0.58
Triglycerides (mg/dl)	130.5±55.7	110.6±52.1	0.31
Apolipoprotein A-I (mg/dl)	102.1±23.1	100.9±23.8	0.88
Apolipoprotein A-II (mg/dl)	29.5±5.6	29.2±8.4	0.90
Apolipoprotein B (mg/dl)	92.3±21.7	87.3±39.5	0.61
LpA-I (mg/dl)	40.5±10.3	42.2±8.8	0.63
LpA-I:A-II (mg/dl)	61.7±24.7	54.0±17.1	0.35
CER (nmol/ml/h)	38.8±15.9	47.2±15.5	0.14
LCAT α-activity (nmol/ml/h)	19.8±12.1	26.9±15.9	0.14
LCAT (μg/ml)	3.7±1.3	3.7±1.5	1.00

Data are reported as mean±SD

LCAT Gene Mutations and Atherosclerosis

Several prospective studies have clearly established an inverse association between plasma HDL-cholesterol levels and the incidence of coronary heart disease (CHD); even small increases in HDL-cholesterol translate into substantial CHD risk reductions [16]. Theoretically, carriers of *LCAT* gene mutations should have an increased risk of CHD, because of the moderate to severe HDL deficiency. However, the low number of affected subjects, the lack of detailed clinical data on CHD in many of them, and the lack of prospective data on the relationship between plasma LCAT levels/activity and CHD in the population make it difficult to draw general conclusions on the association between LCAT deficiency and CHD risk. A review of cases reported till 1997 indicates that FLD cases generally do not present with premature CHD, which is instead described in a consistent number of FED cases [5]. Out of the 19 cases belonging to the 16 Italian families, only one FED case, with multiple CHD risk factors (severe hypercholesterolemia, hypertension and diabetes) presented with premature CHD.

Carotid intima-media thickness (cIMT) has been established as a surrogate marker for human atherosclerosis [17] and has been applied to the study of human atherosclerosis in HA patients carrying mutations in the *apoA-I*, *ABCA1*, and *GBA* genes. Notably, despite the common HA trait, carriers of different mutations display carotid IMT values that are greater [18, 19], or close [20, 21] to those of controls. We compared cIMT values from 40 carriers of *LCAT* gene mutations (one and two mutated alleles together) with those from 80 age-gender matched healthy controls [7]. On average,

carriers had a 0.07 mm smaller cIMT than controls, a difference that remained statistically significant after adjustment for a variety of CHD risk factors. Notably, cIMT measurements in carriers of *LCAT* gene mutations were strikingly similar to those measured in HA individuals of approximately the same age carrying the atheroprotective apoA-I$_{Milano}$ mutation [20]. Therefore, LCAT deficiency is another monogenic disorder of HDL metabolism leading to a paradoxical phenotype characterized by moderate to severe HDL deficiency without enhanced preclinical atherosclerosis. When all the examined subjects were sub-grouped according to the number of mutant alleles, a highly significant LCAT gene-dose-dependent effect on cIMT was found (Fig. 1) [7]. Finally, we compared cIMT values from carriers of *LCAT* gene mutations causing complete or partial (i.e., FLD and FED) enzyme inactivation. Due to the small number of carriers, data from homozygotes, compound heterozygotes, and heterozygotes with the same phenotype (either FLD or FED) were combined in this analysis; cIMT values were similar in FLD and FED carriers and remained similar after adjustment for a variety of CHD risk factors (Table 3) [7]. The present data demonstrate that a partial or complete dysfunction of the LCAT enzyme associates with reduced preclinical atherosclerosis, despite the moderate to severe HDL deficiency. This unexpected finding merits some speculation. The inheritance of a defective LCAT enzyme may not preclude cholesterol removal from the arterial wall and efficient reverse cholesterol transport. Indeed, sera from these same carriers of *LCAT* gene mutations displayed an enhanced capacity for ABCA1-mediated cell cholesterol efflux than sera from non affected family members (Fig. 2), due to the greater content

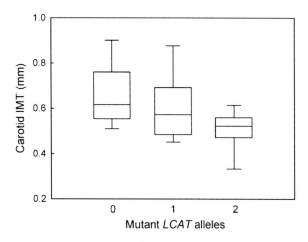

Fig. 1 Carotid IMT values in carriers of one ($n = 28$) or two ($n = 12$) mutant *LCAT* alleles and in control subjects ($n = 80$). The far wall of common carotid artery, bifurcation, and of the first proximal cm of the internal carotid artery were measured in at least three different frames. All measurements were averaged to calculate the average IMT for each subject. IMT measurements were adjusted for age, gender, BMI, smoking status, hypertension, family history of cardiovascular disease, total cholesterol, HDL-C, and triglycerides. The *box plot* displays median values with the 25th and 75th percentiles; *capped bars* indicate the 10th and 90th percentiles

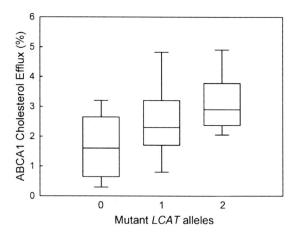

Fig. 2 ABCA1-mediated cholesterol efflux to sera from carriers of one ($n = 27$) or two ($n = 10$) mutant *LCAT* alleles and from non affected family members ($n = 10$). J774 macrophages were labeled with 4 μCi/ml [^{3}H]cholesterol for 24 h in RPMI medium with 1% FCS and 2 μg/ml of an ACAT inhibitor. Cells were then incubated for 18 h with 0.2% BSA in the absence or presence of 0.3 mM cAMP and incubated for 4 h with 5% serum. ABCA1-mediated cholesterol efflux was calculated as the percentage efflux from cAMP-stimulated cells minus the percentage efflux from unstimulated cells. The *box plot* displays median values with the 25th and 75th percentiles; *capped bars* indicate the 10th and 90th percentiles

Table 3 Demographic, clinical, and IMT data in FLD and FED carriers

	FLD	FED	P
n	33	7	
Gender (M/F)	20/13	5/2	0.69
Age (years)	43.0 ± 17.5	35.6 ± 14.3	0.30
BMI (kg/m^2)	24.8 ± 4.6	25.2 ± 2.4	0.86
Smoking status			0.45
Never (n)	22 (66.7%)	6 (85.7%)	
Former (n)	7 (21.2%)	0	
Current (n)	4 (12.1%)	1 (14.3%)	
Hypertension (n)	8 (24.2%)	1 (14.3%)	0.71
Avg-IMT (mm)	0.58 (0.53, 0.64)	0.56 (0.46, 0.69)	0.72
Max-IMT (mm)	0.93 (0.81, 1.07)	0.81 (0.60, 1.10)	0.42
Adjusted Avg-IMT (mm)	0.66 (0.57–0.78)	0.59 (0.54–0.64)	0.15
Adjusted Max-IMT (mm)	0.94 (0.75–1.19)	0.97 (0.86–1.09)	0.84

Data are reported as mean ± SD. IMT data are expressed as geometric mean and 95% confidence intervals. In the adjusted model, IMT values were adjusted for age, gender, BMI, smoking status, hypertension, family history of cardiovascular disease, total cholesterol, HDL-C, and triglycerides

of preβ-HDL particles [22]. The same occurs in LCAT deficient mice, which display a preserved reverse cholesterol transport in vivo despite the severe reduction of HDL cholesterol, mostly due to high plasma content of preβ-HDL and enhanced macrophage cholesterol removal via ABCA1 [23]. The preserved reverse cholesterol transport might not by itself justify the reduced preclinical atherosclerosis observed in the carriers, which may result from delayed cholesterol deposition in the arterial wall, as a consequence of a reduced

CE content of apoB-containing lipoproteins [24], and/or a redistribution of HDL-bound antioxidant enzymes, like paraoxonase-1, to apoB-containing lipoproteins [25].

Conclusions

The availability of a relatively large number of carriers of two and one mutant *LCAT* alleles allowed us to draw some conclusions on the relationships between the inheritance of *LCAT* gene mutations, HDL metabolism, and atherosclerosis. First, we identified a significant *LCAT* gene-dose dependent effect on cholesterol esterification, HDL-related biomarkers, and cIMT. The inheritance of a single mutant *LCAT* allele leads to a biochemical and vascular phenotype intermediate between those of carriers of two or zero copies of mutant alleles. This indicates that both the biochemical and the vascular changes are expressed as codominant traits in families carrying mutations in the *LCAT* gene. Second, despite the different functional defect of the LCAT enzyme in subjects carrying FLD and FED mutations, resulting in clearly distinct cholesterol esterification profiles, changes in HDL biomarkers and cIMT are quite similar, suggesting that FLD and FED are not two distinct syndromes, but the same disease at different levels of LCAT impairment. The clinical presentation of Italian FED and FLD cases supports this concept, with anemia and renal disease being present also in FED cases [6]. Third, the observation that genetically determined low LCAT activity does not associate with enhanced preclinical atherosclerosis despite low HDL cholesterol levels challenges the notion that LCAT is required for effective atheroprotection in humans, and suggests that, despite positive effects on plasma HDL cholesterol concentration, elevating LCAT expression and/or activity is not a promising therapeutic strategy to reduce CHD risk.

Acknowledgments The authors are indebted to Letizia Bocchi, Chiara Candini, and Sebastiano Calandra of the University of Modena and Reggio Emilia for the expression of LCAT mutants in COS-1 cells, and to Elda Favari and Franco Bernini of the University of Parma for the efflux studies. Authors' work described in this article was supported by grants from Telethon-Italy (GGP02264 and GGP07132 to LC) and Fondazione Cariplo (2003-1753 to GF).

References

1. Jonas A (2000) Lecithin cholesterol acyltransferase. Biochim Biophys Acta 1529:245–256
2. Nakamura Y, Kotite L, Gan Y, Spencer TA, Fielding CJ, Fielding PE (2004) Molecular mechanism of reverse cholesterol transport: reaction of pre-beta-migrating high-density lipoprotein with plasma lecithin/cholesterol acyltransferase. Biochemistry 43: 14811–14820
3. Rye KA, Barter PJ (2004) Formation and metabolism of prebeta-migrating, lipid-poor apolipoprotein A-I. Arterioscler Thromb Vasc Biol 24:421–428
4. Santamarina-Fojo S, Hoeg JM, Assmann G, Brewer HB Jr (2001) Lecithin cholesterol acyltransferase deficiency and fish eye disease. In: Scriver CR, Beaudet AL, Sly WS, Valle D (eds) The metabolic and molecular bases of inherited diseases. McGraw-Hill, New York, pp 2817–2833
5. Kuivenhoven JA, Pritchard H, Hill J, Frohlich J, Assmann G, Kastelein J (1997) The molecular pathology of lecithin:cholesterol acyltransferase (LCAT) deficiency syndromes. J Lipid Res 38:191–205
6. Calabresi L, Pisciotta L, Costantin A et al (2005) The molecular basis of lecithin:cholesterol acyltransferase deficiency syndromes: a comprehensive study of molecular and biochemical findings in 13 unrelated Italian families. Arterioscler Thromb Vasc Biol 25: 1972–1978
7. Calabresi L, Baldassarre D, Castelnuovo S et al (2009) Functional LCAT is not required for efficient atheroprotection in humans. Circulation 120(7):628–635
8. Asztalos BF, Schaefer EJ, Horvath KV et al (2007) Role of LCAT in HDL remodeling: investigation of LCAT deficiency states. J Lipid Res 48:592–599
9. Forte TM, Norum KR, Glomset JA, Nichols AV (1971) Plasma lipoproteins in familial lecithin:cholesterol acyltransferase deficiency. Structure of low and high density lipoproteins as revealed by electron microscopy. J Clin Invest 50:1141–1148
10. Ng DS, Xie C, Maguire GF et al (2004) Hypertriglyceridemia in lecithin-cholesterol acyltransferase-deficient mice is associated with hepatic overproduction of triglycerides, increased lipogenesis, and improved glucose tolerance. J Biol Chem 279:7636–7642
11. Song H, Zhu L, Picardo CM et al (2006) Coordinated alteration of hepatic gene expression in fatty acid and triglyceride synthesis in LCAT-null mice is associated with altered PUFA metabolism. Am J Physiol Endocrinol Metab 290:E17–E25
12. Frohlich JJ, McLeod R, Pritchard PH, Fesmire J, McConathy WJ (1988) Plasma lipoprotein abnormalities in heterozygotes for familial lecithin:cholesterol acyltransferase deficiency. Metabolism 37:3–8
13. Franceschini G, Baio M, Calabresi L, Sirtori CR, Cheung MC (1990) Apolipoprotein A-IMilano. Partial lecithin:cholesterol acyltransferase deficiency due to low levels of a functional enzyme. Biochim Biophys Acta 1043:1–6
14. Funke H, von Eckardstein A, Pritchard PH, Karash M, Albers JJ, Assmann G (1991) A frameshift mutation in the human apolipoprotein A-I gene causes high density lipoprotein deficiency, partial lecithin: cholesterol acyltransferase deficiency, and corneal opacities. J Clin Invest 87:371–376
15. The Expert Panel (2001) Executive summary of the third report of the National Cholesterol Education Program (NCEP) expert panel on detection, evaluation, and treatment of high blood cholesterol In adults (Adult Treatment Panel III). JAMA 285:2486–2497
16. Franceschini G (2001) Epidemiologic evidence for high-density lipoprotein cholesterol as a risk factor for coronary artery disease. Am J Cardiol 88:9–13
17. Stein JH, Korcarz CE, Hurst RT et al (2008) Use of carotid ultrasound to identify subclinical vascular disease and evaluate cardiovascular disease risk: a consensus statement from the American Society of Echocardiography Carotid Intima-Media Thickness Task Force. Endorsed by the Society for Vascular Medicine. J Am Soc Echocardiogr 21:93–111
18. van Dam MJ, de Groot E, Clee SM et al (2002) Association between increased arterial-wall thickness and impairment in ABCA1-driven cholesterol efflux: an observational study. Lancet 359:37–42
19. Hovingh GK, Brownlie A, Bisoendial RJ et al (2004) A novel apoA-I mutation (L178P) leads to endothelial dysfunction, increased arterial wall thickness, and premature coronary artery disease. J Am Coll Cardiol 44:1429–1435
20. Sirtori CR, Calabresi L, Franceschini G et al (2001) Cardiovascular status of carriers of the apolipoprotein A-IMilano mutant. The Limone sul Garda Study. Circulation 103:1949–1954
21. de Fost M, Langeveld M, Franssen R et al (2009) Low HDL cholesterol levels in type I Gaucher disease do not lead to an increased risk of cardiovascular disease. Atherosclerosis 204:267–272
22. Calabresi L, Favari E, Moleri E et al (2009) Functional LCAT is not required for macrophage cholesterol efflux to human serum. Atherosclerosis 204:141–146
23. Rader DJ, Alexander ET, Weibel GL, Billheimer J, Rothblat GH (2009) The role of reverse cholesterol transport in animals and humans and relationship to atherosclerosis. J Lipid Res 50 Suppl:S189–S194
24. Glomset JA, Nichols AV, Norum KR, King W, Forte T (1973) Plasma lipoproteins in familial lecithin: cholesterol acyltransferase deficiency. Further studies of very low and low density lipoprotein abnormalities. J Clin Invest 52:1078–1092
25. Ng DS, Maguire GF, Wylie J et al (2002) Oxidative stress is markedly elevated in lecithin:cholesterol acyltransferase-deficient mice and is paradoxically reversed in the apolipoprotein E knockout background in association with a reduction in atherosclerosis. J Biol Chem 277:11715–11720

Human Cholesteryl Ester Transfer Protein in Human HDL Metabolism

Hiroshi Mabuchi and Akihiro Inazu

Introduction

Plasma LDL transports cholesterol from liver to peripheral tissues including the adrenal glands and gonads. On the other hand, HDL transports cholesterol from peripheral tissues including atheroma to the liver, subsequently to bile and feces via the so-called reverse cholesterol transport (RCT) pathway. Cholesterol structure is resistant to enzymatic degradation in the human body, and the only pathway that modifies cholesterol is its hydoxylation for excretion from the body.

In humans, HDL consists of heterogenous particles in size, density, and apolipoprotein composition. HDL is a vehicles for cholesterol, triglyceride, and phospholipids. Also, HDL has several apolipoproteins and enzymes on its surface promoting or inhibiting triglyceride or phospholipids lipolysis, inhibiting hydroperoxidation of lipids, and promoting lipid transfer among lipoproteins. In addition, HDL may be a platform for complement regulation and inflammation.

Plasma HDL levels are usually measured as cholesterol levels, but its particle numbers are better assessed by apolipoprotein A-I levels. As interindividual difference of plasma HDL-cholesterol, HDL2-cholesterol levels appeared to be highly variable, but HDL3 remains constant. One of the determinants of HDL lipid composition is plasma cholesteryl ester transfer protein (CETP).

In incubated human plasma, transfer and equilibration of lecithin:cholesterol acyltransferase (LCAT)-generated CE is found, but the activity of transferring CE among lipoproteins was not found in the rat. Similarly, mice, dogs and pigs were members with a group of low plasma CETP activity, but rabbits and monkeys belong to a group with high CETP activity. Human, hamster, guinea pig, and chicken belong to a group of intermediate CETP activity. Interestingly, more phospho- lipid transfer protein activity is found in plasmas of low CETP activity animals [1, 2].

Plasma CETP binds neutral lipids (CE or TG) and PL on HDL3, but CETP selectively promotes an exchange of CE and TG among lipoproteins. Since HDL–TG can be hydro- lyzed by hepatic lipase, plasma CETP decreases HDL parti- cle size via CE/TG exchange between chylomicron/VLDL and HDL, thereby accelerating a catabolic rate of HDL apolipoproteins [3].

Structure and Function of CETP

Plasma CETP was initially isolated by Pattnaik and Zilversmit et al., then it was highly purified to 74 kD [4]. Human CETP gene is located at chromosome 16q13, near the locus of LCAT gene. The CETP gene consists of 16 exons, spanning 25 kb [5]. The CETP mRNA encodes 476 amino acids [6]. The mature CETP contains four N-linked sugars (88, 240, 341, and 396) with variable glycosylation site of 341 Asn [7]. CETP mRNA is expressed in various tissues, but liver cells, adipocytes, and macrophages are abundant sources. Exon 9 works as a cassette exon to generate short mRNA missing the sequences in frame in addition to full-length mRNA, but the splice variant is not efficiently secreted [8].

The C-terminal 26 amino acids form amphipathic helices, hydrophic residues bind to lipoprotein surfaces, and hydro- phobic residues such as Leu and Phe are essential for binding neutral lipids of CE and TG [9].

A recent paper of crystal structure of CETP suggested that CETP forms a long tunnel occupied by four lipid mole- cules, two of CE or TG located inside of the tunnel and two of PL plugged both sides of tunnel openings. CETP is one of lipopolysaccharide-binding protein (LBP) family members. CETP has an elongated boomerang shape located on lipopro- tein surface. Based on molecular size, CETP prefer CE transfer rather than TG because of steric hindrance of a tunnel neck around residucs of 433, 443, 457, and 459 [10].

H. Mabuchi (✉)
Department of Lipidology, School of Medicine, Institute of Medical, Pharmaceutical and Health Sciences, Kanazawa University, Kanazawa, Japan
e-mail: mabuchi@med.kanazawa.ac.jp

E.J. Schaefer (ed.), *High Density Lipoproteins, Dyslipidemia, and Coronary Heart Disease*, DOI 10.1007/978-1-4419-1059-2_12, © Springer Science+Business Media, LLC 2010

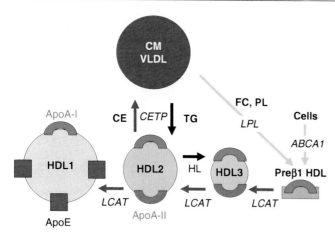

Fig. 1 *Schema for HDL metabolism.* Plasma cholesteryl ester transfer protein (CETP) facilitates the exchange of the neutral lipids CE and TG between chylomicron (CM)/VLDL and HDL2. HDL–TG is provided by CETP, and it is hydrolyzed by hepatic lipase (HL). The synthetic rate of preβ1HDL is positively correlated with lipoprotein lipase (LPL)-mediated lipolysis and increased cholesterol efflux by the ABCA1 transporter. On the other hand, the catabolic rate of preβ1HDL is correlated with the cholesterol esterification rate by lecithin:cholesterol acyltransferase (LCAT)

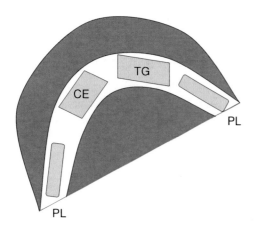

Fig. 2 *Schema for CETP molecule.* CETP is a boomerang-shaped molecule with a long tunnel occupied by CE, TG inside of tunnel and 2 of PC plugged both sides of tunnel openings

Genetics of Human CETP Deficiency

Discovery of Human CETP Deficiency

Plasma CETP deficiency was originally reported in Japanese siblings with hyperalphalipoproteinemia [11]. The first mutation was found in a splice donor site mutation in intron 14 (intron 14 G[+1]-to-A), resulting in exon 14 skipping and producing a stop codon in the fourth codon encoded by exon 15, decreased mRNA levels to one-third of controls, and truncated protein appeared to be rapidly degraded [12, 13].

So far, 20 different mutations were found both in Asian and Caucasian populations but predominantly found in Asians [14]. Two mutations were found in both ethnic groups such as R268X and intron 14 G(+1)-to-A [15], suggesting multiple origins of these mutations (de novo mutations). Both mutations indeed have CpG sequence as hot-spots for deamination of the cytosine. Many mutations were nonsense or splicing mutations. However, four missense mutations were associated with decreased CETP activity (L151P, L261R, R282C, and D442G). Also, one promoter mutation was reported at −69G>A.

Large difference of frequency of CETP deficiency appeared to be related to the frequency of two variants. One is that intron 14 G(+1)-to-A mutation, which is the Japanese-type mutation with a high gene frequency (0.8% in the general population of Japan). Those homozygotes were reported in >50 cases reflecting relatively higher frequency of consanguinity in Japan in the past generations (coefficient of inbreeding, $F=0.005$). The homozygotes have complete CETP deficiency and they have a phenotype of very high HDL-C levels and relatively low LDL-C levels (164 and 77 mg/dl, respectively) [16]. The heterozygotes have a moderate increase in HDL-C (mean 66 mg/dl) and a decrease in plasma CETP levels (mean 1.4 mg/l) as compared to unaffected controls (53 and 2.3 mg/l). The second reason

Fig. 3 *Summary of CETP gene mutations.* Since the first mutations was reported in 1989, 20 different mutations have been found. Only two mutations of Intron 14 +1G>A and R268X have been reported both in Asian and Caucasian populations. Intron 14 +1G>A and D442G mutations are prevalent in the Japanese, and the latter variant is also frequent in other Asian populations

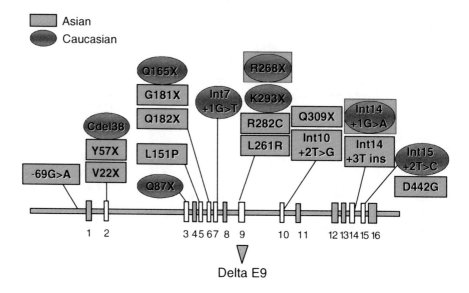

Table 1 Plasma lipoprotein levels in homozygous CETP deficiency with complete and partial deficiency

Genotype	N, Age	CHOL (mg/dl)	TG (mg/dl)	LDL-C (mg/dl)	HDL-C (mg/dl)	CETP (μg/ml)
14A homo	27	275 ± 36	117 ± 64	85 ± 27	167 ± 33	<0.1
14A/14T	1	171	41	57	106	<0.1
14A/R268X	1	316	401	29	207	<0.1
14A/?	2	308 ± 16	54 ± 3	67 ± 25	230 ± 10	<0.1
L261R homo	3	284 ± 26	96 ± 44	118 ± 40	147 ± 17	<0.1
14A/D442G	10	253 ± 52	79 ± 65	112 ± 31	125 ± 20	0.7 ± 0.3
D442G homo	9	231 ± 52	63 ± 21	123 ± 48	96 ± 24	1.0 ± 0.4
All	53, 61 ± 13	264 ± 43	101 ± 72	96 ± 37	148 ± 43	0.2 ± 0.4

L261R, unpublished; ?, undetermined; LDL-C, Friedewald-formula calculated

was the highly prevalent Asp 442 Gly (D442G) mutation in Japan (3.4% in the general population of Japan) as well as in other Asian populations (1.7–5.9%), although it is partially defective in CETP activity [17].

Subjects with homozygous CETP deficiency ($n = 53$) have been identified through 20-year screening efforts of measuring plasma CETP levels and PCR assays for common CETP gene mutations of intron 14 G(+1)-to-A and D442G (Table 1). The 34 cases with complete CETP deficiency have a more severe phenotype of increased HDL and decreased LDL, but less severe phenotype was found in partial CETP deficiency. The combination of intron 14 G(+1)-to-A and D442G produces less severe phenotype of CETP deficiency ($n = 10$, CETP 0.7 ± 0.3 [SD] mg/l, HDL-C 125 ± 20 mg/dl) as compared to mean levels of plasma CETP, which were 1.8 ± 0.6 mg/l (SD) in Japanese men and 2.0 ± 0.5 in women [18].

Phenotype of CETP Deficiency

LCAT Promotes FC Esterification in HDL3 and CETP Transfers Newly Esterified CE from HDL3 to VLDL or Chylomicron

CETP-mediated lipid transfer does not have a unique direction among lipoproteins in a reconstituted system. However, CE is generated in HDL via the LCAT reaction, and a higher CE gradient is found in HDL, and therefore net CE transfer operates from HDL to other lipoproteins. Similarly, TG is rich in chylomicron and VLDL, and net TG transfer occurs from chylomicrons/VLDL to other lipoproteins via hetero-exchange of CE and TG. In addition, some specific apolipoproteins such as apoC-I and apoF and TG lipolysis during postprandial state can modify direction of lipid transfer among lipoproteins.

Since TG-rich LDL became small, dense-LDL after TG lipolysis, large LDL levels and CETP activity were negatively correlated in men in the Framingham Offspring Study [19].

Subjects with complete CETP deficiency have more preβHDL despite less remodeling from large HDL to small

subclasses [20]. Thus, increased preβHDL levels are caused by impaired maturation to large HDL due to decreased endogenous LCAT activity [21] or increased lipolysis of TG-rich lipoproteins. LCAT mass and exogenous LCAT activities remain at normal levels, and impaired LCAT activity is explained by (1) end-product inhibition namely excess CE in large HDL or (2) altered phospholipid composition such as sphingomyelin (SM) levels in HDL. Plasma cholesterol esterification rate (CER) was decreased in CETP deficiency, which is compatible with altered lipid composition found in homozygous CETP deficiency: high CE/TG ratio and low PL/FC ratio [22]. Since CER is inversely associated with SM/PC ratio in HDL, SM level may be the link between low CER and low CETP activity [unpublished data]. Thus, atherogenicity of SM-rich HDL needs to be determined, because HDL with increased SM levels may act as good acceptors in the process of cholesterol efflux from atherosclerotic plaques since SM avidly binds cholesterol [23].

Initially, Ikewaki and Rader et al. reported delayed catabolism of apoA-I and apoA-II in human subjects with CETP deficiency [24]. Also, they reported increased catabolic rate of LDL-apoB in addition to decreased production rate of VLDL-apoB [25]. In a CETP-deficient dog, Ouguerram et al. reported that VLDL and LDL CE metabolism was coupled to apoB catabolism without enrichment of CE during VLDL–LDL conversion and that 60% of HDL CE turnover is mediated by selective uptake pathway [26, 27]. As compared to other CETP-deficient animals, dogs have higher selective uptake of HDL-CE (60% vs. 25–30% in rat and mice). The CER of dog plasma is 160 nmol/ml/h, which is in between 30–80 in human and 300 in rats. Thus, dogs may have an efficient RCT due to high activities of SR-BI and LCAT even in CETP deficiency.

As shown in Fig. 1, Plasma HDL is classified as HDL1 (density 1.08–1.09 g/ml), HDL2 (1.09–1.15), and HDL3 (1.15–1.18). HDL1 is apoE-rich HDL with diameter of 13–19 nm. HDL1 shows α-migration on agarose gel. LCAT activity increased HDL1 levels from HDL2 and HDL3 fractions [28]. HDL1 is also identified in cholesterol-fed CETP-deficient animals such as canine and swine.

In cultured smooth muscle cells, cholesterol from HDLc, lipoprotein with apoE only (density 1.006–1.02), which is found in cholesterol-fed dogs, was as efficiently delivered to cells as was LDL [29]. ApoE-rich HDL appeared in various situations such as genetic dyslipidemia, but its characteristics are not uniform. In cholesterol fed canines, plasma cholesterol increases, and HDL loses apoA-I but gains apoE. HDLc appears when plasma cholesterol levels exceed 700 mg/dl, coinciding with the appearance of β-migrating VLDL. Thus, HDL1 and HDLc appeared to suppress apoB-containing lipoprotein formation in the liver (LDL and β-VLDL), thereby inhibiting atherogenesis in canine models.

Characteristics of ApoE-rich HDL have dual roles in atherogenicity. ApoE can serve as an LRP ligand, and therefore canine HDLc decreases clearance of chylomicrons [30]. An adverse role of apoE-rich HDL in chylomicron clearance probably does not occur in humans, because post-prandial lipemia is suppressed and remnant lipoprotein formation is diminished in CETP deficiency [31]. However, apoE-rich HDL reduces LPL-mediated retention of LDL by subendothelial matrix; therefore, it plays antiatherogenic role in artery walls.

Atherogenicity of Plasma CETP

Relation to TG Metabolism

HDL-cholesterol could be excreted from bile as a consequence of reverse cholesterol transport (RCT) involving HDL maturation from preβHDL to apoE-rich HDL. CETP would bypass the cholesterol flow from HDL to VLDL–LDL without mediating liver. CETP-mediated CE transfer would increase indirect cholesterol transport to the liver via VLDL–IDL–LDL through LDL receptor or remnant receptor pathways. In addition, HDL-cholesterol is directly transported to the liver by selective uptake of HDL-CE or FC via hepatic lipase and/or SR-BI pathway.

Thus, the role of the CETP pathway appears to be antiatherogenic when LDL levels are low and TRL clearance is rapid as observed with low fat diets. Indeed, subjects with high CETP activity may manifest lower coronary risk when plasma TG levels are low [32].

However, western type high saturated-fat diets suppress LDL receptor expression, and therefore the flow of HDL derived cholesterol back to the liver via the LDL pathway is reduced.

CETP Gene Mutations and Polymorphisms on Coronary Heart Disease Risk

Meta-analysis including CETP gene SNPs of TaqIB2, −629C > A and Ile 405 Val (I405V) showed that the genotypes with low CETP may have antiatherogenic effects

[33]. Our data suggested that −1337C > T is responsible for the antiatherogenicity of the well-investigated TaqIB2 allele in the Japanese population [34, 35]. Thus, antiatherogenicity of lower CETP levels was also suggested in heterozygous CETP deficiency [36]. In contrast, increased plasma CETP levels are positively associated with coronary artery calcium and intima-media thickness in middle-aged Japanese men [37].

Coronary heart disease (CHD) prevalence appeared to be low in homozygous CETP deficiency, which is compatible with findings of the Kochi Study of cross-sectional survey of disease prevalence stratified by increased HDL-cholesterol levels >80 and >100 mg/dl [38]. More than 300 subjects with HDL-C > 100 mg/dl were found in that paper, but coronary heart disease was not found. Accordingly, high HDL-cholesterol and intron 14 G(+1) > A variant may increase odds for healthy aging in the Honolulu Heart Program Study [39]. Consistently, recent case reports of Caucasian CETP deficiency showed the rarity of atherosclerotic disease even though they consumed western diets [40, 41]. However, some investigators believe CHD to be present in some cases with homozygous CETP deficiency [14]. In contrast, no definite CAD has been found in our cohort of homozygous CETP deficiency (n = 53), thus CHD risk needs to be clarified in a larger cohort of homozygous CETP deficiency by a national survey.

Development of CETP Inhibitor and Its Phenotypic Similarity to Human CETP Deficiency

There are three compounds that have been developed in clinical trials; these are torcetrapib (CP-529,414), anacetrapib (MK-859), and dalcetrapib (JTT-705/Roche R1658). The phase III of torcetrapib was terminated in December 2006 due to unexpected excess of mortality in the torcetrapib arm. The early termination was partially explained by hypertension due to aldosterone excess. However, the role of CETP inhibition on the increased mortality was not clearly shown, but it may be rather associated with infection or malignancy than coronary heart disease [42].

However, vascular endpoints of carotid atherosclerosis and coronary atheroma volume assessed by intravascular ultrasound showed no further benefit from torcetrapib on a background of atorvastatin despite increased levels of HDL and decreased levels of LDL and TG [43, 44].

HDL-cholesterol could be excreted from bile as consequence of reverse cholesterol transport (RCT) involving HDL maturation from preβHDL to apoE-rich HDL. By using CETP inhibitor, CE uptake of liver was not decreased in rabbits, but fecal sterol excretion was not increased in patients taking torcetrapib, indicating overall RCT was not significantly induced [45–47]. However, torcetrapib could increase overall RCT assessed by cholesterol and bile acids in feces of hamsters [48]. A metabolic difference in the response to CETP inhibitors has not been defined yet, but it is an important objective to be investigated.

Effects on Cholesterol Efflux

Hyperalphalipoproteinemia (HALP) caused by prednisone plus cyclosporine results in HDL that is not effective for cholesterol efflux. The ABCA1-dependent efflux was maintained, but the non-ABCA1-dependent route appeared to be impaired [49].

CETP inhibition may disturb apoA-I liberation from HDL in atherosclerotic lesions. Therefore, ABCA1-mediated cholesterol efflux activity could be compromised. However, recent studies suggest that the ABCG1 transporter induces cholesterol efflux from cells to large HDL [50]. Torcetrapib would increase this large HDL level, which is an active cholesterol acceptor for ABCG1 or SR-BI-mediated efflux, although the role of SR-BI-mediated cholesterol efflux remains controversial [51].

Effects on ApoB-Containing Lipoproteins

By inhibiting neutral lipid transfer among lipoproteins, CE transfer to VLDL in exchange with TG was diminished. Therefore, relatively CE-poor, TG-rich VLDLs were lipolyzed to LDL and VLDL–IDL–LDL were rapidly removed from the circulation probably due to LDL-receptor upregulation [52]. In LDL subclasses, small-and-dense LDL levels were decreased but large LDL levels were increased in patients with torcetrapib [53]. Decreased palms Lp(a) levels are found in genetic CETP deficiency, and about 50% reductions in plasma Lp(a) levels were achieved with anacetrapib treatment [54].

Prospective (Table 2)

CETP would enhance HDL remodeling from large HDL to small subclasses including preβHDL. However, CETP deficiency would decrease cholesterol esterification rate, thereby inhibiting maturation of preβHDL to α-migrating spherical HDL. Therefore, in CETP deficiency, large-to small HDL remodeling is disturbed but preβHDL catabolism via LCAT reaction is also decreased. Such a balance appears to be dependent on the magnitude of CETP deficiency. Indeed, the

Table 2 Summary of anti- and proatherogenic aspects in CETP deficiency. Since phenotypic difference is found between homozygous and heterozygous CETP deficiency, the atherogenicity of apoE-rich HDL has been under debate

	Heterozygote	Homozygote
LDL-C (mg/dl)	110	80
LDL size	Large	Polydispersed
Cholesterol esterification rate	Low	Very low
Preβ1HDL	Decreased	Increased
ApoE-rich HDL	High	Very high
ABCA1-mediated cholesterol efflux acceptor	Preserved	Decreased

levels of preβHDL were increased in homozygous CETP deficiency, but those were decreased in the heterozygotes [20], indicating that maturation of the small HDL subclass is preserved in heterozygotes but not in homozygotes.

As mentioned, conventional HDL-C measurements such as a precipitation method or a homogenous method underscore that total HDL-C can contain apoE-rich HDL. Thus, the apoB/apoA-I ratio appeared to be a better marker than the LDL-C/HDL-C ratio when epidemiological surveys including extreme cases of increased HDLs such as CETP deficiency was conducted, because apolipoprotein measurements provide more accurate assessment than LDL- or HDL-C.

Recent studies suggested PAF-AH (lipoprotein-associated phospholipase A2) inhibitors could inhibit sdLDL, thereby preventing atherosclerosis both in animal model and human. Plasma paraoxonase activity was decreased in HALP with hepatic lipase deficiency [55], but both paraoxonase and PAF-AH activity were not decreased in CETP deficiency (unpublished data), suggesting that antioxidant activity of HDL is less important than antiatherogenicity of CETP deficiency.

Therefore, we considered that rate of net cholesterol catabolism or its excretion is a major factor for antiatherogenicity of CETP deficiency. However, the functional assessment of overall RCT need to be established in vivo in human as shown in a method of macrophage-specific RCT using radiolabeled cholesterol in experimental animals [56].

In hyperlipidemic patients, increased production of VLDL and/or decreased catabolism of LDL are major risk factors in addition to low HDL-C. Since decreased production rate of VLDL appears to be associated with decreased CETP activity in patients with metabolic syndrome treated by fenofibrate [57], CETP inhibitor may be especially useful for combined hyperlipidemia of high VLDL and low HDL state. LDL catabolic rate is increased in CETP inhibitor, but the effect on VLDL production rate has been less established. Clinical trials of an antisense oligonucleotide drug might give a confidential an answer as to whether or not hepatic

CETP inhibition is important for VLDL secretion. Thus, it is important to investigate whether or not CETP antisense therapy is more beneficial than medicinal CETP inhibitor.

References

1. Ha YC, Barter PJ (1982) Differences in plasma cholesteryl ester transfer activity in sixteen vertebrate species. Comp Biochem Physiol 71B:265–269
2. Cheung MC, Wolfbauer G, Albers JJ (1996) Plasma phospholipids mass transfer rate: relationship to plasma phospholipid and cholesteryl ester transfer activities and lipid parameters. Biochim Biophys Acta 1303:103–110
3. Lemarche B, Uffelman KD, Carpentier A, Cohn JS, Steiner G, Barrett PH, Lewis GF (1999) Triglyceride enrichment of HDL enhances in vivo metabolic clearance of HDL apoA-I in healthy men. J Clin Invest 103:1191–1199
4. Pattnaik NM, Montes A, Hughes LB, Zilversmit DB (1978) Cholesteryl ester exchange protein in human plasma isolation and characterization. Biochim Biophys Acta 530:428–438
5. Agellon LB, Quinet EM, Gillette TG, Drayna DT, Brown ML, Tall AR (1990) Organization of the human cholesteryl ester transfer protein gene. Biochemistry 29:1372–1376
6. Drayna D, Jarnagin AS, McLean J et al (1987) Cloning and sequencing of human cholesteryl ester transfer protein cDNA. Nature 327:632–634
7. Stevenson S, Wang S, Deng L, Tall AR (1993) Human plasma cholesteryl ester transfer protein consists of a mixture of two forms reflecting variable glycosylation at asparagine 341. Biochemistry 32:5121–5126
8. Inazu A, Quinet EM, Wang S, Brown ML, Stevenson S, Barr M, Moulin P, Tall AR (1992) Alternative splicing of the mRNA encoding the human cholesteryl ester transfer protein. Biochemistry 31(8):2352–2358
9. Wang S, Wang X, Deng L, Rassart E, Milne RW, Tall AR (1993) Point mutagenesis of carboxyl-terminal amino acids of cholesteryl ester transfer protein. J Biol Chem 268:1955–1959
10. Qiu X, Mistry A, Ammirati MJ et al (2007) Crystal structure of cholesteryl ester transfer protein reveals a long tunnel and four bound lipid molecules. Nat Struct Mol Biol 14(2):106–113
11. Koizumi J, Mabuchi H, Yoshimura A, Michishita I, Takeda M, Itoh H, Sakai Y, Sakai T, Ueda K, Takeda R (1985) Deficiency of serum cholesteryl-ester transfer activity in patients with familial hyperalphalipoproteinaemia. Atherosclerosis 58:175–186
12. Brown ML, Inazu A, Hesler CB, Agellon LB, Mann C, Whitlock ME, Marcel YL, Milne RW, Koizumi J, Mabuchi H, Takeda R, Tall AR (1989) Molecular basis of lipid transfer protein deficiency in a family with increased high-density lipoproteins. Nature 342(6248):448–451
13. Gotoda T, Kinoshita M, Ishibashi S, Inaba T, Harada K, Shimada M, Osuga J, Teramoto T, Yazaki Y, Yamada N (1997) Skipping of exon 14 and possible instability of both the mRNA and the resultant truncated protein underlie a common cholesteryl ester transfer protein deficiency in Japan. Arterioscler Thromb Vasc Biol 17:1376–1381
14. Nagano M, Yamashita S, Hirano KI et al (2004) Molecular mechanisms of cholesteryl ester transfer protein deficiency in Japanese. J Atheroscler Thromb 11:110–121
15. Ai M, Tanaka A, Shimokado K, Inazu A, Kobayashi J, Mabuchi H, Nakano T, Nakajima K (2009) A deficiency of cholesteryl ester transfer protein whose serum remnant-like particle -triglyceride significantly increased, but serum remnant-like particle-cholesterol did not after an oral fat load. Ann Clin Biochem 46(Pt 6):457–463
16. Inazu A, Brown ML, Hesler CB, Agellon LB, Koizumi J, Takata K, Maruhama Y, Mabuchi H, Tall AR (1990) Increased high-density lipoprotein levels caused by a common cholesteryl-ester transfer protein gene mutation. N Engl J Med 323(18):1234–1238
17. Inazu A, Jiang XC, Haraki T, Yagi K, Kamon N, Koizumi J, Mabuchi H, Takeda R, Takata K, Moriyama Y, Doi M, Tall A (1994) Genetic cholesteryl ester transfer protein deficiency caused by two prevalent mutations as a major determinant of increased levels of high density lipoprotein cholesterol. J Clin Invest 94(5):1872–1882
18. Kiyohara T, Kiriyama R, Zamma S, Inazu A, Koizumi J, Mabuchi H, Chichibu K (1998) Enzyme immunoassay for cholesteryl ester transfer protein in human serum. Clin Chim Acta 271(2):109–118
19. Ordovas JM, Cupples LA, Corella D, Otvos JD, Osgood D, Martinez A, Lahoz C, Coltell O, Wilson PW, Schaefer EJ (2000) Association of cholesteryl ester transfer protein-TaqIB polymorphism with variations in lipoprotein subclasses and coronary heart disease risk: the Framingham study. Arterioscler Thromb Vasc Biol 20(5):1323–1329
20. Asztalos B, Horvath KV, Kajinami K, Nartsupha C, Cox CE, Batista M, Schaefer EJ, Inazu A, Mabuchi H (2004) Apolipoprotein composition of HDL in cholesteryl ester transfer protein deficiency. J Lipid Res 45:448–455
21. Oliveira HCF, Ma L, Milne R, Marcovina SM, Inazu A, Mabuchi H, Tall AR (1997) Cholesteryl ester transfer protein (CETP) activity enhances plasma cholesteryl ester formation: studies in CETP transgenic mice and human genetic CETP deficiency. Arterioscler Thromb Vasc Biol 17(6):1045–1052
22. Koizumi J, Inazu A, Yagi K, Koizumi I, Uno Y, Kajinami K, Miyamoto S, Moulin P, Tall AR, Mabuchi H, Takeda R (1991) Serum lipoprotein lipid concentration and composition in homozygous and heterozygous patients with cholesteryl ester transfer protein deficiency. Atherosclerosis 90(2–3):189–196
23. Fournier N, Paul JL, Atger V, Cogny A, Soni T, de la Llera-Moya M, Rothblat G, Moatti N (1997) HDL phospholipid content and composition as a major factor determining cholesterol efflux capacity from Fu5AH cells to human serum. Arterioscler Thromb Vasc Biol 17:2685–2691
24. Ikewaki K, Rader DJ, Sakamoto T et al (1993) Delayed catabolism of high density lipoprotein apolipoprotein A-I and A-II in human cholesteryl ester transfer protein deficiency. J Clin Invest 92:1650–1658
25. Ikewaki K, Nishiwaki M, Sakamoto T, Ishikawa T, Fairwell T, Zech LA, Nagano M, Nakamura H, Brewer HB Jr, Rader DJ (1995) Increased catabolic rate of low density lipoproteins in humans with cholesteryl ester transfer protein deficiency. J Clin Invest 96:1573–1581
26. Bailhache E, Briand F, Nguyen P, Krempf M, Magot T, Ouguerram K (2004) Metabolism of cholesterol ester of apolipoprotein B100-containing lipoproteins in dogs: evidence for disregarding cholesterol ester transfer. Eur J Clin Invest 34:527–534
27. Ouguerram K, Nguyen P, Krempf M, Pouteau E, Briand F, Bailhache E, Magot T (2004) Selective uptake of high density lipoproteins cholesteryl ester in the dog, a species lacking in cholesteryl ester transfer protein activity. An in vivo approach using stable isotopes. Comp Biochem Physiol B Biochem Mol Biol 138:339–345
28. Schmitz G, Assmann G (1982) Isolation of human serum HDL1 by zonal ultracentrifugation. J Lipid Res 23:903–910
29. Mahley RW, Innerarity TL, Weisgraber KH, Fry DL (1977) Canine hyperlipoproteinemia and atherosclerosis. Am J Pathol 87:205–226
30. Hussain MM, Innerarity TL, Brecht WJ, Mahley RW (1995) Chylomicron metabolism in normal, cholesterol-fed, and Watanabe heritable hyperlipidemic rabbits. J Biol Chem 270:8578–8587
31. Inazu A, Nakajima K, Nakano T, Niimi M, Kawashiri M, Nohara A, Kobayashi J, Mabuchi H (2008) Decreased post-prandial triglyceride response and diminished remnant lipoprotein formation in cholesteryl ester transfer protein (CETP) deficiency. Atherosclerosis 196:953–957

32. Borggreve SE, Hillege HL, Dallinga-Thie GM, de Jong PE, Wolffenbuttel BHR, Grobbee DE, van Tol A (2007) on behalf of the PREVEND Study Group. High plasma cholesteryl ester transfer protein levels may favour reduced incidence of cardiovascular events in men with low triglycerides. Eur Heart J 28(8):1012–1018

33. Thompson A, Angelantonio ED, Sarwar N, Erqou S, Saleheen D, Dullaart RPF, Keavney B, Ye Z, Danesh J (2008) Association of cholesteryl ester transfer protein genotypes with CETP mass and activity, lipid levels, and coronary risk. JAMA 299:2777–2788

34. Lu H, Inazu A, Moriyama Y, Higashikata T, Kawashiri MA, Yu W, Huang Z, Okamura T, Mabuchi H (2003) Haplotype analyses of cholesteryl ester transfer protein gene promoter: a clue to an unsolved mystery of TaqIB polymorphism. J Mol Med 81(4):246–255

35. Takata M, Inazu A, Katsuda S, Miwa K, Kawashiri M, Nohara A, Higashikata T, Kobayashi J, Mabuchi H, Yamagishi M (2006) *CETP* (cholesteryl ester transfer protein) promoter -1337 C>T polymorphism protects against coronary atherosclerosis in Japanese patients with heterozygous familial hypercholesterolaemia. Clin Sci (Lond) 111(5):325–331

36. Curb JD, Abbott RD, Rodriguez BL, Masaki K, Chen R, Sharp DS, Tall AR (2004) A prospective study of HDL-C and cholesteryl ester transfer protein gene mutations and the risk of coronary heart disease in the elderly. J Lipid Res 45:948–953

37. Okamura T, Sekikawa A, Kadowaki T et al (2009) Cholesteryl ester transfer protein, coronary calcium and intima-media thickness of the carotid artery in middle-aged Japanese men. Am J Cardiol 104(6):818–822

38. Moriyama Y, Okamura T, Inazu A, Doi M, Iso H, Mouri Y, Ishikawa Y, Suzuki H, Iida M, Koizumi J, Mabuchi H, Komachi Y (1998) A low prevalence of coronary heart disease in subjects with increased high-density lipoprotein cholesterol levels including those with plasma cholesteryl ester transfer protein deficiency. Prev Med 27(5 Pt 1):659–667

39. Koropatnick TA, Kimbell J, Chen R, Grove JS, Donlon TA, Masaki KH, Rodriguez BL, Willcox BJ, Yano K, Curb JD (2008) A prospective study of high-density lipoprotein cholesterol, cholesteryl ester transfer protein gene variants, and healthy aging in very old Japanese-American men. J Gerontol 63A:1235–1240

40. Teh EM, Dolphin PJ, Breckenridge WC, Tan MH (1998) Human plasma CETP deficiency: identification of a novel mutation in exon 9 of the CETP gene in a Caucasian subject from North America. J Lipid Res 39:442–456

41. Rhyne J, Ryan MJ, White C, Chimonas T, Miller M (2006) The two novel CETP mutations Gln87X and Gln165X in a compound heterozygous state are associated with marked hyperalphalipoproteinemia and absence of significant coronary artery disease. J Mol Med 84(8):647–650

42. Barter PJ, Caulfield M, Eriksson M et al; ILLUMINATE Investigators (2007) Effects of torcetrapib in patients at high risk for coronary events. N Engl J Med 357:2109–2122

43. Nissen SE, Tardif JC, Nicholls SJ, Revkin JH, Shear CL, Duggan WT, Ruzyllo W, Bachinsky WB, Lasala GP, Tuzcu EM; ILLUSTRATE Investigators (2007) Effects of torcetrapib on the progression of coronary atherosclerosis. N Engl J Med 356:1304–1316

44. Kastelein JJ, van Leuven SI, Burgess L et al; RADIANCE 1 Investigators (2007) Effects of torcetrapib on carotid atherosclerosis in familial hypercholesterolemia. N Engl J Med 356:1620–1630

45. Brousseau ME, Diffenderfer MR, Millar JS et al (2005) Effects of cholesteryl ester transfer protein inhibition on high-density lipoprotein subspecies, apolipoprotein A-I metabolism, and fecal sterol excretion. Arterioscler Thromb Vasc Biol 25:1–8

46. Kee P, Caiazza D, Rye KA, Barrett PHR, Morehouse LA, Barter PJ (2006) Effects of inhibiting cholesteryl ester transfer protein on the kinetics of high-density lipoprotein cholesteryl ester transport in plasma. In vivo studies in rabbits. Arterioscler Thromb Vasc Biol 26:884–890

47. Catalano G, Julia Z, Frisdal E, Vedie B, Fournier N, Le Goff W, Chapman MJ, Guerin M (2009) Torcetrapib differentially modulates the biological activities of HDL2 and HDL3 particles in the reverse cholesterol transport pathway. Arterioscler Thromb Vasc Biol 29(2): 268–275

48. Tchoua U, D'Souza W, Mukhamedova N, Blum D, Niesor E, Mizrahi J, Maugeais C, Sviridov D (2008) The effect of cholesteryl ester transfer protein overexpression and inhibition on reverse cholesterol transport. Cardiovasc Res 77:732–739

49. Sviridov D, Chin-Dusting J, Nestel P, Kingwell B, Hoang A, Olchawa B, Starr J, Dart A (2006) Elevated HDL cholesterol is functionally ineffective in cardiac transplant recipients: evidence for impaired reverse cholesterol transport. Transplantation 81:361–366

50. Yvan-Charvet L, Matsuura F, Wang N, Bamberger MJ, Nguyen T, Rinninger F, Jiang XC, Shear CL, Tall AR (2007) Inhibition of cholesteryl ester transfer protein by torcetrapib modestly increases macrophage cholesterol efflux to HDL. Arterioscler Thromb Vasc Biol 27:1132–1138

51. Yvan-Charvet L, Pagler TA, Wang N, Senokuchi T, Brundert M, Li H, Rinninger F, Tall AR (2008) SR-BI inhibits ABCG1-stimulated net cholesterol efflux from cells to plasma HDL. J Lipid Res 49:107–114

52. Millar JS, Brousseau ME, Diffenderfer MR et al (2006) Effects of cholesteryl ester transfer protein inhibitor torcetrapib on apolipoprotein B100 metabolism in humans. Arterioscler Thromb Vasc Biol 26:1350–1356

53. Brousseau ME, Schaefer EJ, Wolfe ML, Bloedon LT, Digenio AG, Clark RW, Mancuso JP, Rader DJ (2004) Effects of an inhibitor of cholesteryl ester transfer protein on HDL cholesterol. N Engl J Med 350:1505–1515

54. Bloomfield D, Carlson GL, Sapre A, Tribble D, McKenney JM, Littlejohn TW, Sisk CM, Mitchel Y, Pasternak RC (2009) Efficacy and safety of the cholesteryl ester transfer protein inhibitor anacetrapib as monotherapy and coadministered with atorvastatin in dyslipidemic patients. Am Heart J 157:352–360

55. Kontush A, de Faria EC, Chantepie S, Chapman MJ (2004) Antioxidative activity of HDL particle subspecies is impaired in hyperalphalipoproteinemia: relevance of enzymatic and physicochemical properties. Arterioscler Thromb Vasc Biol 24:526–533

56. Tanigawa H, Billheimer JT, Tohyama J, Zhang Y, Rothblat G, Rader DJ (2007) Expression of cholesteryl ester transfer protein in mice promotes macrophage reverse cholesterol transport. Circulation 116(11):1267–1273

57. Watts GF, Ji J, Chan DC, Ooi EMM, Johnson AG, Rye KA, Barrett PHR (2006) Relationships between changes in plasma lipid transfer proteins and apolipoprotein B-100 kinetics during fenofibrate treatment in the metabolic syndrome. Clin Sci 111:193–199

The HDL Receptor SR-BI

Attilio Rigotti and Monty Krieger

High density lipoproteins (HDL) are cholesterol transport particles whose plasma concentrations are inversely correlated with risk for atherosclerosis [1]. Several underlying mechanisms by which HDL protects against atherosclerotic cardiovascular disease have been proposed, including both lipid transport- and nonlipid transport-related activities of HDL [2]. The most well-known and studied hypothesis for the protective effect of HDL against atherosclerosis is its participation in a process called reverse cholesterol transport [2–4]. This hypothesis postulates that HDL counteracts the proatherogenic activity of low density lipoproteins (LDL) by mobilizing excess cholesterol from cells of the arterial intima and delivering this cholesterol to the liver for excretion into the bile [5].

There appear to be two main pathways by which HDL cholesterol is delivered to the liver in humans (Fig. 1). Humans and many other mammals, but not rodents, synthesize the key protein cholesteryl ester transfer protein (CETP), that mediates the exchange of cholesteryl esters in HDL with triglycerides in apoB containing lipoproteins (VLDL, IDL, LDL) [6]. In the presence of CETP, a significant fraction of HDL cholesteryl esters (HDL-CE) is transferred to these lipoproteins for delivery to the liver by receptor-mediated endocytosis, primarily via the LDL receptor. In addition to the "indirect" CETP-mediated pathway, there is a "direct" pathway for the uptake of HDL cholesterol by the liver and other tissues, called selective HDL lipid uptake [7, 8] (direct uptake via endocytic processes is also possible, but at this time less well-understood [9]). Selective HDL lipid uptake is an important pathway for HDL metabolism in vivo [7, 8], which involves cholesterol delivery from circulating HDL to cells via the scavenger receptor class B type I (SR-BI) that was reported in 1996 as the first molecularly well-defined and functionally active cell surface HDL receptor to be described [10]. Selective lipid uptake is a multistep process involving: (1) high affinity binding of spherical, cholesteryl ester-rich HDL particles to SR-BI, (2) SR-BI-mediated transfer of the core cholesteryl esters to the cell via poorly understood molecular mechanisms, and (3) subsequent dissociation of the lipid-depleted HDL particles from the receptor and their release into the extracellular fluid [11]. SR-BI-mediated selective lipid uptake can take place at the extracellular face of the plasma membrane of cells without the requirement for endocytosis [12] although it is possible that endocytosis may play a role in SR-BI-mediated selective lipid uptake in some types of cells in vivo [13–15].

The HDL Receptor SR-BI Controls HDL Cholesterol Metabolism

SR-BI is a high affinity HDL receptor that is expressed most abundantly in liver and nonplacental steroidogenic tissues [10, 16] (Fig. 1), precisely those tissues that previously had been shown to exhibit the bulk of selective uptake of HDL cholesterol in vivo [7, 8].

Gene targeting and transgenic studies demonstrated that murine SR-BI plays an important role in hepatic HDL cholesterol clearance: deletion of SR-BI expression by homozygous gene targeting (SR-BI knockout (KO) mice) results in the accumulation in the plasma of abnormally large, cholesterol-rich HDL particles with altered lipid and apolipoprotein composition [17, 18]. This is accompanied by impaired biliary cholesterol secretion [19, 20]. Conversely, hepatic SR-BI overexpression can dramatically reduce circulating HDL cholesterol levels and increase cholesterol output into the bile [21, 22]. Furthermore, metabolic studies using HDL radiolabeled in both the protein and lipid components demonstrated that reduced hepatic SR-BI expression was associated with a decrease in selective uptake of cholesteryl esters by the liver, and a corresponding reduction in the selective removal of HDL cholesteryl esters from plasma [23, 24], indicating that SR-BI is the major cell surface receptor mediating selective cholesteryl ester uptake by the liver. Taken together these findings

M. Krieger (✉)
Biology Department, Massachusetts Institute of Technology,
Room 68-483, 77 Massachusetts Ave, Cambridge, MA 02139, USA
e-mail: krieger@mit.edu

E.J. Schaefer (ed.), *High Density Lipoproteins, Dyslipidemia, and Coronary Heart Disease*,
DOI 10.1007/978-1-4419-1059-2_13, © Springer Science+Business Media, LLC 2010

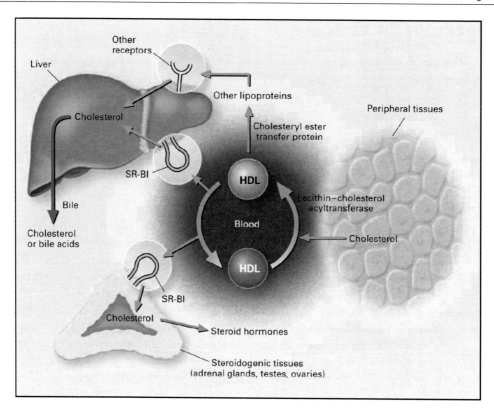

Fig. 1 Role of the HDL receptor SR-BI in the metabolism of HDL in vivo. Rigotti A, Krieger M. Getting a handle on "good" cholesterol with the high-density lipoprotein receptor. N Engl J Med 1999;341:2011–2013. © 1999 Massachusetts Medical Society. All rights reserved

also suggested that SR-BI plays a key role in the hepatic phase of reverse cholesterol transport, including the transhepatic flux of HDL cholesterol from plasma into the bile (Fig. 1). A recent study has established that in mice SR-BI can mediate biliary cholesterol secretion independently of ATP-binding cassette transporters ABCG5 and ABCG8 [25].

A wide variety of studies clearly suggest that hepatic SR-BI expression, which is inversely related to plasma HDL cholesterol concentrations [18, 22], is an important positive regulator of the rate of reverse cholesterol transport in vivo. For instance, mice overexpressing SR-BI in the liver have significantly increased transport of cholesterol from peritoneal macrophages into feces [25], whereas mice deficient in SR-BI have markedly reduced fecal excretion of cholesterol derived from peripheral cells [26]. SR-BI is also expressed in macrophages [27, 28] and it has been shown to promote cholesterol efflux to extracellular acceptors in cultured cells [28, 29]. However, studies [30–33], including those involving the injection of radioactive cholesterol-labeled macrophages lacking of SR-BI into the peritoneum of mice and monitoring the appearance of the label in the feces [34], have suggested that its expression in this cell type may not contribute significantly to reverse cholesterol transport.

Other Functions of SR-BI

SR-BI-Mediated Signaling and Endothelial Function

HDL can influence endothelial cell metabolism and function via pathways that may mediate atheroprotection. Among other activities, HDL facilitates the production of nitric oxide (NO) by stimulating endothelial NO synthase (reviewed by Mineo and Shaul [35]). This effect of HDL on endothelial cells is mediated by SR-BI and involves the activation of an intracellular kinase cascade [36, 37]. HDL also promotes endothelial cell growth and migration via SR-BI-initiated signaling [38]. There is also evidence for a variety of mechanisms by which HDL is antithrombotic, and thereby protects against arterial and venous thrombosis [39–43], including through the activation of prostacyclin synthesis [44, 45]. Thus, in addition to its cholesterol-transporting activity, HDL favorably regulates endothelial cell phenotype and function in an SR-BI dependent manner, which may lead to novel preventive and therapeutic approaches against atherosclerosis.

SR-BI and Adrenal Physiology

Selective cholesterol uptake has also been suggested to play a role in maintaining normal adrenal cholesterol pools and thus the availability of cholesterol for steroid hormone synthesis [46]. In cultured adrenal cells, SR-BI functions as a major route for selective uptake of HDL cholesteryl esters and delivery of HDL cholesterol for steroidogenesis [47]. Initial studies in SR-BI knockout mice also showed a significant reduction in adrenal cholesterol levels [18]. Under basal conditions (e.g., in the absence of stress), SR-BI-independent sources of cholesterol are apparently sufficient for normal adrenal (and other steroidogenic tissue) steroidogenesis – there are no apparent signs of adrenal insufficiency [18]. However, without SR-BI, mice are incapable of adequately responding to different physiological stress conditions (e.g., lipopolysaccharide-induced endotoxic shock and fasting) as a result of primary adrenal glucocorticoid insufficiency [48, 49]. These combined findings demonstrate the importance of SR-BI-mediated HDL uptake in the adrenals for maintaining an appropriate corticosteroid-dependent stress response (Fig. 1).

SR-BI and Microbial Pathogens

SR-BI has been shown in many studies to be a coreceptor for human hepatitis C virus (reviewed by Burlone and Budkowska [50]). Small molecule inhibitors of SR-BI-mediated lipid transport [51] can interfere with hepatitis C virus infection of cultured hepatocytes [52]. There have also been two independent reports that SR-BI may play a role in the entrance of malaria into hepatocytes [53, 54].

SR-BI and Atherosclerosis

Because of its key activity in the hepatic phase of reverse cholesterol transport (Fig. 1), SR-BI expression has been postulated to be critical in mediating at least some of the antiatherogenic effects of HDL.

Experiments using transgenic and KO animals have established that SR-BI expression protects against atherosclerosis in mice. Transgene or adenovirus-mediated hepatic overexpression of SR-BI markedly reduces atherosclerosis in various murine models of the disease [55–57]. In addition, complete disruption of the SR-BI gene in chow-fed apoE-deficient (SR-BI/apoE double-KO mice) [20, 58], Western diet-fed LDL receptor-deficient (SR-BI/LDLR dKO) [59], and Paigen-diet (high fat, high cholesterol, cholic acid) fed,

low apoE (SR-BI KO/apoER61[h/h]) [60] models substantially accelerates the onset of atherosclerosis, as does attenuated SR-BI expression in LDLR-deficient mice [61]. Bone marrow transplantation experiments have established that expression of SR-BI in bone marrow-derived cells is responsible, in part, for the atheroprotective effects of SR-BI [59, 62–64]. Furthermore, SR-BI KO mice develop atherosclerosis when fed a Western-type high-fat/high-cholesterol diet [60, 63]. Taken together, these studies clearly demonstrated the multifaceted antiatherogenic activity of SR-BI in the mouse.

Remarkably, chow-fed SR-BI/apoE dKO and high fat, high cholesterol diet-fed SR-BI KO/apoER61[h/h] mice develop severe hypercholesterolemia, complex aortic and coronary artery disease, myocardial infarction, heart dysfunction, and premature death [20, 58, 60], resembling human ischemic heart disease and its complications. These two animal models can be used for the preclinical testing of potential pharmacological therapies for coronary heart disease. Indeed, treatments with probucol (a hypocholesterolemia and antioxidant agent), ezetimibe (an FDA approved cholesterol absorption inhibitor), or SC-435 (a bile acid absorption inhibitor under development) prevent or attenuate the early onset atherosclerosis and cardiac disease in SR-BI/apoE dKO mice [17, 65].

The exact mechanisms by which SR-BI expression modulates atherogenesis in these murine models remain to be elucidated, but it may involve enhanced reverse cholesterol transport via HDL [21, 22, 26], facilitated uptake of plasma cholesterol transported in apolipoprotein-B containing lipoproteins [66, 67], modulation of macrophage biology [27, 28, 30–34], increased vascular delivery of α-tocopherol [68, 69], HDL-dependent endothelial NO synthase activation [36–38, 68, 69], and/or other activities of SR-BI (maintenance of normal structure, function and levels of red blood cells and platelets) [70–72].

PDZK1-Dependent Regulation of SR-BI

Adaptor proteins that bind to lipoprotein receptors apparently are critical for their normal function, including their influence on lipoprotein metabolism.

PDZK1, a PDZ domain containing protein, interacts with SR-BI [73], playing an essential role in maintaining hepatic SR-BI levels and controlling HDL metabolism [74] as well as mediating SR-BI-dependent regulation of endothelial cell biology by HDL [75]. In mice without PDZK1 (PDZK1 KO mice), hepatic SR-BI protein levels are reduced to less than 5% of normal [74]. This PDZK1-dependence of SR-BI is a tissue-specific phenomenon [74]. In the intestines of PDZK1

KO mice, SR-BI levels in absorptive epithelial cells are reduced by 50%, while the normally high expression of SR-BI in steroidogenic cells is not altered, nor is the expression in endothelial cells or macrophages [74–76]. Thus, PDZK1 is an adaptor protein that can regulate cellular SR-BI activity in a tissue-specific fashion.

Given the importance of PDZK1 for hepatic SR-BI activity, it is not surprising that inactivation of the PDZK1 gene promotes the development of aortic root atherosclerosis in apoE KO mice fed a high fat/high cholesterol diet [75]. However, unlike complete SR-BI-deficiency in SR-BI/apoE double KO mice [20, 58], PDZK1 deficiency in apoE knockout mice does not lead to occlusive coronary artery disease or myocardial infarction when these mice are fed a Western-type, atherogenic diet [76]. This is presumably because of the residual expression of SR-BI [74] or the expression of a spliced isoform of this receptor, SR-BII [77] that is not dependent on PDZK1 for its expression in the liver [74]. However, when these double KO mice are fed a Paigen diet (high fat, high cholesterol, cholic acid), they do develop occlusive atherosclerosis and myocardial infarctions [78]. These findings indicate that several effects of SR-BI on HDL metabolism and function, as well as pathophysiology, may depend on the protein–protein interaction between PDZK1 and this receptor.

Human SR-BI

SR-BI is expressed in humans at high levels in precisely those tissues that exhibit most of selective uptake of HDL cholesterol in vivo [79]. In addition, human SR-BI (which has also been called "CLA-1") [80] mediates selective HDL cholesterol uptake when expressed in cultured cells [81, 82], suggesting that it may also play a key role on HDL metabolism in humans.

The human SR-BI gene (SCARB1) was mapped to human chromosome 12 by PCR analysis of human–hamster hybrids [83], and additional work localized the gene to 12q24.2-qter by FISH [79]. Interestingly, this chromosomal region has been linked to type 2 diabetes [84] and abdominal obesity, a risk factor for type 2 diabetes [85–87].

Genetic variation in the SCARB1 gene has been associated with an increased risk of obesity [88, 89], metabolic syndrome [90], triglycerides [88, 91–93], LDL cholesterol [93], and HDL-cholesterol [88, 91–93, 95–99], although these associations are not very strong. Hsu et al. have reported an association between an 11-base pair deletion in the promoter of SCARB1 and plasma HDL cholesterol levels in Taiwanese Chinese [96]. A preliminary report of a link of a heterozygous mutation in the extracellular domain of human SR-BI and increased plasma HDL and apoA-I levels in a large Caucasian family has appeared [100]. West et al. have reported that SR-BI can independently influence HDL cholesterol levels in women with hyperalphalipoproteinemia (two polymorphisms in the SCARB1 gene were reported to be significantly associated with lower SR-BI protein levels) [101]. However, a causal relationship between human SR-BI gene variations and plasma HDL cholesterol levels and metabolism remains to be established.

In agreement with animal studies, the association of SR-BI variants and triglycerides [88, 91–93] are consistent with the role of this receptor in the metabolism of apolipoprotein B-containing lipoproteins in humans. It has been suggested that the SR-BI-mediated pathway may represent a backup process to LDL receptor-mediated metabolism of non HDL lipoproteins with particular importance in subjects with high levels of apoB-containing lipoproteins, such as those occurring in patients with familial hypercholesterolemia.

In addition, direct evidence for association of SCARB1 polymorphisms with diabetes traits has been reported [102, 103]. Furthermore, there is evidence that diabetes status may modify the SCARB1 association with HDL-cholesterol [104]. Further research is needed in additional populations to reproduce these findings as well as to elucidate a potential role of SR-BI in the development of insulin resistance and diabetes.

SCARB1 gene is in close proximity to a site 161 cM from the tip of the short arm of chromosome 12 that has been mapped to a QTL for internal carotid artery intimal medial thickness [105]. On the other hand, combined SCARB1 gene polymorphisms are predictive of peripheral vascular disease after correction for traditional risk factors [94]. In addition, genetic variation in the SCARB1 gene has also been associated with an increased risk of coronary artery disease [106, 107].

Given the multiple pathophysiological consequences of inactivation of the SR-BI gene in mice and the human studies reported to date, it seems likely that human SR-BI will play a significant role in normal physiology and alterations in its function will likely have pathophysiological consequences.

Conclusion

It has been 14 years since SR-BI was discovered to be an HDL receptor [10]. Numerous studies in vitro and in mice have established that SR-BI is a physiologically relevant HDL receptor that controls HDL metabolism, including the delivery of HDL cholesterol to cells (Fig. 1). SR-BI influences a wide variety of processes, particularly HDL cholesterol metabolism, and cell types (e.g., hepatocytes, steroidogenic cells, endothelial cells, macrophages). Further exploration of the structure, mechanism of action and function of SR-BI is likely to provide new insights into cholesterol metabolism in general and may ultimately lead to new strategies for the prevention and/or treatment of cardiovascular diseases.

Acknowledgments The work from the authors' labs has been supported by grants from the U.S. National Institutes of Health and Fondo de Desarrollo Científico y Tecnológico (Chile). The authors are grateful for the many important contributions to this work by their many collaborators.

References

1. Gordon DJ, Probstfield JL, Garrison RJ et al (1989) High-density lipoprotein cholesterol and cardiovascular disease. Four prospective American studies. Circulation 79(1):8–15

2. Rohrer L, Hersberger M, von Eckardstein A (2004) High density lipoproteins in the intersection of diabetes mellitus, inflammation and cardiovascular disease. Curr Opin Lipidol 15(3):269–278

3. Florentin M, Liberopoulos EN, Wierzbicki AS, Mikhailidis DP (2008) Multiple actions of high-density lipoprotein. Curr Opin Cardiol 23(4):370–378

4. Glomset JA (1968) The plasma lecithins:cholesterol acyltransferase reaction. J Lipid Res 9(2):155–167

5. Lewis GF, Rader DJ (2005) New insights into the regulation of HDL metabolism and reverse cholesterol transport. Circ Res 96(12):1221–1232

6. Bruce C, Tall AR (1995) Cholesteryl ester transfer proteins, reverse cholesterol transport, and atherosclerosis. Curr Opin Lipidol 6(5):306–311

7. Glass C, Pittman RC, Weinstein DB, Steinberg D (1983) Dissociation of tissue uptake of cholesterol ester from that of apoprotein A-I of rat plasma high density lipoprotein: selective delivery of cholesterol ester to liver, adrenal, and gonad. Proc Natl Acad Sci USA 80(17):5435–5439

8. Stein Y, Dabach Y, Hollander G, Halperin G, Stein O (1983) Metabolism of HDL-cholesteryl ester in the rat, studied with a non-hydrolyzable analog, cholesteryl linoleyl ether. Biochim Biophys Acta 752(1):98–105

9. Fidge NH (1999) High density lipoprotein receptors, binding proteins, and ligands. J Lipid Res 40(2):187–201

10. Acton S, Rigotti A, Landschulz KT, Xu S, Hobbs HH, Krieger M (1996) Identification of scavenger receptor SR-BI as a high density lipoprotein receptor. Science 271(5248):518–520

11. Rigotti A, Miettinen HE, Krieger M (2003) The role of the high-density lipoprotein receptor SR-BI in the lipid metabolism of endocrine and other tissues. Endocr Rev 24(3):357–387

12. Nieland TJ, Ehrlich M, Krieger M, Kirchhausen T (2005) Endocytosis is not required for the selective lipid uptake mediated by murine SR-BI. Biochim Biophys Acta 1734(1):44–51

13. Pagler TA, Rhode S, Neuhofer A et al (2006) SR-BI-mediated high density lipoprotein (HDL) endocytosis leads to HDL resecretion facilitating cholesterol efflux. J Biol Chem 281(16):11193–11204

14. Zhang Y, Ahmed AM, Tran TL et al (2007) The inhibition of endocytosis affects HDL-lipid uptake mediated by the human scavenger receptor class B type I. Mol Membr Biol 24(5–6):442–454

15. Ahras M, Naing T, McPherson R (2008) Scavenger receptor class B type I localizes to a late endosomal compartment. J Lipid Res 49(7):1569–1576

16. Landschulz KT, Pathak RK, Rigotti A, Krieger M, Hobbs HH (1996) Regulation of scavenger receptor, class B, type I, a high density lipoprotein receptor, in liver and steroidogenic tissues of the rat. J Clin Invest 98(4):984–995

17. Braun A, Zhang S, Miettinen HE et al (2003) Probucol prevents early coronary heart disease and death in the high-density lipoprotein receptor SR-BI/apolipoprotein E double knockout mouse. Proc Natl Acad Sci USA 100(12):7283–7288

18. Rigotti A, Trigatti BL, Penman M, Rayburn H, Herz J, Krieger M (1997) A targeted mutation in the murine gene encoding the high density lipoprotein (HDL) receptor scavenger receptor class B type I reveals its key role in HDL metabolism. Proc Natl Acad Sci USA 94(23):12610–12615

19. Mardones P, Quinones V, Amigo L et al (2001) Hepatic cholesterol and bile acid metabolism and intestinal cholesterol absorption in scavenger receptor class B type I-deficient mice. J Lipid Res 42(2):170–180

20. Trigatti B, Rayburn H, Vinals M et al (1999) Influence of the high density lipoprotein receptor SR-BI on reproductive and cardiovascular pathophysiology. Proc Natl Acad Sci USA 96(16):9322–9327

21. Ji Y, Wang N, Ramakrishnan R et al (1999) Hepatic scavenger receptor BI promotes rapid clearance of high density lipoprotein free cholesterol and its transport into bile. J Biol Chem 274(47):33398–33402

22. Kozarsky KF, Donahee MH, Rigotti A, Iqbal SN, Edelman ER, Krieger M (1997) Overexpression of the HDL receptor SR-BI alters plasma HDL and bile cholesterol levels. Nature 387(6631): 414–417

23. Brundert M, Ewert A, Heeren J et al (2005) Scavenger receptor class B type I mediates the selective uptake of high-density lipoprotein-associated cholesteryl ester by the liver in mice. Arterioscler Thromb Vasc Biol 25(1):143–148

24. Out R, Hoekstra M, Spijkers JA et al (2004) Scavenger receptor class B type I is solely responsible for the selective uptake of cholesteryl esters from HDL by the liver and the adrenals in mice. J Lipid Res 45(11):2088–2095

25. Wiersma H, Gatti A, Nijstad N, Oude Elferink RP, Kuipers F, Tietge UJ (2009) Scavenger receptor class B type I mediates biliary cholesterol secretion independent of ATP-binding cassette transporter g5/g8 in mice. Hepatology 50(4)):1263–1272

26. Zhang Y, Da Silva JR, Reilly M, Billheimer JT, Rothblat GH, Rader DJ (2005) Hepatic expression of scavenger receptor class B type I (SR-BI) is a positive regulator of macrophage reverse cholesterol transport in vivo. J Clin Invest 115(10):2870–2874

27. Hirano K, Yamashita S, Nakagawa Y et al (1999) Expression of human scavenger receptor class B type I in cultured human monocyte-derived macrophages and atherosclerotic lesions. Circ Res 85(1):108–116

28. Ji Y, Jian B, Wang N et al (1997) Scavenger receptor BI promotes high density lipoprotein-mediated cellular cholesterol efflux. J Biol Chem 272(34):20982–20985

29. Gu X, Kozarsky K, Krieger M (2000) Scavenger receptor class B, type I-mediated [3H]cholesterol efflux to high and low density lipoproteins is dependent on lipoprotein binding to the receptor. J Biol Chem 275(39):29993–30001

30. Brundert M, Heeren J, Bahar-Bayansar M, Ewert A, Moore KJ, Rinninger F (2006) Selective uptake of HDL cholesteryl esters and cholesterol efflux from mouse peritoneal macrophages independent of SR-BI. J Lipid Res 47(11):2408–2421

31. Chen W, Silver DL, Smith JD, Tall AR (2000) Scavenger receptor-BI inhibits ATP-binding cassette transporter 1- mediated cholesterol efflux in macrophages. J Biol Chem 275(40):30794–30800

32. Duong M, Collins HL, Jin W, Zanotti I, Favari E, Rothblat GH (2006) Relative contributions of ABCA1 and SR-BI to cholesterol efflux to serum from fibroblasts and macrophages. Arterioscler Thromb Vasc Biol 26(3):541–547

33. Yvan-Charvet L, Pagler TA, Wang N et al (2008) SR-BI inhibits ABCG1-stimulated net cholesterol efflux from cells to plasma HDL. J Lipid Res 49(1):107–114

34. Wang X, Collins HL, Ranalletta M et al (2007) Macrophage ABCA1 and ABCG1, but not SR-BI, promote macrophage reverse cholesterol transport in vivo. J Clin Invest 117(8):2216–2224

35. Mineo C, Shaul PW (2003) HDL stimulation of endothelial nitric oxide synthase: a novel mechanism of HDL action. Trends Cardiovasc Med 13(6):226–231

36. Mineo C, Yuhanna IS, Quon MJ, Shaul PW (2003) High density lipoprotein-induced endothelial nitric-oxide synthase activation is mediated by Akt and MAP kinases. J Biol Chem 278(11): 9142–9149

37. Yuhanna IS, Zhu Y, Cox BE et al (2001) High-density lipoprotein binding to scavenger receptor-BI activates endothelial nitric oxide synthase. Nat Med 7(7):853–857

38. Seetharam D, Mineo C, Gormley AK et al (2006) High-density lipoprotein promotes endothelial cell migration and reendothelialization via scavenger receptor-B type I. Circ Res 98(1):63–72

39. Deguchi H, Pecheniuk NM, Elias DJ, Averell PM, Griffin JH (2005) High-density lipoprotein deficiency and dyslipoproteinemia associated with venous thrombosis in men. Circulation 112(6):893–899

40. Eichinger S, Pecheniuk NM, Hron G et al (2007) High-density lipoprotein and the risk of recurrent venous thromboembolism. Circulation 115(12):1609–1614

41. Griffin JH, Kojima K, Banka CL, Curtiss LK, Fernandez JA (1999) High-density lipoprotein enhancement of anticoagulant activities of plasma protein S and activated protein C. J Clin Invest 103(2):219–227

42. Li D, Weng S, Yang B et al (1999) Inhibition of arterial thrombus formation by ApoA1 Milano. Arterioscler Thromb Vasc Biol 19(2):378–383

43. Naqvi TZ, Shah PK, Ivey PA et al (1999) Evidence that high-density lipoprotein cholesterol is an independent predictor of acute platelet-dependent thrombus formation. Am J Cardiol 84(9):1011–1017

44. Calabresi L, Rossoni G, Gomaraschi M, Sisto F, Berti F, Franceschini G (2003) High-density lipoproteins protect isolated rat hearts from ischemia-reperfusion injury by reducing cardiac tumor necrosis factor-alpha content and enhancing prostaglandin release. Circ Res 92(3):330–337

45. Fleisher LN, Tall AR, Witte LD, Miller RW, Cannon PJ (1982) Stimulation of arterial endothelial cell prostacyclin synthesis by high density lipoproteins. J Biol Chem 257(12):6653–6655

46. Connelly MA (2009) SR-BI-mediated HDL cholesteryl ester delivery in the adrenal gland. Mol Cell Endocrinol 300(1–2):83–88

47. Temel RE, Trigatti B, DeMattos RB, Azhar S, Krieger M, Williams DL (1997) Scavenger receptor class B, type I (SR-BI) is the major route for the delivery of high density lipoprotein cholesterol to the steroidogenic pathway in cultured mouse adrenocortical cells. Proc Natl Acad Sci USA 94(25):13600–13605

48. Cai L, Ji A, de Beer FC, Tannock LR, van der Westhuyzen DR (2008) SR-BI protects against endotoxemia in mice through its roles in glucocorticoid production and hepatic clearance. J Clin Invest 118(1):364–375

49. Hoekstra M, Meurs I, Koenders M et al (2008) Absence of HDL cholesteryl ester uptake in mice via SR-BI impairs an adequate adrenal glucocorticoid-mediated stress response to fasting. J Lipid Res 49(4):738–745

50. Burlone ME, Budkowska A (2009) Hepatitis C virus cell entry: role of lipoproteins and cellular receptors. J Gen Virol 90(Pt 5):1055–1070

51. Nieland TJ, Penman M, Dori L, Krieger M, Kirchhausen T (2002) Discovery of chemical inhibitors of the selective transfer of lipids mediated by the HDL receptor SR-BI. Proc Natl Acad Sci USA 99(24):15422–15427

52. Voisset C, Callens N, Blanchard E, Op De Beeck A, Dubuisson J, Vu-Dac N (2005) High density lipoproteins facilitate hepatitis C virus entry through the scavenger receptor class B type I. J Biol Chem 280(9):7793–7799

53. Rodrigues CD, Hannus M, Prudencio M et al (2008) Host scavenger receptor SR-BI plays a dual role in the establishment of malaria parasite liver infection. Cell Host Microbe 4(3):271–282

54. Yalaoui S, Huby T, Franetich JF et al (2008) Scavenger receptor BI boosts hepatocyte permissiveness to Plasmodium infection. Cell Host Microbe 4(3):283–292

55. Arai T, Wang N, Bezouevski M, Welch C, Tall AR (1999) Decreased atherosclerosis in heterozygous low density lipoprotein receptor-deficient mice expressing the scavenger receptor BI transgene. J Biol Chem 274(4):2366–2371

56. Kozarsky KF, Donahee MH, Glick JM, Krieger M, Rader DJ (2000) Gene transfer and hepatic overexpression of the HDL receptor SR-BI reduces atherosclerosis in the cholesterol-fed LDL receptor-deficient mouse. Arterioscler Thromb Vasc Biol 20(3):721–727

57. Ueda Y, Gong E, Royer L, Cooper PN, Francone OL, Rubin EM (2000) Relationship between expression levels and atherogenesis in scavenger receptor class B, type I transgenics. J Biol Chem 275(27):20368–20373

58. Braun A, Trigatti BL, Post MJ et al (2002) Loss of SR-BI expression leads to the early onset of occlusive atherosclerotic coronary artery disease, spontaneous myocardial infarctions, severe cardiac dysfunction, and premature death in apolipoprotein E-deficient mice. Circ Res 90(3):270–276

59. Covey SD, Krieger M, Wang W, Penman M, Trigatti BL (2003) Scavenger receptor class B type I-mediated protection against atherosclerosis in LDL receptor-negative mice involves its expression in bone marrow-derived cells. Arterioscler Thromb Vasc Biol 23(9):1589–1594

60. Zhang S, Picard MH, Vasile E et al (2005) Diet-induced occlusive coronary atherosclerosis, myocardial infarction, cardiac dysfunction, and premature death in scavenger receptor class B type I-deficient, hypomorphic apolipoprotein ER61 mice. Circulation 111(25):3457–3464

61. Huszar D, Varban ML, Rinninger F et al (2000) Increased LDL cholesterol and atherosclerosis in LDL receptor-deficient mice with attenuated expression of scavenger receptor B1. Arterioscler Thromb Vasc Biol 20(4):1068–1073

62. Van Eck M, Bos IS, Hildebrand RB, Van Rij BT, Van Berkel TJ (2004) Dual role for scavenger receptor class B, type I on bone marrow-derived cells in atherosclerotic lesion development. Am J Pathol 165(3):785–794

63. Van Eck M, Twisk J, Hoekstra M et al (2003) Differential effects of scavenger receptor BI deficiency on lipid metabolism in cells of the arterial wall and in the liver. J Biol Chem 278(26):23699–23705

64. Zhang W, Yancey PG, Su YR et al (2003) Inactivation of macrophage scavenger receptor class B type I promotes atherosclerotic lesion development in apolipoprotein E-deficient mice. Circulation 108(18):2258–2263

65. Braun A, Yesilaltay A, Acton S et al (2008) Inhibition of intestinal absorption of cholesterol by ezetimibe or bile acids by SC-435 alters lipoprotein metabolism and extends the lifespan of SR-BI/apoE double knockout mice. Atherosclerosis 198(1):77–84

66. Ueda Y, Royer L, Gong E et al (1999) Lower plasma levels and accelerated clearance of high density lipoprotein (HDL) and non-HDL cholesterol in scavenger receptor class B type I transgenic mice. J Biol Chem 274(11):7165–7171

67. Wang N, Arai T, Ji Y, Rinninger F, Tall AR (1998) Liver-specific overexpression of scavenger receptor BI decreases levels of very low density lipoprotein ApoB, low density lipoprotein ApoB, and high density lipoprotein in transgenic mice. J Biol Chem 273(49):32920–32926

68. Goti D, Hrzenjak A, Levak-Frank S et al (2001) Scavenger receptor class B, type I is expressed in porcine brain capillary endothelial cells and contributes to selective uptake of HDL-associated vitamin E. J Neurochem 76(2):498–508

69. Mardones P, Strobel P, Miranda S et al (2002) Alpha-tocopherol metabolism is abnormal in scavenger receptor class B type I (SR-BI)-deficient mice. J Nutr 132(3):443–449

70. Dole VS, Matuskova J, Vasile E et al (2008) Thrombocytopenia and platelet abnormalities in high-density lipoprotein receptor-deficient mice. Arterioscler Thromb Vasc Biol 28(6):1111–1116

71. Holm TM, Braun A, Trigatti BL et al (2002) Failure of red blood cell maturation in mice with defects in the high-density lipoprotein receptor SR-BI. Blood 99(5):1817–1824

72. Meurs I, Hoekstra M, van Wanrooij EJ et al (2005) HDL cholesterol levels are an important factor for determining the lifespan of erythrocytes. Exp Hematol 33(11):1309–1319

73. Ikemoto M, Arai H, Feng D et al (2000) Identification of a PDZ-domain-containing protein that interacts with the scavenger receptor class B type I. Proc Natl Acad Sci USA 97(12):6538–6543

74. Kocher O, Yesilaltay A, Cirovic C, Pal R, Rigotti A, Krieger M (2003) Targeted disruption of the PDZK1 gene in mice causes tissue-specific depletion of the high density lipoprotein receptor scavenger receptor class B type I and altered lipoprotein metabolism. J Biol Chem 278(52):52820–52825

75. Zhu W, Saddar S, Seetharam D et al (2008) The scavenger receptor class B type I adaptor protein PDZK1 maintains endothelial monolayer integrity. Circ Res 102(4):480–487

76. Kocher O, Yesilaltay A, Shen CH et al (2008) Influence of PDZK1 on lipoprotein metabolism and atherosclerosis. Biochim Biophys Acta 1782(5):310–316

77. Webb NR, Connell PM, Graf GA et al (1998) SR-BII, an isoform of the scavenger receptor BI containing an alternate cytoplasmic tail, mediates lipid transfer between high density lipoprotein and cells. J Biol Chem 273(24):15241–15248

78. Yesilaltay A, Daniels K, Par R et al. (2009) Lors of PDZK1 causes coronary artery occlusion and myocardial infarction in paigen diet-fed apolipoprotein E deficient mice. PLOS One 4(12):e8103.

79. Cao G, Garcia CK, Wyne KL, Schultz RA, Parker KL, Hobbs HH (1997) Structure and localization of the human gene encoding SR-BI/CLA-1. Evidence for transcriptional control by steroidogenic factor 1. J Biol Chem 272(52):33068–33076

80. Calvo D, Vega MA (1993) Identification, primary structure, and distribution of CLA-1, a novel member of the CD36/LIMPII gene family. J Biol Chem 268(25):18929–18935

81. Imachi H, Murao K, Sato M, Hosokawa H, Ishida T, Takahara J (1999) CD36 LIMPII analogous-1, a human homolog of the rodent scavenger receptor B1, provides the cholesterol ester for steroidogenesis in adrenocortical cells. Metabolism 48(5):627–630

82. Murao K, Terpstra V, Green SR, Kondratenko N, Steinberg D, Quehenberger O (1997) Characterization of CLA-1, a human homologue of rodent scavenger receptor BI, as a receptor for high density lipoprotein and apoptotic thymocytes. J Biol Chem 272(28):17551–17557

83. Calvo D, Dopazo J, Vega MA (1995) The CD36, CLA-1 (CD36L1), and LIMPII (CD36L2) gene family: cellular distribution, chromosomal location, and genetic evolution. Genomics 25(1):100–106

84. Florez JC, Hirschhorn J, Altshuler D (2003) The inherited basis of diabetes mellitus: implications for the genetic analysis of complex traits. Annu Rev Genomics Hum Genet 4:257–291

85. Lewis CE, North KE, Arnett D et al (2005) Sex-specific findings from a genome-wide linkage analysis of human fatness in non-Hispanic whites and African Americans: the HyperGEN study. Int J Obes (Lond) 29(6):639–649

86. Norris JM, Langefeld CD, Scherzinger AL et al (2005) Quantitative trait loci for abdominal fat and BMI in Hispanic-Americans and African-Americans: the IRAS Family study. Int J Obes (Lond) 29(1):67–77

87. Wilson SG, Adam G, Langdown M et al (2006) Linkage and potential association of obesity-related phenotypes with two genes on chromosome 12q24 in a female dizygous twin cohort. Eur J Hum Genet 14(3):340–348

88. Acton S, Osgood D, Donoghue M et al (1999) Association of polymorphisms at the SR-BI gene locus with plasma lipid levels and body mass index in a white population. Arterioscler Thromb Vasc Biol 19(7):1734–1743

89. Koumanis DJ, Christou NV, Wang XL, Gilfix BM (2002) Pilot study examining the frequency of several gene polymorphisms in a morbidly obese population. Obes Surg 12(6):759–764

90. Junyent M, Arnett DK, Tsai MY et al (2009) Genetic variants at the PDZ-interacting domain of the scavenger receptor class B type

I interact with diet to influence the risk of metabolic syndrome in obese men and women. J Nutr 139(5):842–848

91. McCarthy JJ, Lehner T, Reeves C et al (2003) Association of genetic variants in the HDL receptor, SR-B1, with abnormal lipids in women with coronary artery disease. J Med Genet 40(6):453–458

92. McCarthy JJ, Lewitzky S, Reeves C et al (2003) Polymorphisms of the HDL receptor gene associated with HDL cholesterol levels in diabetic kindred from three populations. Hum Hered 55(4):163–170

93. Tai ES, Adiconis X, Ordovas JM et al (2003) Polymorphisms at the SRBI locus are associated with lipoprotein levels in subjects with heterozygous familial hypercholesterolemia. Clin Genet 63(1):53–58

94. Ritsch A, Sonderegger G, Sandhofer A et al (2007) Scavenger receptor class B type I polymorphisms and peripheral arterial disease. Metabolism 56(8):1135–1141

95. Hong SH, Kim YR, Yoon YM, Min WK, Chun SI, Kim JQ (2002) Association between HaeIII polymorphism of scavenger receptor class B type I gene and plasma HDL-cholesterol concentration. Ann Clin Biochem 39(Pt 5):478–481

96. Hsu LA, Ko YL, Wu S et al (2003) Association between a novel 11-base pair deletion mutation in the promoter region of the scavenger receptor class B type I gene and plasma HDL cholesterol levels in Taiwanese Chinese. Arterioscler Thromb Vasc Biol 23(10):1869–1874

97. Morabia A, Ross BM, Costanza MC et al (2004) Population-based study of SR-BI genetic variation and lipid profile. Atherosclerosis 175(1):159–168

98. Richard E, von Muhlen D, Barrett-Connor E, Alcaraz J, Davis R, McCarthy JJ (2005) Modification of the effects of estrogen therapy on HDL cholesterol levels by polymorphisms of the HDL-C receptor, SR-BI: the Rancho Bernardo Study. Atherosclerosis 180(2):255–262

99. Roberts CG, Shen H, Mitchell BD, Damcott CM, Shuldiner AR, Rodriguez A (2007) Variants in scavenger receptor class B type I gene are associated with HDL cholesterol levels in younger women. Hum Hered 64(2):107–113

100. Vergeer M, Hovingh K, Vissers MN, Kastelein JJ, Kuivenhoven JA (2006) Heterozygosity for a mutation in the extracellular domain of SR-BI is associated with high HDL cholesterol levels in a family of Caucasian descent. Circulation 114(18):254

101. West M, Greason E, Kolmakova A et al (2009) Scavenger receptor class B type I protein as an independent predictor of high-density lipoprotein cholesterol levels in subjects with hyperalphalipoproteinemia. J Clin Endocrinol Metab 94(4):1451–1457

102. McCarthy JJ, Somji A, Weiss LA et al (2009) Polymorphisms of the scavenger receptor class B member 1 are associated with insulin resistance with evidence of gene by sex interaction. J Clin Endocrinol Metab 94(5):1789–1796

103. Perez-Martinez P, Perez-Jimenez F, Bellido C et al (2005) A polymorphism exon 1 variant at the locus of the scavenger receptor class B type I (SCARB1) gene is associated with differences in insulin sensitivity in healthy people during the consumption of an olive oil-rich diet. J Clin Endocrinol Metab 90(4):2297–2300

104. Osgood D, Corella D, Demissie S et al (2003) Genetic variation at the scavenger receptor class B type I gene locus determines plasma lipoprotein concentrations and particle size and interacts with type 2 diabetes: the Framingham study. J Clin Endocrinol Metab 88(6):2869–2879

105. Fox CS, Cupples LA, Chazaro I et al (2004) Genomewide linkage analysis for internal carotid artery intimal medial thickness: evidence for linkage to chromosome 12. Am J Hum Genet 74(2):253–261

106. Rodriguez-Esparragon F, Rodriguez-Perez JC, Hernandez-Trujillo Y et al (2005) Allelic variants of the human scavenger receptor class B type 1 and paraoxonase 1 on coronary heart disease: genotype-phenotype correlations. Arterioscler Thromb Vasc Biol 25(4):854–860

107. Yoon Y, Song J, Hong SH, Kim JQ (2003) Analysis of multiple single nucleotide polymorphisms of candidate genes related to coronary heart disease susceptibility by using support vector machines. Clin Chem Lab Med 41(4):529–534

Genetic Loci Influencing Plasma High Density Lipoprotein Cholesterol Concentrations in Humans

Margaret E. Brousseau

Introduction

Numerous population studies have shown that a strong inverse relationship exists between plasma high density lipoprotein (HDL) cholesterol concentrations and coronary heart disease (CHD) risk [1–4]. HDL cholesterol level is a heritable characteristic, with the majority of studies reporting heritability estimates in the range of 40–60% [5]. As discussed elsewhere within this atlas, a significant portion of our knowledge of the HDL metabolic pathway has evolved from analysis of patients having rare, monogenic inborn errors of metabolism. However, the majority of variation in HDL cholesterol observed at the population level is of polygenic origin and is the result of the complex interaction between genetic and environmental factors. For many years, genotype–phenotype associations were explored by evaluating a single common variant in a candidate gene. Although important genetic determinants of HDL cholesterol variation have been identified in such studies, this approach does not take into account the multifactorial nature of this complex trait. With the advent of genome-wide association (GWA) technology, it is now possible to study relationships between complex genetic traits, such as HDL cholesterol, and common variants in numerous loci in large populations. Over the past few years, GWA analysis has led to the discovery of novel, as well as confirmation of previously known, common genetic determinants of plasma lipoproteins (reviewed in refs. [6, 7]). This review summarizes the results of GWA studies (GWAS) reported from 2007 to present that have identified common genetic loci associated with plasma HDL cholesterol concentrations in humans.

M.E. Brousseau (✉)
Novartis Institutes for Biomedical Research, Inc,
100 Technology Square, Rm 6402, Cambridge,
MA 02139, USA
e-mail: margaret.brousseau@novartis.com

Single Cohort GWAS for HDL Cholesterol

In 2007, Kathiresan et al. [8] reported the results of a GWAS for blood lipid phenotypes, which included HDL cholesterol concentration, in 1,087 subjects from the Framingham Heart Study (FHS) Offspring cohort. The long-term average of up to seven measurements of HDL cholesterol, over a ~30 year span, was included among the primary phenotypes. All genotype data for this study were derived from an Affymetrix 100K GeneChip analysis of the FHS cohort [9]. Generalized estimating equations (GEE), family-based association tests (FBAT), and variance components linkage were used to investigate the relationships between single nucleotide polymorphisms (SNPs) and multivariable-adjusted residuals. In order to minimize false positive associations, analyses were limited to SNPs meeting the following criteria: (1) a genotyping call rate of ≥80%, (2) a Hardy–Weinberg Equilibrium (HWE) $P \geq 0.001$, and (3) a minor allele frequency (MAF) of ≥10%. Moreover, a three-stage replication strategy was also employed. Despite this careful analysis and the availability of long-term phenotypic data, the results of this study were largely negative. Although GEE and FBAT analysis revealed some statistically significant associations for SNPs with HDL cholesterol in the FHS cohort, none of these associations were significant in the replication cohorts. The lack of replication may have been due, in part, to inadequate statistical power to detect modest effects on HDL cholesterol.

Since the report of this initial negative study, a number of GWAS have successfully identified common genetic determinants of HDL cholesterol levels. The key characteristics of GWAS for the HDL cholesterol trait conducted in a single cohort, and replicated in at least one additional cohort, are summarized in Table 1. The results of a genome-wide quantitative trait analysis for 25 biochemical parameters, including HDL cholesterol, in hypertensive subjects from the MRC British Genetics of Hypertension (BRIGHT) study were reported by Wallace and colleagues in 2008 [10]. Enrollment criteria for this study included blood pressure readings of >145/95 (mean of three readings) or 150/100 (single reading). Genotype data were generated by Affymetrix

Table 1 Summary of recent single-cohort GWAS for HDL cholesterol[a]

Study	Cohort, n	Genotyping platform	SNP	Nearest gene(s) or region	MAF	Effect size	P[b]	P[c]
Wallace et al. [10]	*GWAS cohort* BRIGHT, 1,955	Affymetrix 500K	rs11017236	Chr 10	A, 0.16	1.1[d]	5.7×10^{-7}	NS
			rs11826048	Chr 11	T, 0.09	0.9	9.7×10^{-7}	NS
			rs905648	*COLQ*	T, 0.34	1.0	4.6×10^{-6}	NS
	Replication cohorts GRAPHIC, 2,033	Taqman						
	TwinsUK	Illumina 317K						
	Registry, 1,461							
Chasman et al. [12]	*GWAS cohort* WGHS, 6,382	Illumina Infinium II	rs1532085	*LIPC*	A, 0.37	1.8[d]	1.3×10^{-10}	0.03
			rs3764261	*CETP*	A, 0.31	4.0	1.0×10^{-41}	0.03
	Replication cohorts PRINCE, 671	Illumina 317K						
	CAP, 299	Illumina 317K						
Sabatti et al. [15]	*GWAS cohort* NFBC1966, 4,763	Illumina Infinium 370cnvDuo array	rs2167079	*NR1H3*	A, 0.42	0.04[e]	5.1×10^{-8}	NS
	Replication cohorts		rs7120118	*NR1H3*	G, 0.42	0.04	3.6×10^{-8}	NS
	Compared their GWAS	NA	rs1532085	*LIPC*	A, 0.44	0.05	1.8×10^{-10}	NS
	data to those generated		rs3764261	*CETP*	A, 0.28	0.09	7.0×10^{-29}	5.0×10^{-7}
	by Kathiresan et al. [14]		rs255049	*LCAT*	G, 0.22	0.05	3.1×10^{-8}	5.0×10^{-7}
	and Willer et al. [13]		rs9891572	Chr 17	A, 0.16	0.05	2.3×10^{-7}	NS
Lanktree et al. [17]	*GWAS cohort* SHARE, 906	Illumina Human CVD gene chip	rs9939224	*CETP*	A, 0.19	−0.09	6.2×10^{-7}	NA[f]
	– European, 272							
	– South Asian, 330				0.22			
	– Chinese, 304				0.14			

BRIGHT MRC British genetics of hypertension; *CAP* cholesterol and pharmacogenetics; *CETP* cholesteryl ester transfer protein; *Chr* chromosome; *COLQ* collagen-like tail subunit of asymmetric acetylcholinesterase; *CVD* cardiovascular disease; *GRAPHIC* genetic regulation of arterial pressure of humans in the community; *GWAS* genome-wide association study; *HDL* high density lipoprotein; *LCAT* lecithin: cholesteryl acyltransferase; *LIPC* hepatic lipase gene; *LPL* lipoprotein lipase; *MAF* minor allele frequency; *n* number of subjects; *NA* not applicable; *NFBC* Northern Finnish Birth Cohort; *NR1H3* nuclear receptor subfamily 1, group H, member 3; *NS* not statistically significant; *PRINCE* pravastatin inflammation/CRP evaluation; *SHARE* Study of Health Assessment and Risk in Ethnic Groups; *SNP* single nucleotide polymorphism; *WGHS* Women's Genome Health Study

[a]Studies published from January 1, 2007 to July 31, 2009
[b]*P* value for primary test of association
[c]*P* value observed in replication cohort(s)
[d]Effect size in mg/dL
[e]Beta (the effect on the untransformed trait for each copy of the minor allele)
[f]This study was conducted to replicate previously reported genetic associations with plasma lipids in a multi-ethnic cohort

500K GeneChip analysis. Primary associations with HDL cholesterol having a significance value of $P < 1 \times 10^{-5}$ in BRIGHT subjects included rs11017236 ($P = 5.7 \times 10^{-7}$), rs11826048 ($P = 9.7 \times 10^{-7}$), and rs905648 ($P = 4.6 \times 10^{-6}$), which are located on chromosome 10, chromosome 11, and within the *COLQ* (acetylcholinesterase collagenic tail peptide precursor) gene, respectively. However, in a meta-analysis that included genome-wide data from a type 2 diabetes scan [11], these associations were not replicated.

The GWAS of Chasman et al. [12], which was conducted in the Women's Genome Health Study (WGHS) cohort, examined genetic associations with HDL cholesterol, as well as with plasma apolipoprotein (apo) A-I, concentrations in 6,382 women. Replication analysis was conducted in a total

of 970 subjects from two independent cohorts (Table 1). In the primary analysis, SNPs within or near the genes encoding cholesteryl ester transfer protein (*CETP*, rs3764261) and hepatic lipase (*LIPC*, rs1532085) were significantly associated with both plasma apoA-I and HDL cholesterol concentrations, while SNPs within or near the genes encoding lipoprotein lipase (*LPL*, rs331) and *APOA5/APOA1* (rs12225230) were associated with apoA-I but not HDL cholesterol. The most significant association ($P = 1.1 \times 10^{-41}$) observed in the primary analysis was that between the rs3764261 SNP in *CETP* and HDL cholesterol, with an increase in HDL cholesterol of 4 mg/dL associated with the minor allele. Only two of the six genome-wide associations with HDL cholesterol identified in the primary analysis (rs3764261 and rs1532085) were replicated in the independent cohorts. These investigators also compared their results to those of studies that were published during preparation of their manuscript. Replication of the association reported between HDL cholesterol and rs255052 in lecithin:cholesterol acyltransferase (*LCAT*) [13] was observed in the WGHS cohort, while apoA-I, rather than HDL cholesterol [14], was significantly associated with rs4939883 in the region near the endothelial lipase (*LIPG*)/acetyl-Coenzyme A acyltransferase 2 (*ACAA2*) genes. In addition, an alternative SNP near the mevalonate kinase (*MVK*)/methylmalonic aciduria cblB type (*MMAB*) loci confirmed the association with HDL cholesterol reported by Willer et al. [13].

In 2009, Sabatti et al. [15] published GWAS results for nine quantitative metabolic traits, one of which was HDL cholesterol, in subjects from the Northern Finland Birth Cohort 1966 (NFBC1966). Participants in this study were born in the same year and derived from a relatively homogeneous genetic background. All genomic DNA samples were analyzed by Illumina Infinium 370cnvDuo array, and a conservative threshold of significance [16], $P < 5 \times 10^{-7}$, was employed. After applying exclusion criteria and quality control procedures, genotypes on 329,091 SNPs in 4,763 individuals were obtained. Five associations with P values of $< 5 \times 10^{-7}$ were identified with HDL cholesterol. These included SNPs in genes previously known to be associated with HDL cholesterol, rs3764261 ($P = 7.0 \times 10^{-29}$), rs255049 ($P = 3.1 \times 10^{-8}$), and rs1532085 ($P = 1.8 \times 10^{-10}$) in *CETP*, *LCAT*, and *LIPC*, respectively. Two novel associations were also identified: (1) rs2167079 ($P = 5.1 \times 10^{-8}$) and rs7120118 ($P = 3.6 \times 10^{-8}$) in the liver-X-receptor-alpha (*NR1H3*) gene and (2) rs9891572 ($P = 2.3 \times 10^{-7}$) on chromosome 17. Replication of two of the three known, but not the two novel, associations was reported. Genotype data from the NFBC1966 cohort were further evaluated in an attempt to replicate previously reported genetic associations with HDL cholesterol [13, 14]. In addition to the SNPs listed above, SNP associations with UDP-*N*-acetyl-alpha-D-galactosamine:polypeptide *N*-acetylgalactosaminyl-transferase 2 (*GALNT2*), *LPL*, and ATP-binding cassette transporter A1 (*ABCA1*) were replicated at a significance level of $P < 5 \times 10^{-7}$, whereas an association with the *APOA1/C3/A4/A5* gene complex was not observed.

The recent study of Lanktree et al. [17] was designed to address the important issue of replication of genetic associations with plasma lipid traits in subjects of different ethnicities. Samples from subjects in the Study of Health Assessment and Risk in Ethnic Groups (SHARE) were genotyped using the new Illumina cardiovascular disease (CVD) beadchip, which contains ~50,000 SNPs densely mapping ~2,100 genes with a potential role in CVD [18]. The samples consisted of individuals with European ($n = 272$), South Asian ($n = 330$), and Chinese ($n = 304$) ancestry. After false discovery rate correction and permutation analysis, rs9939224 in the *CETP* gene was the only SNP strongly associated ($P = 6.2 \times 10^{-7}$) with HDL cholesterol concentration in SHARE participants. The lack of statistically significant findings in this study was likely due to small sample sizes.

Multiple Cohort GWAS for HDL Cholesterol

Given the complex nature of HDL regulation, the identification of common genetic variants that influence the HDL trait is likely to be facilitated by the evaluation of large sample sizes. GWAS for the HDL cholesterol trait conducted in multiple cohorts are discussed in this section and are summarized in Table 2. In early 2008, Willer et al. [13] reported the results of a combined analysis of three GWA scans involving a total of 8,816 subjects from the Finland–United States Investigation of NIDDM Genetics (FUSION) [19], the SardiNIA Study of Aging [20], and the Diabetes Genetics Initiative (DGI) [11] studies, as well as follow-up analysis in ~11,000 subjects from additional cohorts. In FUSION, 304,581 SNPs with an MAF of >1% from the HumanHap300 Bead Chip and a GoldenGate panel were genotyped in 1,874 Finnish individuals, while genotype data for 4,184 subjects in SardiNIA were generated with the Affymetrix 500K Mapping Array Set. To increase statistical power, data for 347,010 SNPs that had been genotyped in 2,758 participants of the DGI study, the results of which were published in a companion paper and are described in detail below [11], were also included in the analysis. However, only 44,998 SNPs overlapped across the three studies. In order to address this limitation, HapMap data from Utah residents with ancestry from northern and western Europe (CEU) were used to infer missing genotypes *in silico* and to facilitate comparison between the studies. As shown in Table 2, seven loci, all of which have known associations with HDL cholesterol levels, were identified in this study. Of these seven SNPs, those in *CETP* (rs3764261, $P = 2.8 \times 10^{-19}$) and *LPL* (rs12678919, $P = 1.3 \times 10^{-11}$) had the greatest effects on HDL cholesterol concentrations, with increases of 2.4 mg/dL associated with both SNPs. Follow-up analysis of a subset of SNPs in six additional cohorts of European ancestry was next conducted in two stages. After adjustment for multiple testing, the strongest evidence for association with HDL cholesterol was observed with SNPs in the genes encoding *CETP*, *LIPC*, and *LPL*. Novel SNPs associated with HDL cholesterol were also identified in this study, including those in the *LIPG* gene and near the *GALNT2* and *MVK/MMAB* loci.

In the same issue of *Nature Genetics*, Kathiresan et al. [14] reported the results of their GWAS for plasma LDL- and HDL-cholesterol and triglycerides, which was conducted in the same three cohorts (FUSION, SardiNIA, and DGI) as

Table 2 Summary of recent multiple-cohort GWAS for HDL cholesterol[a]

Study	Cohort, n	Genotyping platform	SNP	Nearest gene(s) or region	MAF	Effect size	P
Willer et al. [13]	*GWAS cohorts*						
	FUSION, 1,874	Illumina 317K	rs3764261	*CETP*	A, 0.29	2.4[b]	2.8×10^{-19c}
	SardiNIA, 4,184	Affymetrix 500K	rs12678919	*LPL*	G, 0.12	2.4	1.3×10^{-11}
	DGI, 2,758	Affymetrix 500K	rs10468017	*LIPC*	T, 0.32	1.8	8.6×10^{-11}
			rs1323432	*GRIN3A/PPP3R2*	A, 0.87	1.9	2.5×10^{-8}
	Replication cohorts						
	FUSION, 2,219	Sequenom	rs3764261[d]	*CETP*	A, 0.69	3.5	2.3×10^{-57}
	ISIS, 2,506	Sequenom	rs1864163	*CETP*	G, 0.80	4.1	6.9×10^{-39}
	HAPI, 861	Affymetrix 500K	rs9989419	*CETP*	G, 0.65	1.7	3.2×10^{-31}
	SUVIMAX, 1,551	Illumina 317K	rs12596776	*CETP*	G, 0.13	1.3	2.8×10^{-8}
	BWHHS, 3,358	KASPar	rs1566439	*CETP*	C, 0.45	1.0	3.3×10^{-8}
	Caerphilly, 1,074	KASPar	rs4775041	*LIPC*	C, 0.67	1.4	3.2×10^{-20}
			rs261332	*LIPC*	A, 0.19	1.4	2.3×10^{-15}
			rs10503669	*LPL*	A, 0.10	2.1	4.1×10^{-19}
			rs2197089	*LPL*	A, 0.42	1.4	1.0×10^{-11}
			rs6586891	*LPL*	A, 0.34	1.0	2.9×10^{-9}
			rs2144300	*GALNT2*	T, 0.40	1.1	2.6×10^{-14}
			rs2156552	*LIPG*	T, 0.84	1.2	6.4×10^{-12}
			rs4149268	*ABCA1*	C, 0.36	0.8	1.2×10^{-10}
			rs2338104	*MVK/MMAB*	G, 0.45	0.5	3.4×10^{-8}
Kathiresan et al. [14]	*GWAS cohorts*						
	DGI, 2,758	Affymetrix 500K	rs4846914[d]	*GALNT2*	G, 0.40	−0.07[f]	$2 \times 10^{-13d,f}$
	FUSION, 1,874	Illumina 317K	rs3890182	*ABCA1*	A, 0.13	−0.10	3×10^{-10}
	SardiNIA, 4,184	Affymetrix 500K	rs28927680	*APOA1/C3/A4/A5*	G, 0.07	−0.13	2×10^{-5}
			rs1800775	*CETP*	C, 0.51	−0.18	1×10^{-73}
	Replication cohorts						
	MDC-CC, 5,519	Sequenom, TaqMan	rs1800588	*LIPC*	T, 0.21	+0.14	2×10^{-32}
	FINRISK97, 7,940	Sequenom, TaqMan	rs2156552	*LIPG/ACAA2*	A, 0.18	−0.07	2×10^{-7}
	NORDIL, 5,095	Sequenom, TaqMan	rs328	*LPL*	G, 0.09	+0.17	9×10^{-23}
Kathiresan et al. [21]	*GWAS cohorts*						
	FHS, 7,423	Affymetrix 500K,	rs174547	*FADS1/2/3*	C, 0.33	−0.09[f,g]	2×10^{-12}
		Supplemental 50K	rs2271293	*LCAT*	A, 0.11	+0.07	9×10^{-13}
	LOLIPOP, 1,050	Affymetrix 500K	rs471364	*TTC39B*	C, 0.12	−0.08	3×10^{-10}
	SUVIMAX, 1,551	Illimina 317K	rs1800961	*HNF4A*	T, 0.03	−0.19	8×10^{-10}
	InCHIANTI, 1,132	Illumina 550K	rs7679	*PLTP*	C, 0.19	−0.07	4×10^{-9}
	DGI, 2,626	Affymetrix 500K	rs2967605	*ANGPTL4*	T, 0.16	−0.12	1×10^{-8}
	FUSION, 1,874	Illumina 317K	rs173539	*CETP*	T, 0.32	+0.25	4×10^{-75}
	SardiNIA, 4,184	Affymetrix 500K	rs12678919	*LPL*	G, 0.10	+0.23	2×10^{-34}
			rs10468017	*LIPC*	T, 0.30	+0.10	8×10^{-23}
	Replication cohorts						
	MDC-CC, 5,519	Sequenom, TaqMan	rs4939883	*LIPG*	T, 0.17	−0.14	7×10^{-15}
	FINRISK97, 7,940	Sequenom	rs964184	*APOA1/C3/A4/A5*	G, 0.14	−0.17	1×10^{-12}
	FUSION, 2,224	Sequenom	rs2338104	*MMAB/MVK*	C, 0.45	−0.07	1×10^{-10}
	METSIM, 3,764	Sequenom	rs1883025	*ABCA1*	T, 0.26	−0.08	1×10^{-9}
	ISIS, 2,497	TaqMan	rs4846914	*GALNT2*	G, 0.40	−0.05	4×10^{-8}
Kooner et al. [23]	*GWAS cohorts*						
	Northern Europeans, 1,005	Affymetrix custom array	rs711752	*CETP*			
	Indian Asians, 1,006	Affymetrix custom array					
	Replication cohorts						
	European women, 859	Custom array	rs326	*LPL*	G, 0.70[h]	−2.2[j]	7×10^{-5}
	Indian Asian	Custom array	rs9282541	*ABCA1*	C, 0.00[i]	−3.2	1.1×10^{-5d}
	women, 1,181	Custom array	rs11858164	*LIPC*	T, 0.55	−1.9	3.2×10^{-5}
	Mexican women, 1,560	Custom array	rs2217332	*CETP*	C, 0.14	−1.8	4.6×10^{-5}
	Mexican men, 968	TaqMan	rs711752	*CETP*	A, 0.58	−3.5	5.7×10^{-3}
	TNT women, 1,132	TaqMan	rs7205804	*CETP*	A, 0.56	−3.4	5.2×10^{-38}
	TNT men, 4,836		rs5880	*CETP*	G, 0.05	−6.3	3.1×10^{-44}
			rs5882	*CETP*	G, 0.68	−1.5	2.0×10^{-18}
			rs1800777	*CETP*	G, 0.03	−6.9	5.1×10^{-6}
							1.8×10^{-15}

(continued)

Table 2 (continued)

Study	Cohort, n	Genotyping platform	SNP	Nearest gene(s) or region	MAF	Effect size	P
Heid et al. [25]	*GWAS cohorts*						
	KORA S3/F3, 1,643	Affymetrix 500K	rs9989419	*CETP*	A, 0.39	-2.7^h	8.5×10^{-27k}
	DGI, 2,631	Affymetrix 500K	rs17482753	*LPL*	T, 0.10	+3.7	2.8×10^{-11}
			rs7240405	*LIPG*	A, 0.15	−2.8	4.7×10^{-10}
	Replication cohorts						
	KORA S4, 4,037	iPLEX (Sequenom), Taqman					
	Copenhagen City Heart Study, 9,205	Taqman					
Aulchenko et al. [26]	*GWAS cohorts*						
	ENGAGE cohort, ~17,798–22,562		rs2083637	*LPL*	G, 0.26	+0.11	5.5×10^{-18}
			rs10096633	*LPL*	G, 0.88	−0.14	6.1×10^{-16}
	– ATR	Illumina 318K	rs3905000	*ABCA1*	G, 0.86	+0.11	8.6×10^{-13}
	– DK-TWIN	Illumina 318K	rs7395662	*MADD/FOLH1*	G, 0.61	−0.07	6.0×10^{-11}
	– ERF	Illumina 318K	rs1532085	*LIPC*	G, 0.59	−0.13	9.7×10^{-36}
	– FTC	Illumina 318K	rs1532624	*CETP*	C, 0.57	−0.21	9.4×10^{-94}
	– KORA	Affymetrix 500K	rs2271293	*CTCF/PRMT7*	G, 0.87	−0.13	8.3×10^{-16}
	– MICROS	Illumina 318K	rs4939883	*LIPG*	G, 0.83	+0.10	1.6×10^{-11}
	– NFBC1966	Illumina 370K	rs6754295	*APOB*	C, 0.25	+0.07	4.4×10^{-8}
	– 1966 NSPHS	Illumina 318K					
	– NTR	Illumina 318K					
	– NTRNESDA	Affymetrix 600K					
	– ORCADES	Illumina 318K					
	– Rotterdam Study	Illumina 550K					
	– STR	Illumina 318K					
	– Twin-UK	Illumina 318K					
	– UK-Twin	Illumina 318K					
	– Vis Study	Illumina 318K					

ABCA1 ATP-binding cassette transporter A1; *ACAA2* acetyl-CoA acyltransferase; *APO* apolipoprotein; *ANGPTL4* angiopoietin-like 4; *ATR* Australian Twin Registry; *BWHHS* British Women's Heart and Health Study; *CETP* cholesteryl ester transfer protein; *CTCF* CCCTC-binding factor; *DGI* diabetes genetics initiative; *DK-TWIN* Danish Twin Registry; *ERF* Erasmus Ruchpen Family study; *FADS* fatty acid desaturase; *FHS* Framingham Heart Study; *FOLH1* folate hydrolase 1; *FTC* Finnish Twin Cohort; *FUSION* Finland-United States Investigation of NIDDM Genetics; *GALNT2* UDP-*N*-acetyl-alpha-D-galactosamine:polypeptide *N*-acetylgalactosaminyltransferase 2; *GRIN3A* glutamate receptor, ionotropic, *N*-methyl-D-aspartate 3A; *GWAS* genome-wide association study; *HAPI* heredity and phenotype intervention heart; *HDL* high density lipoprotein ; *HNF4A* hepatocyte nuclear factor 4, alpha; *InCHIANTI* Invecchiare in Chianti; *ISIS* International Study of Infarct Survival; *KASPar* fluorescence-based competitive allele-specific PCR technology (KBiosciences); *KORA* Cooperative Health Research in the Region Augsburg; *LCAT* lecithin:cholesteryl acyltransferase; *LIPC* hepatic lipase gene; *LIPG* endothelial lipase gene; *LOLIPOP* London Life Sciences Population; *LPL* lipoprotein lipase; *MADD* MAP-kinase activating death domain; *MAF* minor allele frequency; *MDC-CC* Malmo Diet and Cancer Study-Cardiovascular Cohort; *METSIM* metabolic syndrome in men; *MICROS* Study of Microisolates in South Tyrol; *MMAB* methylmalonic aciduria cblB type; *MVK* mevalonate kinase; *n* number of subjects; *NFBC* Northern Finnish Birth Cohort; *NORDIL* Nordic Diltiazem Study; *NSPHS* Northern Swedish Population Health Study; *NTR* Netherlands Twin Register; *NTRNESDA* Netherlands Twin Register and the Netherlands Study of Depression and Anxiety; *ORCADES* Orkney Complex Disease Study; *PLTP* phospholipid transfer protein; *PPP3R2* protein phosphatase 3, regulatory subunit B, beta isoform; *PRMT7* protein arginine methyltransferase 7; *SardiNIA* SardiNIA Study of Aging; *SNP* single nucleotide polymorphism; *STR* Swedish Twin Registry; *SUVIMAX* supplementation in vitamins and mineral antioxidants; *TNT* treating to new targets; *TTC39B* tetratricopeptide repeat domain 39B

[a] Studies published from January 1, 2007 to July 31, 2009

[b] Effect size, mg/dL

[c] *P* values exceeding a threshold of 5×10^{-8} (corresponds to a false-positive rate of 0.05 after adjustment for 1 million independent tests)

[d] *P* value for combined analysis

[e] Effect size, beta-coefficient (represents the proportion of 1 standard deviation change)

[f] *P* value for variance-weighted meta-analysis of data from up to four samples (DGI, MDC-CC, FINRISK, and NORDIL)

[g] Effect size and direction from the FHS cohort, the largest of the primary studies

[h] Minor allele frequency data from stage 3 analysis

[i] SNP identified only in subjects of Mexican ancestry (MAF=0.09)

[j] Effect size for the high-risk allele, expressed as percentage change per allele copy (stage 3 analysis)

[k] Pooled probability values for KORA S3/F3, KORA S4, and DGI)

those described by Willer et al. [13]. A targeted replication analysis of 226 SNPs was also conducted in up to 18,554 individuals from three independent cohorts. In addition to confirming known genetic associations with HDL cholesterol (Table 2), a novel association with rs4846914 ($P=2\times10^{-13}$) in the *GALNT2* gene was observed.

In late 2008, the identification of six novel loci associated with HDL cholesterol was reported by Kathiresan et al. [21]. This study involved a meta-analysis of data from seven GWAS for blood lipid phenotypes, as well as follow-up replication analyses in five additional studies. A total of ~2.6 million SNPs that were directly genotyped or imputed were tested for association with lipoprotein traits. Statistical significance was set at $P<5\times10^{-8}$, which is currently defined as the genome-wide significance threshold [22]. This value corresponds to $P<0.05$, after adjusting for ~1 million independent tests. As described in Table 2, newly identified common SNPs associated with HDL cholesterol included those in/near the genes encoding fatty acid desaturases (*FADS1–FADS2–FADS3*), *LCAT*, tetratricopeptide repeat domain 39B (*TTC39B*), hepatic nuclear factor 4-alpha (*HNF4A*), phospholipid transfer protein (*PLTP*), and angiopoietin-like 4 (*ANGPTL4*). With the exception of the rs2271293 SNP in *LCAT*, the minor allele of each SNP was associated with increased HDL cholesterol relative to major allele homozygotes. To better understand the biological significance of their findings, these investigators further explored whether these SNPs, the majority of which are noncoding, might influence gene expression as *cis*-acting regulators of nearby genes. In an elegant set of experiments, genotyping of DNA and RNA expression profiling of >39,000 transcripts was performed in 957 human liver tissue samples. Quantitative trait locus analysis was conducted by relating each SNP with liver transcripts located within 500 kb to either side of the SNP. In most instances, consistency between the direction of effect on transcript levels and HDL cholesterol concentration was observed, providing strong evidence that, when conducted carefully, GWA has the capacity to generate biologically meaningful data.

In an attempt to identify SNPs associated with components of the metabolic syndrome, Kooner et al. [23] genotyped ~267,000 SNPs in 1,005 Northern Europeans and ~248,000 SNPs in 1,006 Indian Asians who had metabolic syndrome, as defined by Adult Treatment Panel III guidelines [24]. Of the ~200,000 SNPs that were successfully genotyped in these cohorts, only a single SNP in the *CETP* gene, rs711752, showed genome-wide significance with HDL cholesterol in Europeans, but not Indian Asians, after correction for multiple testing. In stage 2 of their analysis, these investigators selected SNPs that showed equivocal significance in the original GWA ($<10^{-4}$ in either scan or $<10^{-2}$ in either scan if in the vicinity of known genes having potential functional significance) for further testing in larger cohorts. A total of 656 SNPs were successfully genotyped in a total of 4,568 individuals from four different cohorts. In stage 3, 15 SNPs associated with HDL cholesterol were genotyped in ~6,000 subjects. Nine SNPs, six of which are located in or near the *CETP* gene, were significantly ($P<8\times10^{-5}$) associated with HDL cholesterol. The other three SNPs were located in the genes encoding *ABCA1*, *LIPC*, and *LPL* (Table 2). Novel genetic associations with HDL cholesterol were not identified in this study.

Novel SNPs in two genes known to play important roles in HDL metabolism, *CETP* and *LIPG*, were identified in the GWA study of Heid et al. [25], which was conducted in 1,643 subjects from the Cooperative Health Research Region of Augsburg study and complemented by publicly available data from the DGI study [11]. Replication analysis was conducted in >13,000 individuals from two independent cohorts. Consistent associations were observed between HDL cholesterol and rs9989419 ($P=8.5\times10^{-27}$), which is located ~10 kb upstream of the *CETP* gene, and rs7240405 ($P=4.7\times10^{-10}$), which is located ~40 kb downstream of the *LIPG* gene. In addition, an SNP previously shown to be associated with HDL cholesterol, rs17482753 in *LPL*, was also identified.

In the most extensive GWA analysis conducted to date, Aulchenko et al. [26] conducted a meta-analysis of GWA data generated from 16 population-based cohorts (≤22,562 individuals, aged 18–104). In most cases, genotyping data for these studies was generated using the Infinium II assay on HumanHap300-Duo Genotyping BeadChips. As shown in Table 2, eight regions showed genome-wide significance ($P<5\times10^{-8}$) with HDL, including two novel loci near the CCCTC-binding factor (*CTCF*)/protein arginine methyltransferase (*PRMT7*) (rs2271293, $P=8.3\times10^{-16}$) and map kinase-activating death domain (*MADD*)/folate hydrolase 1 (*FOLH1*) (rs7395662, $P=6.0\times10^{-11}$) genes. The potential role that these loci may play in HDL metabolism is not immediately obvious. With respect to the *MADD/FOLH1* locus on chromosome 11p, the *NR1H3* gene, in which a SNP was associated with HDL cholesterol in the NFBC cohort [15], is located 0.5 kb telomeric of the *MADD* gene. Included among the known genes associated with HDL cholesterol in this study are those encoding for *ABCA1*, *CETP*, *LIPC*, *LIPG*, and *LPL*.

Summary and Conclusions

SNPs within/near genes known to play important roles in HDL metabolism, such as those encoding *ABCA1*, *CETP*, and *LIPC*, are consistently identified in GWAS as having highly significant associations with HDL cholesterol concentrations (Table 3, Figs. 1–8). In each of the multiple cohort GWAS

Table 3 Summary of previously known genetic associations with HDL cholesterol identified by GWAS

Gene	Role in HDL metabolism	Comments
ABCA1 (see Fig. 1)	Promotes net cholesterol efflux to lipid-poor apoA-I Essential for *de novo* HDL synthesis	Identified in five GWAS for HDL cholesterol [13, 14, 21, 23, 26]
APOA1/C3/A4/A5 (see Fig. 2)	Apolipoproteins are important structural components of lipoproteins ApoA-I is an activator of LCAT activity ApoC-III inhibits LPL activity	Identified in two GWAS for HDL cholesterol [14, 21]
CETP (see Fig. 3)	Facilitates the transfer of cholesteryl esters from HDL to apoB-containing lipoproteins in exchange for triglycerides Decreased CETP activity is associated with increased HDL cholesterol levels	The most statistically significant genetic association with HDL cholesterol observed in the majority of GWAS [12–15, 17, 21, 23, 25, 26]
LCAT (see Fig. 4)	Converts free cholesterol into cholesteryl ester Key enzyme in the HDL maturation process Decreased LCAT activity is associated with reduced HDL cholesterol levels	Identified in two GWAS for HDL cholesterol [15, 21]
LIPC (see Fig. 5)	Hydrolyzes triglyceride and phospholipids on lipoproteins Serves as a ligand/bridging factor for receptor-mediated lipoprotein uptake Decreased hepatic lipase (*LIPC*) activity is associated with increased HDL cholesterol levels	Consistently identified as having genome-wide significance for HDL cholesterol [12–15, 21, 23, 26]
LIPG (see Fig. 6)	Primarily hydrolyzes phospholipids with little triglyceride lipase activity Serves as a ligand/bridging factor for receptor-mediated lipoprotein uptake Decreased endothelial lipase (*LIPG*) activity is associated with increased HDL cholesterol levels	Consistently identified as having genome-wide significance for HDL cholesterol [13, 14, 21, 25, 26] Deep resequencing of *LIPG* exons in cases with elevated HDL cholesterol (≥95th percentile for age and gender) and controls with decreased HDL cholesterol (≤25th percentile for age and gender) demonstrated that loss-of-function mutations in *LIPG* lead to increased HDL cholesterol levels [27]
LPL (see Fig. 7)	Primarily hydrolyzes triglycerides with little phospholipase activity Serves as a ligand/bridging factor for receptor-mediated lipoprotein uptake Decreased LPL activity is associated with decreased HDL cholesterol levels	Consistently identified as having genome-wide significance for HDL cholesterol [13, 14, 21, 23, 25, 26]
PLTP (see Fig. 8)	Transfers phospholipids from triglyceride-rich lipoproteins to HDL Generates pre-beta-HDL during conversion of HDL Decreased PLTP activity is associated with increased HDL cholesterol levels	Identified in one GWAS for HDL cholesterol [21]

ABCA1 ATP-binding cassette transporter A1; *apo* apolipoprotein; *CETP* cholesteryl ester transfer protein; *GWAS* genome-wide association study; *HDL* high density lipoprotein; *LCAT* lecithin:cholesterol acyltransferase; *LIPC* hepatic lipase gene; *LIPG* endothelial lipase gene; *LPL* lipoprotein lipase; *PLTP* phospholipid transfer protein

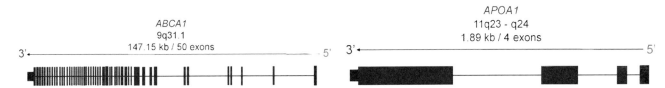

Fig. 1 Schematic representation of the ATP-binding cassette transporter A1 (*ABCA1*) gene. The *ABCA1* gene, located on chromosome 9, consists of 50 exons. Translated regions (exons) are depicted by *blue boxes*. Untranslated regions are indicated by *red boxes*

Fig. 2 Schematic representation of the apolipoprotein A-I (*APOA1*) gene. The *APOA1* gene, located on chromosome 11, consists of four exons. Translated regions (exons) are depicted by *blue boxes*. Untranslated regions are indicated by *red boxes*

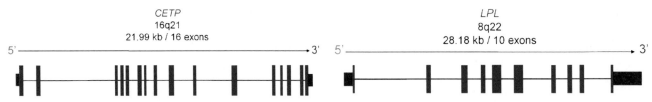

Fig. 3 Schematic representation of the cholesteryl ester transfer protein (*CETP*) gene. The *CETP* gene, located on chromosome 15, consists of 16 exons. Translated regions (exons) are depicted by *blue boxes*. Untranslated regions are indicated by *red boxes*

Fig. 7 Schematic representation of the lipoprotein lipase (*LPL*) gene. The *LPL* gene, located on chromosome 8, consists of ten exons. Translated regions (exons) are depicted by *blue boxes*. Untranslated regions are indicated by *red boxes*

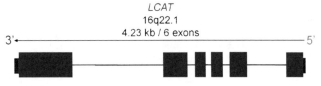

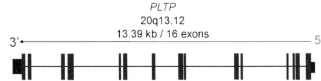

Fig. 4 Schematic representation of the lecithin:cholesterol acyltransferase (*LCAT*) gene. The *LCAT* gene, located on chromosome 16, consists of six exons. Translated regions (exons) are depicted by *blue boxes*. Untranslated regions are indicated by *red boxes*.

Fig. 8 Schematic representation of the phospholipid transfer protein (*PLTP*) gene. The *PLTP* gene, located on chromosome 20, consists of 16 exons. Translated regions (exons) are depicted by *blue boxes*. Untranslated regions are indicated by *red boxes*

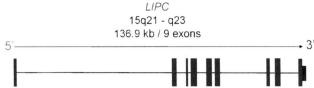

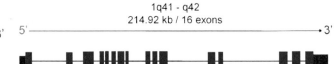

Fig. 5 Schematic representation of the hepatic lipase (*LIPC*) gene. The *LIPC* gene, located on chromosome 15, consists of nine exons. Translated regions (exons) are depicted by *blue boxes*. Untranslated regions are indicated by *red boxes*

Fig. 9 Schematic representation of the *N*-acetylgalactosaminyltransferase 2 (*GALNT2*) gene. The *GALNT2* gene, located on chromosome 1, consists of 16 exons. Translated regions (exons) are depicted by *blue boxes*. Untranslated regions are indicated by *red boxes*

summarized in Table 2, SNPs within/near the *CETP* gene have the most statistically significant associations with HDL cholesterol. This finding not only validates GWA methodology but also highlights the impact that CETP has in the regulation of HDL cholesterol concentrations at the population level. Only a few novel genetic associations with HDL cholesterol have been identified in GWAS (Table 4, Fig. 9). Of these, SNPs in *GALNT2* [13, 14, 21] and near *MVK/MMAB* [13, 21] have been identified in at least two studies. The lack of novel loci identified thus far, together with the relatively small effect sizes associated with both known and novel loci, suggest that much remains to be discovered about the genetic determinants of HDL cholesterol concentrations.

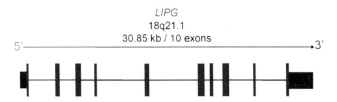

Fig. 6 Schematic representation of the endothelial lipase (*LIPG*) gene. The *LIPG* gene, located on chromosome 18, consists of ten exons. Translated regions (exons) are depicted by *blue boxes*. Untranslated regions are indicated by *red boxes*

Table 4 Summary of novel genetic associations with HDL cholesterol identified by GWAS

Gene	Proposed role in HDL metabolism	Comments
ANGPTL4	ANGPTL4 appears to inhibit LPL activity; decreased LPL activity is associated with decreased HDL cholesterol levels	Identified in 1 GWAS for HDL cholesterol [21] Inhibits LPL in mice [28], leading to increased triglycerides Population-based resequencing of ANGPTL4 in >3,000 subjects identified common genetic variants associated with reduced triglycerides and increased HDL [29]
CTCF/PRMT7	Unknown Located on chromosome 16q22.1, the CTCF and PRMT7 genes encode a transcriptional regulator potentially involved in hormone-dependent gene silencing and an arginine methyltransferase, respectively	Identified in 1 GWAS for HDL cholesterol [26] Not associated with HDL cholesterol in any other GWAS
FADS1/2/3	Fatty acids desaturases convert polyunsaturated fatty acids into cell signaling metabolites, such as arachidonic acid Omega-3 polyunsaturated fatty acids, key substrates for FADS1, can reduce plasma triglycerides, which may, in turn, increase HDL cholesterol	Showed association with both HDL cholesterol and triglycerides in the GWAS of Kathiresan et al. [21]
GALNT2 (see Fig. 9)	Encodes UDP-N-acetyl-alpha-D-galactosamine: polypeptide N-acetylgalactosaminyltransferase 2, an enzyme involved in O-linked glycosylation and transfer of N-acetylgalactosamine May modify apolipoproteins, lipoprotein receptors, or transfer proteins/enzymes (i.e., endothelial lipase, hepatic lipase)	Identified in three GWAS for HDL cholesterol [13, 14, 21] Also associated with plasma triglyceride levels [15]
MADD/FOLH1	Unknown	Identified in one GWAS for HDL cholesterol [26]; however, the gene for LXRA (NR1H3), which was associated with HDL cholesterol in the GWAS of Sabatti et al. [15], is located in close proximity to MADD
MVK/MMAB	Unknown Encode enzymes involved in cholesterol synthesis (MVK) and degradation (MMAB) Share a common promoter and are both regulated by by SREBP2	Identified in two GWAS for HDL cholesterol [13, 21]
NR1H3	Encodes liver-X-receptor-alpha (LXRA), which is involved in the transcriptional regulation of many genes involved in HDL metabolism (i.e., ABCA1, CETP)	Not identified in any other GWAS; however, loci near NR1H3 associated with HDL cholesterol in the GWAS of Sabatti et al. [15]
TTC39B	Unknown	Analysis of human liver tissue samples demonstrated that the allele associated with lower TTC39B transcript levels was also associated with higher HDL cholesterol [21]

ANGPTL4 angiopoietin-like 4; CETP cholesteryl ester transfer protein; CTCF CCCTC-binding factor; FADS fatty acid desaturase; FOLH1 folate hydrolase 1; GALNT2 UDP-N-acetyl-alpha-D-galactosamine:polypeptide N-acetylgalactosaminyltransferase 2; GWAS genome-wide association; HDL high density lipoprotein; LPL lipoprotein lipase; MADD MAP-kinase activating death domain; MMAB methylmalonic aciduria cblB type; MVK mevalonate kinase; NR1H3 nuclear receptor subfamily 1, group H, member 3; PRMT7 protein arginine methyltransferase 7; SREBP2 sterol-responsive element-binding protein 2; TTC39B tetratricopeptide repeat domain 39B

References

1. Miller GJ, Miller NE (1975) Plasma high density lipoprotein concentration and development of ischaemic heart-disease. Lancet 1:16–25
2. Gordon DJ, Probstfield JL, Garrison RJ et al (1989) High density lipoprotein cholesterol and cardiovascular disease: four prospective American studies. Circulation 79:8–15
3. Stampfer MJ, Sacks FM, Salvini S, Willett WC, Hennekens CH (1991) A prospective study of cholesterol, apolipoproteins and the risk of myocardial infarction. N Engl J Med 325:373–381
4. Goldbourt U, Yaari S, Medalie JH (1997) Isolated low HDL cholesterol as a risk factor for coronary heart disease. Arterioscler Thromb Vasc Biol 17:107–113
5. Heller DA, DeFaire D, Pedersen NL, Dahlen G, McClearn GE (1993) Genetic and environmental influences on serum lipid levels in twins. N Engl J Med 328:1150–1156
6. Kathiresan S, Musunuru K, Orho-Melander M (2008) Defining the spectrum of alleles that contribute to blood lipid concentrations in humans. Curr Opin Lipid 19:122–127
7. Hegele RA (2009) Plasma lipoproteins: genetic influences and clinical implications. Nat Rev Genet 10:109–121
8. Kathiresan S, Manning AK, Demissie S et al (2007) A genome-wide association study for blood lipid phenotypes in the Framingham Heart Study. BMC Med Genet 8(Suppl 1):S17
9. Herbert A, Gerry NP, McQueen MB et al (2006) A common genetic variant is associated with adult and childhood obesity. Science 312:279–283

10. Wallace C, Newhouse SJ, Braund P et al (2008) Genome-wide association study identifies genes for biomarkers of cardiovascular disease: serum urate and dyslipidemia. Am J Hum Genet 82:139–149

11. Saxena R, Voight BF, Lyssenko V et al (2007) Genome-wide association analysis identifies loci for type 2 diabetes and triglyceride levels. Science 316:1331–1336

12. Chasman DI, Pare G, Zee RYL et al (2008) Genetic loci associated with plasma concentration of low-density lipoprotein cholesterol, high-density lipoprotein cholesterol, triglycerides, apolipoprotein A1, and apolipoprotein B among 6382 white women in genome-wide analysis with replication. Circ Cardiovasc Genet 1:21–30

13. Willer CJ, Sanna S, Jackson AU et al (2008) Newly identified loci that influence lipid concentrations and risk of coronary artery disease. Nat Genet 40:161–169

14. Kathiresan S, Melander O, Guiducci C et al (2008) Six new loci associated with blood low-density lipoprotein cholesterol, high-density lipoprotein cholesterol or triglycerides in humans. Nat Genet 40:189–197

15. Sabatti C, Service SK, Hartikainen AL et al (2009) Genome-wide association analysis of metabolic traits in a birth cohort from a founder population. Nat Genet 41:35–46

16. Benjamini Y, Hochberg Y (1995) Controlling the false discovery rate: a practical and powerful approach to multiple testing. J R Stat Soc Ser 57:289–300

17. Lanktree MB, Anand SS, Yusuf S, Hegele RA (2009) Replication of genetic associations with plasma lipoprotein traits in a multiethnic sample. J Lipid Res 50:1487–1496

18. Keating BJ, Tischfield S, Murray SS et al (2008) Concept, design and implementation of a cardiovascular gene-centric 50 k SNP array for large-scale genomic association studies. PLoS One 3:e3583

19. Scott LJ, Mohlke KL, Bonnycastle LL et al (2007) A genome-wide association study of type 2 diabetes in Finns detects multiple susceptibility variants. Science 316:1341–1345

20. Pilia G, Chen WM, Scuteri A et al (2006) Heritability of cardiovascular and personality traits in 6,148 Sardinians. PLoS Genet 2:e132

21. Kathiresan S, Willer CJ, Peloso GM et al (2009) Common variants at 30 loci contribute to polygenic dyslipidemia. Nat Genet 41:56–65

22. The International HapMap Consortium (2005) A haplotype map of the human genome. Nature 437:1299–1320

23. Kooner JS, Chambers JC, Aguilar-Salinas CA et al (2008) Genome-wide scan identifies variation in MLXIPL associated with plasma triglycerides. Nat Genet 40:149–151

24. Grundy SM, Brewer HB Jr, Cleeman JI, Smith SC Jr, Lenfant C (2004) Definition of metabolic syndrome: report of the National Heart, Lung, and Blood Institute/American Heart Association conference on scientific issues related to definition. Arterioscler Thromb Vasc Biol 24:e13–e18

25. Heid IM, Boes E, Muller M et al (2008) Genome-wide association analysis of high-density lipoprotein cholesterol in the population-based KORA study sheds new light on intergenic regions. Circ Cardiovasc Genet 1:10–20

26. Aulchenko YS, Ripatti S, Lindqvist I et al (2009) Loci influencing lipid levels and coronary heart disease risk in 16 European population cohorts. Nat Genet 41:47–55

27. Edmondson AC, Brown RJ, Kathiresan S et al (2009) Loss-of-function variants in endothelial lipase are a cause of elevated HDL cholesterol in humans. J Clin Invest 119:1042–1050

28. Yoshida K, Shimizugawa T, Ono M, Furukawa H (2002) Angiopoietin-like protein 4 is a potent hyperlipidemia-inducing factor in mice and inhibitor of lipoprotein lipase. J Lipid Res 43:1770–1772

29. Romeo S, Pennacchio LA, Fu Y et al (2007) Population-based resequencing of ANGPTL4 uncovers variations that reduce triglycerides and increase HDL. Nat Genet 39:513–516

Nutritional and Lifestyle Factors and High-Density Lipoprotein Metabolism

Ernst J. Schaefer

Introduction

Much of the cholesterol in plasma is synthesized in the body. Markers of cholesterol synthesis include lathosterol and desmosterol, precursors in the pathway (see Fig. 1). Cholesterol synthesis is increased in obese subjects. Cholesterol is also obtained from the diet via cholesterol absorption, with major diet sources being meats, dairy products, and eggs. Cholesterol is absorbed via the Niemann–Pick C1-Like 1 Protein (NPC1L1) transporter in the intestine, and then can either be transported into the lymph and then into plasma on both chylomicrons and HDL made in the intestine, or be resecreted back into the intestinal lumen via the ATP-binding cassette (ABC) transporters G5 and G8 (see Fig. 2). On average, about 50% of cholesterol is retained in the intestinal cell and placed on lipoproteins, with the remainder being transported back into the intestinal lumen. Dietary fatty acids are very efficiently absorbed by the intestine (about 95%). The essential fatty acids linoleic acid (18:2n6) and alpha linolenic acid (18:3n3) must be obtained from the diet and cannot be synthesized in the body. Linoleic acid can be converted to arachidonic acid (20:4n6), which has thrombotic and inflammatory properties. Alpha linolenic acid can be converted into eicosapentaenoic acid (EPA, 20:5n3) and docosahexaenoic acid (DHA, 22:6n3). EPA has anti-thrombotic and anti-inflammatory properties, while DHA is important for maintaining the fluidity of membranes (see Fig. 3).

An overview of lipoprotein metabolism is shown in Fig. 4. Chylomicrons, very rich in triglycerides enter the lymph, and then the plasma space. The production of intestinal apolipoprotein (apo) B-48 is about 2 mg/kg/day. Once chylomicrons enter the plasma, their triglyceride is rapidly removed via lipolysis in the capillary bed through the action of lipoprotein lipase. The triglyceride in the core of these particles is replaced by cholesteryl ester via the action of

cholesteryl ester transfer protein (CETP). During this process atherogenic chylomicron remnants are formed, which are removed with a residence time of about 5 h. The amount of cholesteryl ester delivered to the liver by chylomicron remnants is dependent about the amount placed in these particles via the intestine (dependent on dietary intake and absorption), and the amount transferred to chylomicrons from HDL via CETP. This amount is increased when lipolysis is impaired or clearance is delayed as in diabetes and/or hypertriglyceridemia. The same thing occurs when very-low-density lipoproteins (VLDLs) are converted into low-density lipoproteins. If HDL cholesteryl ester transfer is enhanced, then HDL never matures from small particles to large particles (see Figs. 5 and 6). Low HDL is usually associated with decreased large HDL and elevated triglyceride-rich lipoproteins. In this situation HDL apoA-I production is normal, but fractional clearance is enhanced.

Effects of Dietary Cholesterol

Nicolosi et al., Stucchi et al., and Hennessy et al. have examined the effects of isolated increased dietary cholesterol in Cebus monkeys [1–3]. They documented that high cholesterol intake was associated with significant increases in: (1) hepatic cholesterol content, (2) hepatic apoA-I mRNA levels, (3) apoA-I production as assessed by tracer studies, and (4) increased HDL cholesterol and apoA-I levels in plasma as compared to low cholesterol diets [1–3]. In human studies, Lichtenstein et al. have documented that increasing dietary cholesterol from less than 200 mg/day to over 400 mg/day results in statistically significant increases in both LDL cholesterol and HDL cholesterol of about 10%, respectively [4]. Studies by Velez-Carrasco have shown that diets restricted in cholesterol and saturated fat in humans are associated with significant reductions in HDL cholesterol and apoA-I levels in plasma, due to decreased apoA-I production rates [5]. The overall data are consistent with the concept that dietary cholesterol increases apoA-I secretion via directly stimulating

E.J. Schaefer (✉)
Lipid Metabolism Laboratory, Tufts University,
711 Washington Street, Boston, MA 02111, USA
e-mail: ernst.schaefer@tufts.edu

Fig. 1 A diagram showing the final steps in cholesterol synthesis from squalene to lanosterol then to either desmosterol or lathosterol, both of which can be converted to cholesterol. Elevated lathosterol and desmosterol levels in plasma serve as markers of increased cholesterol synthesis in the body

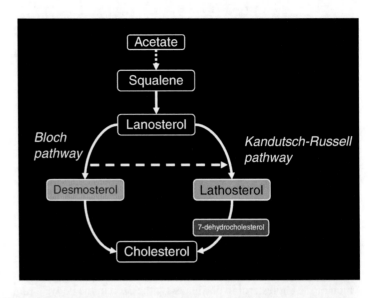

Fig. 2 A diagram showing intestinal cholesterol absorption, with cholesterol entering the intestinal cell via Niemann–Pick C1-Like 1 Protein (NPC1L1), and being excreted back into the lumen of the intestine via the ATP-binding cassette transporters (ABC) ABCG5 and ABCG8 or being placed onto chylomicrons or high-density lipoproteins

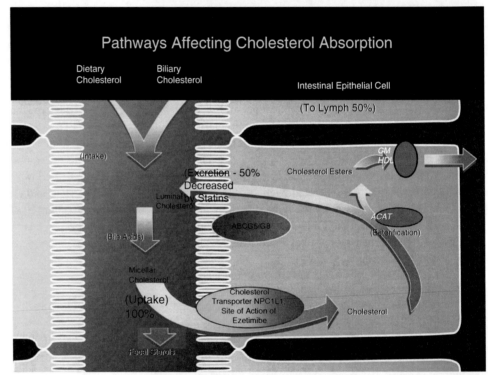

Fig. 3 The conversion of linoleic acid (18:2n6) into arachidonic acid and alpha linolenic acid (18:3n3) into eicosapentaenoic (20:5n3) and docosahexaenoic acid (22:6n3) are shown. The body cannot place a double bond at the n3 or n6 position. Therefore, linoleic acid and alpha linolenic acid must be obtained from the diet. Vegetable oils are rich in these fatty acids. EPA and DHA also can be obtained directly by consuming oily fish or fish oil

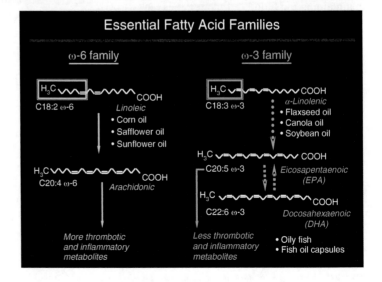

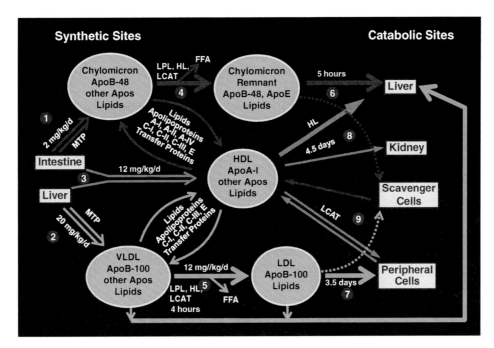

Fig. 4 A model of human lipoprotein metabolism is shown in which chylomicrons are converted to chylomicron remnant particles, which are then taken up by the liver via binding of apoE to the LDL receptor over a 4–5 h period. The liver makes very-low-density lipoproteins which can be converted into large and small LDL, which is cleared from the plasma over about 4 days. LDL is removed from the plasma by the liver and other tissues over about 3.5 days. HDLs are made in both the liver and intestine, and the HDL apoA-I has a plasma residence day of about 4.5 days (see ref. [39])

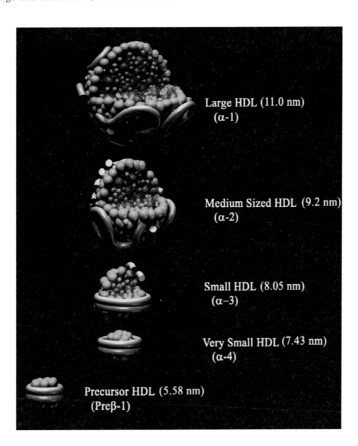

Fig. 5 Models of high-density lipoprotein particles as isolated by two-dimensional gel electrophoresis are shown as separated by charge (pre-beta and alpha mobility) in the horizontal dimension and by size (5.5–11 nm in diameter) in the vertical dimension. Very small discoidal precursor pre-beta-1 HDL (5.58 nm in diameter), very small discoidal alpha-4 HDL (7.43 nm in diameter), small spherical alpha-3 HDL (8.05 nm in diameter), medium-sized spherical alpha-2 HDL (9.2 nm), and large spherical 1 alpha-1 HDL (11.0 nm) particles are shown. All particles contain apoA-I, but small alpha-3 and medium-sized alpha-2 HDL also contain apoA-II. Patients with coronary heart disease often have elevated levels of precursor pre-beta-1 and very small alpha-4 HDL, and decreased levels of medium-sized alpha-2 and large spherical alpha-1 HDL. Created by Mr. Martin Jacob. Courtesy of Boston Heart Lab Corporation, Framingham, MA, USA

Fig. 6 An overview of HDL
particle metabolism documenting
the conversion of very small
pre-beta-1 HDL to larger HDL
particles, and the potential for
cholesteryl ester on larger HDL
to either be transferred to
triglyceride-rich lipoproteins
(TRL) or to be taken up by the
liver via scavenger receptor B1
(SR-B1). The apoA-I can then
recycle back to smaller particles
or be catabolized via the kidney

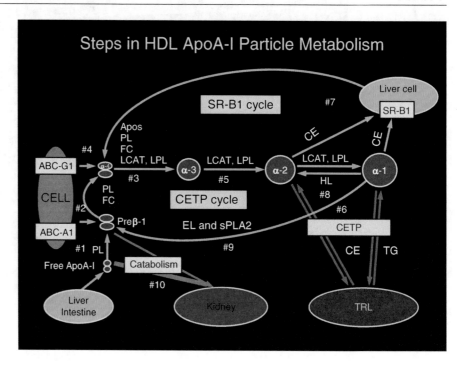

increases in hepatic apoA-I mRNA levels, which in turn were
linked to increased hepatic cellular cholesteryl ester content
[1–3]. These data suggest that there is upregulation of hepatic
apoA-I mRNA when there is an increased need for cellular
cholesterol efflux [1–5].

Effects of Dietary Fatty Acids

Information about fatty acids is provided in the introductory
chapter by Dr. Schaefer. Schaefer et al. reported marked
reductions in both LDL cholesterol and HDL cholesterol in
humans when saturated fat was replaced by polyunsaturated
fat [6]. Lichtenstein et al. reported similar results when saturated fat-rich oil was replaced by polyunsaturated fat-rich oil
in humans [7]. Brousseau et al. examined the effects of diets
high in saturated fat, monounsaturated fat, and polyunsaturated fat (constant dietary cholesterol content) on plasma
HDL cholesterol and apoA-I levels, hepatic apoA-I mRNA
levels, and plasma apoA-I kinetics in cynomolgus monkeys
[8, 9]. HDL cholesterol and apoA-I levels were lowest on the
high polyunsaturated fat diet, highest on the saturated fat
diet, with intermediate levels on the high monounsaturated
fat diet. There were no differences in hepatic cholesterol or
apoA-I mRNA levels, and kinetic studies revealed significant
differences in plasma apoA-I fractional catabolic rates to
account for these differences [8, 9]. The data discussed
pertain mainly to the n6 fatty acids, particularly linoleic acid
(18:2n6) and arachidonic acid (20:4n6).

Spady et al. have examined the effects of a control chow diet,
a high saturated fat (coconut) diet , a high polyunsaturated
fat (safflower oil) diet, and then the same latter diets also

high in cholesterol (0.08%) in hamsters [10]. Animals on the
high polyunsaturated fat diet had significantly lower HDL
cholesterol levels and about 50% higher liver SR-BI mRNA
and protein levels, higher relative delivery of HDL cholesteryl esters to the liver than animals on the high saturated fat
diets [10]. Their major conclusion was that substituting
polyunsaturated fatty acids for saturated fat lowered HDL
cholesterol, and increased HDL cholesterol delivery to the
liver and liver cholesterol content, but had no effect on overall reverse cholesterol transport in this animal model under
the conditions tested [10]. The overall data are consistent
with the concept that replacing saturated fatty acids with
omega 6 polyunsaturated fatty acids in the diet lowers HDL
levels, by upregulating HDL apoA-I fractional catabolic rate
and SR-B1 gene expression, which may account for the beneficial effects of polyunsaturated fats in CHD risk reduction,
along with LDL reduction [8–10].

Randomized dietary trials support the concept that replacing saturated fat with polyunsaturated in the diet – as was
done in the Oslo Diet Heart Study, the Los Angeles Veterans
Affairs Study, and the Finnish Mental Hospital Study – can
significantly reduce the risk of coronary heart disease (CHD)
morbidity and mortality [11–13]. The overall data in animals and humans suggest that restricting dietary cholesterol
lowers LDL apoB by enhancing its fractional catabolism,
and lowers HDL apoA-I by decreasing its production.
Replacing saturated fat with polyunsaturated fat (mainly the
omega-6 fatty acid linoleic acid) will lower both LDL apoB-
100 and HDL apoA-I by enhancing their fractional catabolism. Replacing animal fat with vegetable fat is a powerful
modality for CHD risk reduction even though HDL cholesterol levels may be reduced.

The effects of omega-3 fatty acids on HDL metabolism appear to be somewhat different than those of omega-6 fatty acids. Frenais et al. have reported in six diabetic subjects that six 1-g omega-3 fatty acid capsules (MaxEpa) per day significantly lowered plasma triglyceride levels, with no effect on apoA-I or apoA-II plasma levels, but significant reductions in both the production of HDL apoA-I and apoA-II, as well as their fractional catabolism [14]. Chan et al. reported similar findings for fish oil in 12 men with increased waist circumference studied on placebo and on fish oil (Omacor 4 capsules/day) [15]. These data indicate that in contrast to omega-6 fatty acids, such as linoleic acid which enhance HDL apoA-I fractional clearance, omega-3 fatty acids, specifically eicosapentaenoic acid and docosahexaenoic acid, have the opposite effect of delaying fractional clearance, but also lowering apoA-I production [14, 15]. Moreover, we have recently observed that omega-3 fatty acid supplements have very beneficial effects in increasing large protective HDL particles.

Effects of Dietary Carbohydrates

Schaefer et al. examined the effects of a virtually fat-free, high carbohydrate diet in humans relative to an average American diet in humans, and reported the low-fat, high carbohydrate diet lowered LDL cholesterol and HDL cholesterol each by approximately 30%, respectively [6]. Schaefer et al. subsequently reported similar finding with diets restricted in total fat, saturated fat, and cholesterol, even along with weight loss [16–19]. Dansinger et al. have reported that diets restricted in calories that promote weight loss, will raise HDL cholesterol provided there is carbohydrate restriction [20].

Blum et al. carried out kinetic studies in humans and reported that high carbohydrate, low-fat diets reduced HDL cholesterol and apoA-I levels significantly, associated with significant increases in the HDL apoA-I fractional catabolic rate, with no effect on HDL apoA-I production [21]. Brinton et al., in contrast, reported that low-fat, high carbohydrate diets lowered HDL apoA-I by decreasing production [22]. However, this diet was also low in cholesterol [22]. Velez-Carrasco et al., reported that a National Cholesterol Education Program step 2 diet containing less than 200 mg/day of cholesterol, less than 7% of calories as saturated fat, and less than 30% of calories as total fat, significantly lowered plasma apoA-I levels as compared to an average American diet (higher in cholesterol, saturated fat, and total fat, due to decreased production (22).

Just as there are differences in fatty acids, there are also differences in dietary carbohydrate. Absorbed glucose tends to be utilized in the periphery, while absorbed fructose is taken up by the liver and generally utilized for fatty acid synthesis or triglyceride storage in the liver [23]. Therefore, high-fructose diets appear to have an even more deleterious effect on increasing abdominal adiposity, insulin resistance, and triglyceride levels and lowering HDL levels, than does dietary glucose [24].

In animal studies, Woolett et al. examined the effects of control chow diets, diets high in carbohydrate and low in cholesterol and saturated fat, the same diet supplemented with fiber, as well as a diet high in saturated fat and cholesterol (Western diet) in hamsters [25, 26]. In these studies, the Western diet was associated with 46% higher plasma HDL cholesteryl esters and 25% higher apoA-I levels than the control diet, and 86 and 45% higher values than the high-fiber diet. These differences were all due to differences in HDL cholesteryl ester and apoA-I entry into plasma versus differences in plasma clearance rates [25, 26]. Woolett et al. concluded that the dietary modifications studies altered plasma HDL cholesterol levels due to changes in production, and not due alterations in the transport of HDL cholesteryl esters to the liver [25, 26].

The combined data suggest that when there is no change in dietary cholesterol or fatty acid content in the diet, and when a substantial amount of fat in the diet is replaced isocalorically by carbohydrate, there are usually elevation in TRL, and HDL apoA-I decreases due to enhanced fractional catabolism, associated with increased HDL cholesteryl ester transfer to TRL. These data are consistent with observations that HDL apoA-I fractional catabolic rates are increased in patients with hypertriglyceridemia. In contrast, when there is only modest replacement of fat with carbohydrate, and significant restriction of dietary cholesterol and saturated fat, the primary mechanism whereby plasma apoA-I is reduced is by decreased apoA-I production, with little or no change in TRL concentration. This latter effect is probably mediated by less need for reverse cellular cholesterol efflux in the setting of dietary cholesterol restriction.

Effects of Diets Restricted in Cholesterol and Saturated Fat

Schaefer et al. has reported that diets restricted in cholesterol and saturated fat in humans reduce HDL cholesterol, almost as much as LDL cholesterol [6, 16–18]. Velez-Carrasco et al. related such changes to decreased HDL apoA-I production, as did Brinton et al. [5, 22]. Asztalos et al. reported that such diets were associated with reductions in the large protective HDL apoA-I concentrations only in those with normal HDL cholesterol concentrations, but not those with decreased HDL cholesterol values [27]. As previously mentioned, the plasma apoA-I levels in this setting are reduced because of decreased apoA-I production, and it may be that those with normal levels of HDL on an atherogenic diet, have been able to upregulate apoA-I production, while those with low HDL are unable to do so [5].

Effects of Weight Loss

Weight loss can have variable effects on HDL cholesterol and apoA-I levels. If there is no change in dietary composition, and only restriction in calories, HDL cholesterol and apoA-I levels decrease during the hypocaloric phase, and then increases significantly above the baseline value when the subjects are in a new steady state with substantially lower body weight [28]. Dattilo et al. have developed precise equations for predicting the rise in HDL cholesterol based on weight reduction, when a new lower stable body weight is achieved [28].

It should be noted that in the Framingham Offspring Study, the most important determinants of low HDL cholesterol were elevated triglycerides, elevated body mass index, lack of alcohol intake, and cigarette smoking [29, 30]. The relationship between triglyceride levels and HDL cholesterol is curvilinear [29]. Moreover, if one selects for men with CHD and low HDL as was done in the Veterans Affairs High-Density Lipoprotein Intervention Trial (VA-HIT), one finds men who are overweight or obese with high insulin levels [31]. Most recently, when we have carefully examined the effects of marked weight loss induced by gastric bypass surgery over 1 year, we have observed marked increases in HDL cholesterol and in large apoA-I-containing HDL particles associated with reductions in body weight, body fat, plasma insulin levels, and increases in the mass of lecithin:cholesterol acyltransferase or LCAT [32].

Effects of Exercise

Exercise has variable effects on HDL cholesterol and apoA-I levels. If there is no significant change in body composition or weight, increased exercise has little effect on HDL levels [33, 34]. However, if the exercise intervention is substantial and prolonged, and if there is associated weight loss, with increased muscle mass and decreased body fat, HDL cholesterol levels can increase quite significantly, along with lowering of TRL, less HDL cholesteryl ester transfer to TRL, and a decrease in HDL apoA-I fractional catabolic rate [35]. Intensive aerobic exercise over 7 years of follow-up has been associated with significant benefit in terms of heart disease morbidity and mortality in patients sustaining a myocardial infarction [36].

Conclusions

Dietary restriction of animal fat high in saturated fat and its replacement with vegetable oils rich in polyunsaturated fatty acids remains the cornerstone of CHD risk reduction and

disease prevention, and such interventions have been shown to reduce CHD morbidity and mortality [11–13]. Lowering dietary cholesterol is also important in this regard, even though this intervention reduces apoA-I production [2, 3]. In contrast, exchanging saturated fat with polyunsaturated fat lowers HDL cholesterol by enhancing HDL cholesteryl ester delivery to the liver by upregulation of hepatic SR-BI mRNA and protein [8–10]. Replacing total fat with carbohydrate also enhances apo-A-I fractional catabolism [21]. Weight loss with calorie restriction and exercise will raise HDL cholesterol and apoA-I significantly due to lowering of TRL, and delayed HDL apoA-I fractional catabolism. The most effective strategies for raising HDL cholesterol and apoA-I are caloric restriction and weight loss if indicated, restriction of sugars and refined high glycemic index carbohydrates, and increased physical activity. While restriction of dietary saturated fat and cholesterol as well as increased intake of essential fatty acids will lower HDL cholesterol, such interventions have been shown to substantially reduce CHD morbidity and mortality. Equations have been developed to quantitate dietary effects on HDL cholesterol, but there is a wide variability in response [37, 38]. Moreover, those individuals who cannot increase their HDL levels on an atherogenic diet may be at the greatest risk [27]. Optimal lifestyle and diet goals are shown in Fig. 7. These include: (1) not smoking, (2) replacement of animal fat with vegetable oils, (3) replacement of butter, whole milk, and eggs with trans fat-free soft margarine, skimmed milk, and egg whites or egg substitutes, (4) replacement of meat with chicken, turkey, or fish, (5) increasing the consumption of fatty fish or fish oil, (6) keeping body mass index <25 kg/m², (7) avoidance of high-fat, high-sugar desserts, (8) not adding salt or sugar to your food, (9) by increasing consumption of vegetables, fruits, and whole grains, and (10) daily exercise for at least 30 min [39].

Ideal Lifestyle and Dietary Goals

1. Do Not Smoke
2. Replace Animal Fat with Vegetable Oils
3. Replace Butter, Whole Milk, and Eggs with Trans Fat Free Soft Margarine, Skimmed Milk, and Egg Whites or Egg Substitutes
4. Replace Meat with Chicken, Turkey, or Fish
5. Increase Consumption of Fatty Fish or Fish oil
6. Try to Keep Body Mass Index < 25 kg/m²
7. Avoid High Fat, High Sugar Desserts
8. Do Not Add Salt or Sugar to your Food
9. Increase Consumption of Vegetables, Fruits, and Whole Grains
10. Exercise Daily for at least 30 minutes

Fig. 7 Our view of optimal lifestyle and diet goals for the prevention of CHD (see ref. [39])

References

1. Nicolosi RJ, Stucchi AF, Kowala MC et al (1990) Effect of dietary fat saturation and cholesterol on low density lipoprotein composition and metabolism. I. In vivo studies of receptor and non-receptor mediated catabolism of LDL in Cebus monkeys. Arteriosclerosis 10:119–128

2. Hennessy LK, Osada J, Ordovas JM et al (1992) Effects of dietary fatty acids and cholesterol on liver lipid content and hepatic apolipoprotein A-I, B and E and LDL receptor mRNA levels in Cebus monkeys. J Lipid Res 33:351–360

3. Stucchi AF, Hennessy LK, Vespa DB et al (1991) Effect of corn and coconut oil-containing diets with and without cholesterol on high density lipoprotein apoprotein A-I metabolism and hepatic apoprotein A-I mRNA levels in Cebus monkeys. Arterioscler Thromb 11:1719–1729

4. Lichtenstein AH, Ausman LM, Carrasco W et al (1994) Hypercholesterolemic effect of dietary cholesterol in diets enriched in polyunsaturated and saturated fat. Arterioscler Thromb 14:168–175

5. Velez-Carrasco W, Lichtenstein AH, Welty FK et al (1999) Dietary restriction of saturated fat and cholesterol decreases HDL apoA-I secretion. Arterioscler Thromb Vasc Biol 19:918–924

6. Schaefer EJ, Levy RI, Ernst ND et al (1981) The effects of low cholesterol, high polyunsaturated fat, and low fat diets on plasma lipid and lipoprotein cholesterol levels in normal and hypercholesterolemic subjects. Am J Clin Nutr 34:1758–1763

7. Lichtenstein AH, Carrasco W, Jenner JL et al (1993) Effects of canola, corn, olive, and rice bran oil on fasting and post-prandial lipoproteins in humans as part of a National Cholesterol Education Program Step 2 diet. Arterioscler Thromb 13:1533–1542

8. Brousseau ME, Schaefer EJ, Stucchi AF et al (1995) Diets enriched in unsaturated fatty acids enhance apolipoprotein A-I catabolism but do not affect either its production or hepatic mRNA abundance in cynomolgus monkeys. Atherosclerosis 15:107–119

9. Brousseau ME, Ordovas J, Osada J et al (1995) Dietary monounsaturated and polyunsaturated fatty acids are comparable in their effects on hepatic apolipoprotein mRNA abundance and liver lipid concentrations when substituted for saturated fatty acids in cynomolgus monkeys. J Nutr 125:425–436

10. Spady DK, Kearney DM, Hobbs HH (1999) Polyunsaturated fatty acids upregulate hepatic scavenger receptor B1 (SR-B1) expression and HDL cholesteryl ester uptake in the hamster. J Lipid Res 40:1384–1394

11. Leren P (1966) The effect of plasma cholesterol lowering diet in male survivors of myocardial infarction. Acta Med Scand 466:1–92

12. Dayton S, Pearce ML, Goldman H et al (1968) Controlled trial of a diet high in unsaturated fat for prevention of atherosclerotic complications. Lancet 2:1060–1062

13. Turpeinen O (1979) Effect of a cholesterol lowering diet on mortality from coronary heart diseases and other causes. Circulation 59:1–7

14. Frenais R, Ouguerram K, Maugeais C et al (2001) Effect of dietary omega-3 fatty acids on high density lipoprotein apolipoprotein AI kinetics in type II diabetes mellitus. Atherosclerosis 157:131–135

15. Chan DC, Watts GF, Barrett PHR (2006) Factorial study of the effect of n-3 fatty acid supplementation and atorvastatin on the kinetics of HDL apolipoproteins A-I and A-II in men with abdominal obesity. Am J Clin Nutr 84:37–43

16. Schaefer EJ, Lichtenstein AH, Lamon-Fava S et al (1995) Efficacy of a National Cholesterol Education Program Step 2 Diet in normolipidemic and hyperlipidemic middle aged and elderly men and women. Arterioscler Thromb Vasc Biol 15:1079–1085

17. Schaefer EJ, Lichtenstein AH, Lamon-Fava S et al (1996) Effects of National Cholesterol Education Program Step 2 diets relatively high or relatively low in fish-derived fatty acids on plasma lipoproteins in middle-aged and elderly subjects. Am J Clin Nutr 63:234–241

18. Schaefer EJ, Lamon-Fava S, Ausman LM et al (1997) Individual variability in lipoprotein cholesterol response to National Cholesterol Education Program Step 2 diets. Am J Clin Nutr 65:823–830

19. Schaefer EJ, Lichtenstein AH, Lamon-Fava S et al (1995) Body weight and low-density lipoprotein cholesterol changes after consumption of a low fat ad libitum diet. JAMA 274:1450–1455

20. Dansinger ML, Gleason JA, Griffith JL et al (2005) Comparison of the Atkins, Ornish, Weight Watchers, and Zone diets for weight loss and heart disease risk reduction. JAMA 293:43–53

21. Blum CB, Levy RI, Eisenberg S et al (1977) High density lipoprotein metabolism in man. J Clin Invest 60:795–807

22. Brinton EA, Eisenberg S, Breslow JL (1990) A low-fat diet decreases high density lipoprotein (HDL) cholesterol by decreasing HDL apolipoprotein transport rates. J Clin Invest 85:144–151

23. Schaefer EJ, Gleason JA, Dansinger ML (2009) Dietary fructose and glucose differentially affect lipid and glucose homeostasis. J Nutr 139(6):1257S–1262S

24. Stanhope KI, Schwartz JM, Keim NL et al (2009) Consuming fructose sweetened, not glucose-sweetened, beverages increases visceral adiposity and lipids, and decreases insulin sensitivity in overweight and obese subjects. J Clin Invest 119:1322–1334

25. Woollett LA, Spady DK (1997) Kinetic parameters for high density lipoprotein apoprotein AI and cholesteryl ester transport in the hamster. J Clin Invest 99:1704–1713

26. Woollett LA, Kearney DM, Spady DK (1997) Diet modification alters HDL cholesterol, but not the transport of HDL cholesteryl ester to the liver in the hamster. J Lipid Res 38:2289–2302

27. Asztalos BF, Lefevre M, Wong L et al (2000) Differential response to low fat diet between low and normal HDL cholesterol subjects. J Lipid Res 41:321–328

28. Dattilo AM, Kris-Etherton PM (1992) Effects of weight reduction on blood lipids and lipoproteins: a meta analysis. Am J Clin Nutr 56:320–328

29. Schaefer EJ, Lamon-Fava S, Ordovas JM et al (1994) Factors associated with low and elevated plasma high density lipoprotein cholesterol and apolipoprotein A-1 levels in the Framingham Offspring Study. J Lipid Res 35:871–882

30. Lamon-Fava S, Wilson PWF, Schaefer EJ (1996) Impact of body mass index on coronary heart risk factors in men and women. The Framingham Offspring Study. Arterioscler Thromb Vasc Biol 16:1509–1515

31. Rubins HB, Robins SJ, Collins D et al. For the VA-HIT Study Group (2002) Diabetes, plasma insulin, and cardiovascular disease. Subgroup Analysis From the Department of Veterans Affairs High-Density Lipoprotein Intervention Trial (VA-HIT). Arch Intern Med 162:2597–2604

32. Asztalos BF, Swarbrick MM, Schaefer EJ et al (2009) Effects of weight loss, induced by gastric bypass surgery, on HDL remodeling in obese women. J Lipid Res in press 2010

33. Lipson LC, Bonow RO, Schaefer EJ et al (1980) Effect of exercise conditioning on plasma high density lipoproteins (HDL) and other lipoproteins. Atherosclerosis 37:529–538

34. Lamon-Fava S, McNamara JR, Farber HW et al (1989) Acute changes in lipid, lipoproteins, apolipoproteins and low density lipoprotein particle size after an endurance triathlon. Metabolism 38:921–925

35. Thompson PD, Jurqalevitch SM, Flynn MM et al (1997) Effects of prolonged exercise training without weight loss on HDL metabolism in overweight men. Metabolism 46:217–223

36. Steffen-Battey L, Nichaman MZ, Goff DC Jr et al (2000) Change in physical activity and risk of all cause mortality: the Corpus Christi Heart Project. Circulation 102:2204–2209

37. Mensink RP, Katan MB (1992) Effect of dietary fatty acids on serum lipids and lipoproteins: a meta analysis of 27 trials. Arterioscler Thromb 12:911–919

38. Kris-Etherton PM, Yu S (1995) Individual fatty acid effects on plasma lipids and lipoproteins: human studies. Am J Clin Nutr 65(Suppl):1628S–1644S

39. Schaefer EJ (2002) E.V. McCollum Award Lecture: Lipoproteins, nutrition, and heart disease. Am J Clin Nutr 75:191–212

Effects of Ethanol Intake on High Density Lipoprotein Metabolism in Humans

Eliot A. Brinton and M. Nazeem Nanjee

Introduction

Moderate ethanol intake consistently has been associated with a decreased risk of cardiovascular disease (CVD) in observational studies [1–3], although the decrease is most pronounced and consistent for coronary heart disease [1] and less so for stroke [1]. Although a few studies have shown increases [4] or no changes [5] in carotid atherosclerosis by ultrasound (carotid intima-media thickness, CIMT) with moderate ethanol intake, most have reported decreased CIMT in men but curiously no change in women [6–8]. Heavy ethanol intake appears to have adverse effects on CIMT [9, 10].

Ethanol appears favorably to affect many risk factors for atherosclerosis and CVD, including antithrombotic/anticoagulant factors (see ref. [11] for a review) and antiinflammatory factors (see ref. [12] for review). The best-studied effect, however, is an increase in plasma concentrations of high density lipoprotein (HDL), and it is estimated that about half of the relationship between ethanol and CVD may be attributed to its effects on HDL [3, 12]. For these reasons, the effects of ethanol on HDL metabolism, as outlined in this chapter, are of clinical, as well as research interest.

Effects of Ethanol Dose, Pattern of Intake, and Beverage Type

Generally, the dose-relationship between ethanol intake and CVD events is J-shaped [13, 14] with lowest CVD rates at about two drinks per day in men [1, 13]. Moderately, higher ethanol intake appears to confer no further decrease in CVD, and, at substantially higher doses, CVD risk may increase [2, 14]. HDL-C increases with a relatively linear relationship to ethanol dose in the moderate to high intake range (up to about 90 g or six drinks per day, Fig. 1). Above that dose, HDL-C effects tend to plateau and become less consistent (Fig. 2), roughly at the dose at which the CVD risk may begin to rise. Women tend to respond similarly to men regarding both HDL and CVD, but at about half the ethanol dose (Fig. 2), and at roughly half as much intake in women [2, 13, 15, 16]. Moderate ethanol intake (generally up to 30 g/day or about two drinks per day) consistently raises HDL-C by about 4 mg/dL in over 40 short-term trials included in a meta-analysis [17]. High or heavy ethanol intake (generally defined as over 60 g/day or more than four drinks per day) appears to have greater effects than moderate intake on several aspects of HDL composition and HDL-related factors, as discussed below. These potentially beneficial effects may be counterbalanced by increased adverse effects at higher intake, such as increased blood pressure and an increase in the inflammatory factor IL-6 seen with higher intake plus a certain genotype (see below) [18]. Most studies of heavy intake have been done in alcoholics admitted for treatment, in whom the effects of ethanol are inferred by the changes during the first few weeks of ethanol withdrawal.

Interestingly, greater frequency of ethanol ingestion is associated with a further decrease in CVD rates at a given average daily intake [19], while the opposite is seen with episodic consumption of large amounts of ethanol ("binge drinking") both for carotid atherosclerosis [20] and CVD events [21]. A mechanism of this lack of protective effect may be the fact that binge drinking appears to attenuate [22] or even eliminate [23] the increase in HDL levels otherwise seen with a given level of ethanol intake, thus suggesting that the pattern of ethanol intake alters CVD risk at least in part via HDL effects.

Considerable attention has been given to the question of whether the type of alcoholic beverage alters the effects on HDL levels or CVD risk. Despite some evidence that wine intake, on account of its polyphenol and flavonoid content, may be more cardioprotective (for example, see ref. [24]) or may increase HDL-C or certain HDL subfractions [25], most reports have concluded that there are similar effects on HDL metabolism and CVD risk across all types of ethanolic beverages [2, 19, 26, 27].

E.A. Brinton (✉)
Metabolism Section, Division of Cardiovascular Genetics, University of Utah Medical Center, 420 Chipeta Way, Room 1160, Salt Lake City, UT 84108, USA
e-mail: eliot.brinton@utah.edu

E.J. Schaefer (ed.), *High Density Lipoproteins, Dyslipidemia, and Coronary Heart Disease*,
DOI 10.1007/978-1-4419-1059-2_16, © Springer Science+Business Media, LLC 2010

Effects of Ethanol Intake on the Composition and Concentration of Plasma HDL

HDL Size Subfractions

HDL consists of two major spherical subfractions, the larger is called HDL_2 and smaller is HDL_3, and interindividual variability in their plasma levels is generally greater in the former than in the latter. Similarly, most therapies for raising HDL levels tend to raise HDL_2 more than HDL_3, but the opposite tends to be true for moderate ethanol intake. Some studies of moderate intake have shown only HDL_3 to be increased, while HDL_2 was decreased [28]. More often, both subfractions increase, but with a greater increase in HDL_3 [28–34], although a few studies have shown comparable increases in HDL_3 and HDL_2 [35, 36], both of which may contribute to reduced CVD event rates [37]. These discrepancies in part seem due to variability in ethanol dose, since 30 g/day increases HDL_3 primarily or solely, while 60 g/day increases both HDL_3 and HDL_2 [38], and over 100 g/day, increases HDL_2 even more strikingly (see Table 1) [39]. Curiously, a study of very heavy ethanol use (average 186 g/day) reported only a small, nonsignificant increase in apo A-I and HDL_3-C but striking increases in apo A-II and HDL_2-C [40].

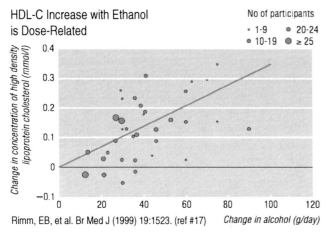

HDL-C Increase with Ethanol is Dose-Related

No of participants
- 1-9   ● 20-24
● 10-19 ● ≥ 25

Rimm, EB, et al. Br Med J (1999) 19:1523. (ref #17) *Change in alcohol (g/day)*

Fig. 1 Weighted regression analysis of alcohol and high density lipoprotein cholesterol concentration from 36 data records abstracted from experimental studies of alcohol intake. Reprinted from Rimm EB, Williams P, Fosher K. Criqui M, Stampfer MJ. Moderate alcohol intake and lower risk of coronary heart disease: meta-analysis of effects on lipids and haemostatic factors. BMJ 1999;319(7224):1523–1528 with permission from BMJ Publishing Group Ltd.

Table 1 Changes in HDL lipid composition/levels with moderate or high ethanol intake

Factor	Moderate	High/heavy
HDL-C	↑	↑↑
HDL2-C	–/↑	↑↑/↑↑↑
HDL3-C	↑↑	↑/↑↑
HDL-TG	–	–
HDL-PL	↑	↑↑

"–" denotes no change and "↑" denotes an increase in the factor listed. Multiple symbols denote greater changes. Presence of more than one type of symbol denotes significant divergence in published findings

"Moderate intake" generally refers to about one to two drinks (15–30 g ethanol) per day. "High" or "heavy" intake generally refers to twice that amount or more

Most changes noted are similar between men and women.

Please refer to the text for abbreviations, descriptions of the changes, and literature references

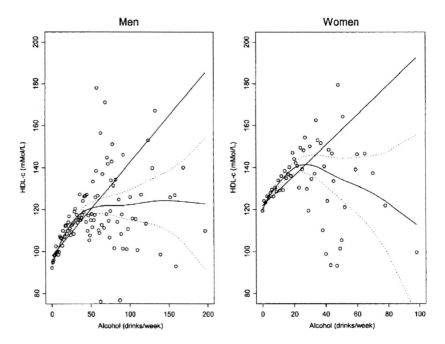

Fig. 2 HDL-C dose-response to ethanol flattens and scatters at high intake in men and women. Reprinted from Johansen D, Andersen PK, Jensen MK, Schnohr P, Gronbaek M. Nonlinear relation between alcohol intake and high-density lipoprotein cholesterol level: results from the Copenhagen City Heart Study. Alcohol Clin Exp Res 2003;27(8):1305–1309

Table 2 Changes in HDL protein composition/levels with moderate or high ethanol intake

Factor	Moderate	High/heavy
Lp A-I	↑	–/↑
Lp A-I/A-II	–/↑	↑
Pre-beta	↑↑	↑↑
Apo A-I	↑↑	↑↑↑
Apo A-II	↑↑	↑↑
Apo A-IV	—	—
Apo E	–/↑	↑↑

"–" denotes no change and "↑" denotes an increase in the factor listed. Multiple symbols denote greater changes. Presence of more than one type of symbol denotes significant divergence in published findings

"Moderate intake" generally refers to about one to two drinks (15–30 g ethanol) per day. "High" or "heavy" intake generally refers to twice that amount or more

Most changes noted are similar between men and women.

Please refer to the text for abbreviations, descriptions of the changes, and literature references

A few HDL particles, consisting of apo A-I without core lipids, have prebeta, instead of the typical alpha, electrophoretic mobility. These are found as two divergent subtypes, either phospholipid-rich, very large discoidal particles, or lipid-poor, very small (<50 kDa) globular particles. Levels of small prebeta HDL increase dramatically with ethanol intake (see Table 2) [41, 42].

HDL Lipid Content

Several studies have shown no change in the triglyceride (TG) content of HDL with ethanol intake [43–45]; in contrast, the phospholipid (PL) content of HDL is increased (see Table 1) [46]. The content of polyunsaturated fatty acids (PUFA), specifically eicosapentaenoic acid and arachidonic acid, are also reported to be increased [45]. These changes would tend to increase the fluidity of HDL, thus, possibly changing some HDL functions.

Finally, ethanol may promote formation of unusual lipids in HDL and other lipoproteins. In the presence of ethanol, phospholipase D metabolizes phosphatidylcholine, the most common HDL phospholipid, to phosphatidylethanol, instead of to phosphatidic acid. Phosphatidylethanol may alter effects of HDL on atherogenesis by affecting activity of various signaling pathways such as MAP kinase, by changing HDL binding to cells, or by altering HDL effects of growth factors and cytokines (see refs. [3, 47] for reviews). Ethanol is also a substrate for production of fatty acid ethyl esters in various tissues, which are carried on HDL or other lipoproteins or on albumin to organs, such as the liver, where they may mediate hepatic fibrosis or possibly other adverse effects (again, see refs. [3, 47] for reviews).

HDL-Related Apolipoprotein Levels

Plasma levels of apo A-I, the most prevalent apolipoprotein on HDL, consistently have been found to be increased with ethanol ingestion (see Table 2) [17, 38, 41, 48–51]. Levels of apo A-II, the second most prevalent HDL apolipoprotein, also consistently increase with ethanol use [38, 49, 50, 52]. With moderate intake, increases in apo A-I and apo A-II tend to be similar, or perhaps are greater in apo A-II [53], while with heavy alcohol use, the increase in apo A-I may be higher [49] or similar to that of apo A-II (see Table 2) [50].

Another important HDL apolipoprotein is apo E (also present on triglyceride-rich lipoproteins, TGRL), which appears to play an important role in facilitating cholesterol efflux from macrophages to HDL. Plasma levels of Apo E are generally reported to be increased with high alcohol intake [49, 54, 55], (especially above 100 g/day [55]) although one study reported much lower plasma apo E in this setting (see Table 2) [50]. Ethanol in moderation may either increase plasma apo E levels [56, 57], or leave them unchanged [51, 58] or possibly even decrease them [50, 59]. The plasma levels of apo A-IV, another common HDL apolipoprotein, are reported to be unchanged with ethanol ingestion [57].

HDL Subfractions by Apolipoprotein Content

Essentially, all HDL particles have apo A-I, whereas most, but not all, have apo A-II (referred to as Lp A-I/A-II, those lacking apo A-II being referred to as Lp A-I). Lp A-I is more prevalent than Lp A-I/A-II among the largest HDL_2 particles, while Lp A-I/A-II predominates among most other HDL sizes, including HDL_3 [3]. One study reported that Lp A-I, but not Lp A-I/A-II, was increased by moderate intake, although both were increased by heavy intake [60]. Another study of moderate intake showed both subfractions to be equally increased [41]. In contrast, a study of relatively high intake (50 g/day) showed an increase in Lp A-I/A-II but not in Lp A-I (see Table 2) [53].

Mechanisms of HDL Increases with Ethanol: Apolipoprotein Turnover

In one of three in vivo human turnover studies published to date, seven healthy lean male volunteers received relatively high ethanol intake (60 g/day vodka or gin, added to their diet) during which turnover of apo A-I was measured [61]. Despite only a 2% increase in HDL-C, the apo A-I level was increased by 12%, resulting from a mean 49% increase in the apo A-I production or transport rate (TR), partially offset by a 30% increase in the apo A-I fractional catabolic rate (FCR) [61]. Apo A-II turnover was not measured.

In a second study, five healthy male subjects had 50 g/day of alcohol as red wine added to their diets, leading to increases of 14, 20, 60%, in HDL-C, apo A-I, apo A-II, respectively [53]. Only very small, nonsignificant changes in apo A-I turnover were seen (a 11% increase and a 6% decrease in TR and FCR, respectively). In contrast, apo A-II TR tended to increase by 18% and its FCR was decreased by 21% [53].

In a third study, nine men and five women ingested differing amounts of ethanol as vodka, with the intake being matched to their usual reported daily average, (from 0.20 to 0.81 g/kg/day, or about 12–60 g/day) substituted isocalorically for carbohydrate in a metabolic diet [52]. HDL-C increased 18%, apo A-I increased 10%, and apo A-II 17%. These changes related to significant 21 and 19% increases in the TR of apo A-I and apo A-II, respectively, while the respective FCR did not change significantly (11 and 3% increases, both NS). Both the increase in the HDL-C and in apo A-I TR correlated significantly with the ethanol dose ($r = 0.66$ and 0.57, $p = 0.01$ and 0.03, respectively, see Fig. 3). The change in HDL-C, in turn, correlated strongly with the change in the apo A-I TR ($r = 0.61$, $p = 0.02$) but not with the change in apo A-I FCR ($r = 0.43$, $p = NS$, Fig. 4), while the increase in apo A-I TR correlated well with ethanol dose (Fig. 3) [52]. No gender differences were observed.

The apparent discrepancies among these kinetics trials might be explained by: (1) small numbers of subjects (all three studies); (2) insufficient compensation for the impact of added alcohol on total caloric intake (first and second studies); and (3) intake of metabolically active nonalcoholic components (second study). Nevertheless, one reasonably consistent finding is that ethanol causes a likely dose-dependent increase in the TR of apo HDL, likely both of A-I and apo A-II and, which relates to the increase in levels of apo A-I and HDL-C. Any changes in FCR are less consistent and seem less likely related to changes in HDL levels. Interestingly, the apparent in vivo increase in apo A-I synthesis has been corroborated by several in vitro studies in which addition of ethanol to cultured transformed human hepatocytes (Hep G2) increased synthesis and secretion of apo A-I by the cells [62–64].

Mechanisms of HDL Increases with Ethanol: Enzymes and Factors Important in HDL Metabolism and Function

Lecithin: cholesterol acyltransferase (LCAT) is carried primarily on HDL and is the enzyme mainly responsible for esterification of cholesterol after its transfer from cellular

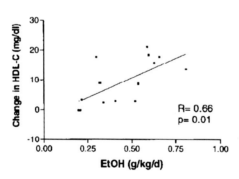
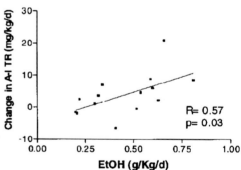

Fig. 3 Ethanol-induced increases in HDL-C and apo A-I TR are dose dependent. Reprinted from De Oliveira E, Silva ER, Foster D, McGee Harper M, et al. Alcohol consumption raises HDL cholesterol levels by increasing the transport rate of apolipoproteins A-I and A-II. Circulation 2000;102(19):2347–2352

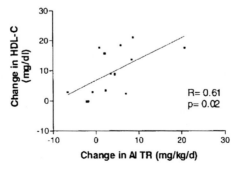
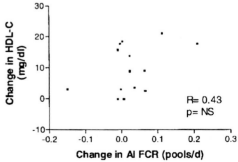

Fig. 4 Ethanol-induced increase in HDL-C correlates with TR, not FCR of apo A-I. Reprinted from De Oliveira E, Silva ER, Foster D, McGee Harper M, et al. Alcohol consumption raises HDL cholesterol levels by increasing the transport rate of apolipoproteins A-I and A-II. Circulation 2000;102(19):2347–2352

sources. Several studies have shown ethanol intake to increase LCAT activity [41, 65, 66], or the ability of whole plasma to esterify cholesterol [45, 67]. Although some studies have failed to detect this increase [28, 46, 68], it remains likely that ethanol intake can and does often raise LCAT activity and cholesterol esterification.

Phospholipid transfer protein (PLTP) mediates transfer of the major surface lipid, phospholipid (PL), between TGRL and HDL, and facilitates fusion of HDL particles with each other, resulting in major changes in HDL particle composition and size. PLTP activity may increase with high ethanol intake (related to increased HDL_2) [39] but it appears to be unchanged with moderate ethanol use (see Table 3) [41, 68].

Another important factor in HDL metabolism and function is cholesteryl-ester transfer protein (CETP), which binds to HDL, LDL, and VLDL, and promotes core lipid exchange of cholesterol ester (CE) out of HDL into VLDL and LDL, in exchange for triglycerides (TG) coming back. This may play an important role in transferring cholesterol from HDL back to the liver (see below) and also tends to result in net lipid depletion of HDL, due to subsequent TG lipolysis by hepatic lipase (see below). Heavy ethanol intake decreases CETP activity [39, 40, 49, 69] in a dose-dependent fashion, [70, 71] which tends to lead to decreased HDL_3 [39] but increased HDL_2 [49]. Moderate alcohol intake also may reduce CETP activity [72] although most reports have found no effect [28, 46, 68].

Lipoprotein lipase (LPL) catalyzes lipolysis of TG, mainly from very large TGRL. In contrast, its impact on HDL metabolism is indirect in that (1) it helps reduce TG levels, which suppresses TG-driven loss of HDL-C (via CETP) that would otherwise lead to hypercatabolism of apo HDL, and (2) by shrinking the TG-rich core of large TGRL, it frees up excess surface lipid (PL and free cholesterol) from TGRL,

which may then transfer to HDL, facilitating growth in HDL particle size. LPL activity clearly increases with moderate [28, 29, 40, 49] and heavy ethanol intake [49].

Hepatic lipase (HL) acts on smaller lipoproteins, including HDL, from which it avidly removes TG and also PL. Although ethanol is reported to increase HL activity [73], or leave it unchanged [28], most studies have found decreased activity [3, 49, 52, 74].

We are not aware of any published material, which addresses the effect of ethanol on the activity of endothelial lipase (EL). Importantly, however, the vast majority of the published studies cited above demonstrate that the ethanol-induced changes in HDL-remodeling factors tend to favor formation of larger, less-dense HDL particles.

Effects of Ethanol on Key Aspects of the Protective Effect of HDL Against Atherosclerosis

Ethanol alters various functions of HDL, which appear to be related to its ability to protect against atherosclerosis. The best established of these mechanisms is reverse cholesterol transport (RCT) in which HDL accepts cholesterol from cells and transports it to the liver, where it can be removed from the body. The effects of ethanol ingestion on each of the several steps in RCT have been studied.

First, ethanol appears to increase the ability of HDL to promote cholesterol efflux from cultured cells. Moderate consumption of ethanol (regardless of beverage type) increases cholesterol transfer from various cell types, including the J774 transformed mouse macrophage, both to smaller and larger HDL particles, [41, 67, 75]. and the same has been shown in heavy alcohol users [76], associated with increased concentrations of larger HDL_2, increased HDL-PL and HDL-sphyngomyelin (SM), increased PLTP, and decreased CETP [77]. This has been documented in some studies specifically to occur via the action of ABCA1 upregulated in skeletal muscle [78] and macrophages [41]. One study, however, reported decreased cholesterol efflux to HDL from alcohol abusers with chronic high intake [59].

The second step of RCT is esterification of cholesterol in HDL, which is important because the cholesterol fluxing to HDL is unesterified, and ongoing flux requires sequestration of cholesterol by esterification. As noted above, this step is catalyzed by LCAT, the activity of which is generally increased by ethanol use.

The third and final step of RCT is transfer of cholesterol ester from HDL to the liver by one of two routes. Some HDL cholesteryl ester is transferred to apo B-containing lipoproteins by CETP, which can then be taken up by the

Table 3 Changes in HDL-related factors with of moderate or high ethanol intake

Factor	Moderate	High/heavy
LCAT	–/↑	–/↑
PLTP	–	↑
CETP	–/↓	↓↓
LPL	↑	↑
HL	–/↓	↓
EL	NA	NA
PON-1	↑	↑↑

"↓" denotes a decrease, "–" denotes no change and "↑" denotes an increase in the factor listed. Double symbols denote greater changes. Presence of more than one type of symbol denotes significant divergence in published findings

"Moderate intake" generally refers to about one to two drinks (15–30 g ethanol) per day. "High" or "heavy" intake generally refers to twice that amount or more

Most changes noted are similar between men and women, but some gender differences are great

Please refer to the text for abbreviations, descriptions of the changes, and literature references

liver via action of the apo B, E receptor. Alternatively, published data from one group suggest that heavy ethanol intake might even promote CETP-mediated CE transfer in the opposite direction, from LDL to HDL [79, 80], which would likely also enhance overall transfer of cholesterol back to the liver. The existence and importance of such a transfer, however, are uncertain. Meanwhile, the main action of CETP, to transfer CE from HDL to apo B lipoproteins, instead has the potential to facilitate its delivery back to the periphery, thus defeating RCT.

On the other hand, the final step in RCT may instead depend on direct transfer of cholesterol ester from HDL to the liver. One study found increased transfer of CE to an SR-B1 model system from HDL from ethanol consuming subjects [46], but other studies reported decreased CE transfer to transformed human hepatoma cells (HepG2) from HDL taken from alcohol abusers [59, 77].

Since the early steps of RCT are likely increased, and the last step might also be facilitated, ethanol use may enhance overall RCT. This, however, remains to be established by further research designed (1) to better understand the net impact of CETP activity on RCT and (2) to more firmly establish the effects of ethanol on the extravascular, intravascular and intrahepatic steps of RCT.

Aside from RCT, an important antiatherosclerotic function of HDL appears to be prevention (or possibly reversal) of oxidation of LDL and other lipoproteins [81]. Ethanol intake increases the levels and activity of the two major HDL-related antioxidant proteins, apo A-I (as noted above) and PON-1, [82–85], proportional to the degree of increase in HDL-C [82]. Interestingly, ethanol intake ablates the decrease in PON-1 activity normally seen with cigarette smoking [85].

Finally, ethanol is reported to decrease many parameters of inflammation, which appear to be proatherosclerotic. These include CRP, LpPLA2, TNFα, IL-6, VCAM-1, e-selectin, p-selectin, CD40L, fibrinogen, and plasma viscosity [86, 87], and this reduction appears to be dose-dependent [88]. Interestingly, this antiinflammatory effect is largely related to increased HDL-C levels, in that adjustment for HDL-C may reduce or eliminate the relationships (e.g., with fibrinogen and LpPLA2, or CRP, respectively) [87, 88]. Thus, much of the apparent antiinflammatory effect of ethanol may be mediated via increased plasma levels of HDL. Of further interest, in individuals with at least one apo E4 allele, the inverse relationship between ethanol dose and inflammatory markers related is reduced or even reversed (again, for fibrinogen or CRP, respectively) [88], possibly related to the blunting of the usual ethanol-induced increase in HDL-C (especially HDL_3-C) [89]. Also, a proinflammatory increase in IL-6 levels may be seen with high ethanol intake in patients with a certain IL-6 promoter genotype (see below) [18].

Evidence for Genetic Modulation of HDL Response to Ethanol Intake

There is considerable interindividual variability in the response of HDL levels to a given dose of ethanol [16], which is likely to be due in large part to genetic differences. Although an understanding of the contributions of individual genes to the response of HDL metabolism to alcohol is beginning to emerge, many of these relationships have been little studied or remain unexplored. Nevertheless, emerging evidence suggests that certain associations between ethanol intake, HDL levels/metabolism, and atherosclerosis/CVD events visible in the general population may be driven by one genetic subset, while other relationships not visible in general may be quite striking and important in a given genetic subgroup.

Alcohol dehydrogenase (ADH) is responsible for metabolic inactivation of ethanol in the body. Individuals with a common allelic variation of the ADH1C (also called ADH3) subunit, γ2, metabolize ethanol slower than do those with γ1. As might be expected, HDL-C levels are higher and CHD events lower in γ2 vs. γ1 homozygotes, among men [90] and postmenopausal women not taking estrogen replacement [91]; but surprisingly, premenopausal women and those taking estrogen had no such effect [91]. Thus, the effect of high estrogen levels to raise HDL-C appears to overcome the interaction of the ADH1C γ2 with ethanol.

The apo E gene has three common alleles, 2, 3, and 4, in the coding-region of the gene, which result in corresponding protein isoforms with structural differences of functional significance. Apo E4 homozygotes or heterozygotes have blunted increases in HDL-C with ethanol intake [89, 92]. Interestingly, in individuals with an Apo E4 allele, increasing ethanol intake is associated with an increase in CRP, instead of the usual decrease in those without an apo E4 allele [88].

The CETP gene has a common point mutation, a polymorphism at a Taq1 restriction site in a noncoding region, which is in strong linkage disequilibrium with a structural mutation related to functional differences in CETP activity. The B2 allele is associated in a codominant fashion with decreased CETP activity and increased HDL-C levels [93]. Several studies have reported the B2 allele to be associated with a more pronounced increase in HDL-C levels at a given level of ethanol intake [70–72, 94], and importantly, with a greater decrease in CVD events with ethanol intake [71, 72, 94, 95]. Curiously, there is a gender interaction in that this effect seems to be greater in women than in men [70, 94].

As noted above, PON-1 is a powerful HDL-related antioxidant factor, the activity of which increases with ethanol intake [82–85]. A prime example of monogenic modulation of the response of HDL-related factors to ethanol is the finding that the increase in PON-1 with ethanol intake is greatly enhanced in carriers of the 107T allele for PON-1 [85] but not three other PON-1-related genetic polymorphisms [83].

The T allele of the C-480T polymorphism of the HL gene associates with decreased HL activity and increased levels of HDL-C and apo A-I [96] and curiously also with increased coronary fatty streaks [97]. One study reported no interaction between this allele and the effect of ethanol intake on HDL-C and apo A-I levels, but mean ethanol intake was less than one drink (~15 g) daily, at which dose there is little or no effect on HL activity [98].

The CC genotype of the interleukin-6 −174 promoter polymorphism has been found not only to associate with increased IL-6 levels (presumably by up regulating IL-6 production) but also to modify the relationship between ethanol intake and carotid artery atherosclerosis. Interestingly, patients with the CC genotype have been found to have increased IL-6 levels, increased CIMT, and increased carotid artery plaque when consuming over 30 g/day of ethanol [18], although the interaction of this finding with HDL levels or function is not clear.

Although the genetic explanations for higher HDL-C levels in Blacks than in Caucasians are not clear, it is interesting to note that both races have a similar ethanol dose–response of increasing HDL-C and apo A-I levels [27].

Summary and Conclusions

Ethanol has many important effects on HDL composition, concentration, and metabolism. Although some of these changes appear to be unfavorable, the majority of effects appear to enhance the probable antiatherosclerosis effects of HDL. These data thus fit with the impression coming from virtually all observational studies that moderate and regular ethanol intake is associated with decreased CVD risk in large part due to effects on HDL.

Major effects of ethanol on HDL include increases in all of its major subfractions and components. Mechanisms of increased HDL levels with ethanol include increased apo A-I synthesis, reduced CETP activity, increased LPL activity, and possibly decreased HL activity, all occurring in a relatively linear dose-dependent fashion. An important genetic predictor of increased response of HDL levels and/or atherosclerosis to ethanol is having at least one copy of the Taq1B allele of the CETP gene. Predictors of decreased or adverse responses to ethanol include the presence of at least one copy of the apo E4 allele, or two copies of the C allele for the IL-6 −174 promoter.

Importantly, although considerable mechanistic data suggest that ethanol intake protects against CVD, the HDL-related mechanisms stimulated by ethanol intake are not uniformly favorable. Further, although a great number of observational studies have consistently shown that regular and moderate ethanol ingestion is associated with lower CVD risk, no randomized prospective clinical trials have been performed as yet to prove the apparent cause–effect relationship between moderate long-term ethanol intake on reduced CVD event rates. In addition to the lack of clinical trial data, there is another reason for tempering enthusiasm for prescription of ethanol as a clinically useful measure for atheroprevention. It is the potential that a "prescription" for moderate ethanol use may harm the patient and others, either due to unintended ethanol abuse and addiction, or due to an adverse event (e.g., an automobile accident), which might result even from "moderate" drinking.

References

1. Gaziano JM, Gaziano TA, Glynn RJ et al (2000) Light-to-moderate alcohol consumption and mortality in the Physicians' Health Study enrollment cohort. J Am Coll Cardiol 35(1):96–105
2. Sesso HD (2001) Alcohol and cardiovascular health: recent findings. Am J Cardiovasc Drugs 1(3):167–172
3. Hannuksela ML, Liisanantti MK, Savolainen MJ (2002) Effect of alcohol on lipids and lipoproteins in relation to atherosclerosis. Crit Rev Clin Lab Sci 39(3):225–283
4. Juonala M, Viikari JS, Kahonen M et al (2009) Alcohol consumption is directly associated with carotid intima-media thickness in Finnish young adults: the Cardiovascular Risk in Young Finns Study. Atherosclerosis 204(2):e93–e98
5. Kitamura A, Iso H, Imano H et al (2004) Prevalence and correlates of carotid atherosclerosis among elderly Japanese men. Atherosclerosis 172(2):353–359
6. Zureik M, Gariepy J, Courbon D et al (2004) Alcohol consumption and carotid artery structure in older French adults: the Three-City Study. Stroke 35(12):2770–2775
7. Fujisawa M, Okumiya K, Matsubayashi K, Hamada T, Endo H, Doi Y (2008) Factors associated with carotid atherosclerosis in community-dwelling oldest elderly aged over 80 years. Geriatr Gerontol Int 8(1):12–18
8. Lee YH, Shin MH, Kweon SS et al (2009) Alcohol consumption and carotid artery structure in Korean adults aged 50 years and older. BMC Public Health 9(1):358
9. Schminke U, Luedemann J, Berger K et al (2005) Association between alcohol consumption and subclinical carotid atherosclerosis: the Study of Health in Pomerania. Stroke 36(8):1746–1752
10. Mukamal KJ, Kronmal RA, Mittleman MA et al (2003) Alcohol consumption and carotid atherosclerosis in older adults: the Cardiovascular Health Study. Arterioscler Thromb Vasc Biol 23(12):2252–2259
11. van Tol A (2001) Moderate alcohol consumption: effects on lipids and cardiovascular disease risk. Curr Opin Lipidol 12:19–23
12. Li JM, Mukamal KJ (2004) An update on alcohol and atherosclerosis. Curr Opin Lipidol 15(6):673–680
13. Corrao G, Rubbiati L, Bagnardi V, Zambon A, Poikolainen K (2000) Alcohol and coronary heart disease: a meta-analysis. Addiction 95(10):1505–1523
14. Standridge JB, Zylstra RG, Adams SM (2004) Alcohol consumption: an overview of benefits and risks. South Med J 97(7):664–672
15. White IR (1999) The level of alcohol consumption at which all-cause mortality is least. J Clin Epidemiol 52(10):967–975
16. Johansen D, Andersen PK, Jensen MK, Schnohr P, Gronbaek M (2003) Nonlinear relation between alcohol intake and high-density lipoprotein cholesterol level: results from the Copenhagen City Heart Study. Alcohol Clin Exp Res 27(8):1305–1309

17. Rimm EB, Williams P, Fosher K, Criqui M, Stampfer MJ (1999) Moderate alcohol intake and lower risk of coronary heart disease: meta- analysis of effects on lipids and haemostatic factors. BMJ 319(7224):1523–1528

18. Jerrard-Dunne P, Sitzer M, Risley P et al (2003) Interleukin-6 promoter polymorphism modulates the effects of heavy alcohol consumption on early carotid artery atherosclerosis: the Carotid Atherosclerosis Progression Study (CAPS). Stroke 34(2):402–407

19. Mukamal KJ, Conigrave KM, Mittleman MA et al (2003) Roles of drinking pattern and type of alcohol consumed in coronary heart disease in men. N Engl J Med 348(2):109–118

20. Kauhanen J, Kaplan GA, Goldberg DE, Salonen R, Salonen JT (1999) Pattern of alcohol drinking and progression of atherosclerosis. Arterioscler Thromb Vasc Biol 19(12):3001–3006

21. Kauhanen J, Kaplan GA, Goldberg DE, Salonen JT (1997) Beer binging and mortality: results from the Kuopio ischaemic heart disease risk factor study, a prospective population based study. BMJ 315(7112):846–851

22. Peasey A, Bobak M, Malyutina S et al (2005) Do lipids contribute to the lack of cardio-protective effect of binge drinking: alcohol consumption and lipids in three eastern European countries. Alcohol Alcohol 40(5):431–435

23. Frohlich JJ (1996) Effects of alcohol on plasma lipoprotein metabolism. Clin Chim Acta 246(1–2):39–49

24. Di Castelnuovo A, Rotondo S, Iacoviello L, Donati MB, De Gaetano G (2002) Meta-analysis of wine and beer consumption in relation to vascular risk. Circulation 105(24):2836–2844

25. Marques-Vidal P, Montaye M, Haas B et al (2001) Relationships between alcoholic beverages and cardiovascular risk factor levels in middle-aged men, the PRIME Study. Prospective Epidemiological Study of Myocardial Infarction Study. Atherosclerosis 157(2):431–440

26. Rimm EB, Klatsky A, Groggee D, Stampfer MJ (1996) Review of moderate alcohol consumption and reduced risk of coronary heart disease: is the effect due to beer, wine, or spirits? BMJ 312:731–736

27. Volcik KA, Ballantyne CM, Fuchs FD, Sharrett AR, Boerwinkle E (2008) Relationship of alcohol consumption and type of alcoholic beverage consumed with plasma lipid levels: differences between Whites and African Americans of the ARIC study. Ann Epidemiol 18(2):101–107

28. Nishiwaki M, Ishikawa T, Ito T et al (1994) Effects of alcohol on lipoprotein lipase, hepatic lipase, cholesteryl ester transfer protein, and lecithin:cholesterol acyltransferase in high-density lipoprotein cholesterol elevation. Atherosclerosis 111(1):99–109

29. Valimaki M, Nikkila EA, Taskinen MR, Ylikahri R (1986) Rapid decrease in high density lipoprotein subfractions and postheparin plasma lipase activities after cessation of chronic alcohol intake. Atherosclerosis 59(2):147–153

30. Haskell WI, Camargo C, Williams PT (1984) The effect of cessation and resumption of moderate alcohol intake on serum high density lipoprotein subfractions: a controlled study. N Engl J Med 310:805–810

31. Diehl AK, Fuller JH, Mattock MB, Salter AM, el-Gohari R, Keen H (1988) The relationship of high density lipoprotein subfractions to alcohol consumption, other lifestyle factors, and coronary heart disease. Atherosclerosis 69(2–3):145–153

32. Sillanaukee P, Koivula T, Jokela H, Myllyharju H, Seppa K (1993) Relationship of alcohol consumption to changes in HDL-subfractions. Eur J Clin Invest 23(8):486–491

33. Sillanaukee P, Koivula T, Jokela H, Pitkajarvi T, Seppa K (2000) Alcohol consumption and its relation to lipid-based cardiovascular risk factors among middle-aged women: the role of HDL(3) cholesterol. Atherosclerosis 152(2):503–510

34. Gardner CD, Tribble DL, Young DR, Ahn D, Fortmann SP (2000) Associations of HDL, HDL(2), and HDL(3) cholesterol and apolipoproteins A-I and B with lifestyle factors in healthy women and men: the Stanford Five City Project. Prev Med 31(4):346–356

35. Hartung GH, Foreyt JP, Reeves RS et al (1990) Effect of alcohol dose on plasma lipoprotein subfractions and lipolytic enzyme activity in active and inactive men. Metabolism 39(1):81–86

36. Clevidence BA, Reichman ME, Judd JT et al (1995) Effects of alcohol consumption on lipoproteins of premenopausal women. A controlled diet study. Arterioscler Thromb Vasc Biol 15:179–184

37. Gaziano JM, Buring JE, Breslow JL et al (1993) Moderate alcohol intake, increased levels of high-density lipoprotein and its subfractions, and decreased risk of myocardial infarction. N Engl J Med 329(25):1829–1834

38. Valimaki M, Taskinen MR, Ylikahri R, Roine R, Kuusi T, Nikkila EA (1988) Comparison of the effects of two different doses of alcohol on serum lipoproteins, HDL-subfractions and apolipoproteins A-I and A-II: a controlled study. Eur J Clin Invest 18(5):472–480

39. Lagrost L, Athias A, Herbeth B et al (1996) Opposite effects of cholesteryl ester transfer protein and phospholipid transfer protein on the size distribution of plasma high density lipoproteins. Physiological relevance in alcoholic patients. J Biol Chem 271(32):19058–19065

40. Valimaki M, Kahri J, Laitinen K et al (1993) High density lipoprotein subfractions, apolipoprotein A-I containing lipoproteins, lipoprotein (a), and cholesterol ester transfer protein activity in alcoholic women before and after ethanol withdrawal. Eur J Clin Invest 23(7):406–417

41. Beulens JW, Sierksma A, van Tol A et al (2004) Moderate alcohol consumption increases cholesterol efflux mediated by ABCA1. J Lipid Res 45(9):1716–1723

42. Atmeh RG, Robenek H (1996) Measurement of small high density lipoprotein subclass by an improved immunoblotting technique. J Lipid Res 37(11):2461–2469

43. Taskinen MR, Valimaki M, Nikkila EA, Kuusi T, Ehnholm C, Ylikahri R (1982) High density lipoprotein subfractions and postheparin plasma lipases in alcoholic men before and after ethanol withdrawal. Metabolism 31(11):1168–1174

44. Savolainen MJ, Hannuksela M, Seppanen S, Kervinen K, Kesaniemi YA (1990) Increased high-density lipoprotein cholesterol concentration in alcoholics is related to low cholesteryl ester transfer protein activity. Eur J Clin Invest 20(6):593–599

45. Perret B, Ruidavets JB, Vieu C et al (2002) Alcohol consumption is associated with enrichment of high-density lipoprotein particles in polyunsaturated lipids and increased cholesterol esterification rate. Alcohol Clin Exp Res 26(8):1134–1140

46. Sierksma A, Vermunt SH, Lankhuizen IM et al (2004) Effect of moderate alcohol consumption on parameters of reverse cholesterol transport in postmenopausal women. Alcohol Clin Exp Res 28(4):662–666

47. Hannuksela ML, Ramet ME, Nissinen AE, Liisanantti MK, Savolainen MJ (2003) Effects of ethanol on lipids and atherosclerosis. Pathophysiology 10(2):93–103

48. Valimaki M, Laitinen K, Ylikahri R, Ehnholm C (1991) The effect of moderate alcohol intake on serum apolipoprotein A-I-containing lipoproteins and lipoprotein (a). Metabolism 40:1168–1172

49. Hirano K, Matsuzawa Y, Sakai N et al (1992) Polydisperse low-density lipoproteins in hyperalphalipoproteinemic chronic alcohol drinkers in association with marked reduction of cholesteryl ester transfer protein activity. Metabolism 41(12):1313–1318

50. Lin RC, Miller BA, Kelly TJ (1995) Concentrations of apolipoprotein AI, AII, and E in plasma and lipoprotein fractions of alcoholic patients: gender differences in the effects of alcohol. Hepatology 21(4):942–949

51. Lecomte E, Herbeth B, Paille F, Steinmetz J, Artur Y, Siest G (1996) Changes in serum apolipoprotein and lipoprotein profile induced by chronic alcohol consumption and withdrawal: determinant effect on heart disease? Clin Chem 42(10):1666–1675

52. De Oliveira E Silva ER, Foster D, McGee Harper M et al (2000) Alcohol consumption raises HDL cholesterol levels by increasing the transport rate of apolipoproteins A-I and A-II. Circulation 102(19):2347–2352

53. Gottrand F, Beghin L, Duhal N et al (1999) Moderate red wine consumption in healthy volunteers reduced plasma clearance of apolipoprotein AII. Eur J Clin Invest 29(5):387–394

54. Wehr H, Bednarska-Makaruk M, Szacka E (1995) Apolipoprotein E in alcoholics. Alcohol Alcohol 30(1):27–30

55. Gueguen S, Herbeth B, Pirollet P, Paille F, Siest G, Visvikis S (2002) Changes in serum apolipoprotein and lipoprotein profile after alcohol withdrawal: effect of apolipoprotein E polymorphism. Alcohol Clin Exp Res 26(4):501–508

56. Braeckman L, De Bacquer D, Rosseneu M, De Backer G (1998) The effect of age and lifestyle factors on plasma levels of apolipoprotein E. J Cardiovasc Risk 5(3):155–159

57. Sun Z, Larson IA, Ordovas JM, Barnard JR, Schaefer EJ (2000) Effects of age, gender, and lifestyle factors on plasma apolipoprotein A-IV concentrations. Atherosclerosis 151(2):381–388

58. Cushman P Jr, Barboriak J, Kalbfleisch J (1986) Alcohol: high density lipoproteins, apolipoproteins. Alcohol Clin Exp Res 10(2): 154–157

59. Rao MN, Liu QH, Marmillot P, Seeff LB, Strader DB, Lakshman MR (2000) High-density lipoproteins from human alcoholics exhibit impaired reverse cholesterol transport function. Metabolism 49(11):1406–1410

60. Branchi A, Rovellini A, Tomella C et al (1997) Association of alcohol consumption with HDL subpopulations defined by apolipoprotein A-I and apolipoprotein A-II content. Eur J Clin Nutr 51(6):362–365

61. Malmendier CL, Delcroix C (1985) Effect of alcohol intake on high and low density lipoprotein metabolism in healthy volunteers. Clin Chim Acta 152(3):281–288

62. Amarasuriya RN, Gupta AK, Civen M, Horng YC, Maeda T, Kashyap ML (1992) Ethanol stimulates apolipoprotein A-I secretion by human hepatocytes: implications for a mechanism for atherosclerosis protection. Metabolism 41(8):827–832

63. Tam SP (1992) Effect of ethanol on lipoprotein secretion in two human hepatoma cell lines, HepG2 and Hep3B. Alcohol Clin Exp Res 16(6):1021–1028

64. Dashti N, Franklin FA, Abrahamson DR (1996) Effect of ethanol on the synthesis and secretion of apoA-I- and apoB-containing lipoproteins in HepG2 cells. J Lipid Res 37(4):810–824

65. Goto A, Sasai K, Suzuki S et al (2003) Plasma concentrations of LPL and LCAT are in putative association with females and alcohol use which are independent negative risk factors for coronary atherosclerosis among Japanese. Clin Chim Acta 329(1–2):69–76

66. Hendriks HF, Veenstra J, van Tol A, Groener JE, Schaafsma G (1998) Moderate doses of alcoholic beverages with dinner and postprandial high density lipoprotein composition. Alcohol Alcohol 33(4):403–410

67. van Der Gaag MS, van Tol A, Vermunt SH, Scheek LM, Schaafsma G, Hendriks HF (2001) Alcohol consumption stimulates early steps in reverse cholesterol transport. J Lipid Res 42(12):2077–2083

68. Riemens SC, van Tol A, Hoogenberg K et al (1997) Higher high density lipoprotein cholesterol associated with moderate alcohol consumption is not related to altered plasma lecithin:cholesterol acyltransferase and lipid transfer protein activity levels. Clin Chim Acta 258(1):105–115

69. Hannuksela M, Marcel YL, Kesaniemi YA, Savolainen MJ (1992) Reduction in the concentration and activity of plasma cholesteryl ester transfer protein by alcohol. J Lipid Res 33:737–744

70. Tsujita Y, Nakamura Y, Zhang Q et al (2007) The association between high-density lipoprotein cholesterol level and cholesteryl ester transfer protein TaqIB gene polymorphism is influenced by alcohol drinking in a population-based sample. Atherosclerosis 191(1):199–205

71. Fumeron F, Betoulle D, Luc G et al (1995) Alcohol intake modulates the effect of a polymorphism of the cholestery ester transfer protein gene on plasma high density lipoprotein and the risk of myocardial infarction. J Clin Invest 96:1664–1671

72. Boekholdt SM, Sacks FM, Jukema JW et al (2005) Cholesteryl ester transfer protein TaqIB variant, high-density lipoprotein cholesterol levels, cardiovascular risk, and efficacy of pravastatin treatment: individual patient meta-analysis of 13, 677 subjects. Circulation 111(3):278–287

73. Taskinen MR, Nikkila EA, Valimaki M et al (1987) Alcohol-induced changes in serum lipoproteins and in their metabolism. Am Heart J 113(2 Pt 2):458–464

74. Goldberg CS, Tall AR, Krumholz S (1984) Acute inhibition of hepatic lipase and increase in plasma lipoproteins after alcohol intake. J Lipid Res 25(7):714–720

75. Senault C, Betoulle D, Luc G, Hauw P, Rigaud D, Fumeron F (2000) Beneficial effects of a moderate consumption of red wine on cellular cholesterol efflux in young men. Nutr Metab Cardiovasc Dis 10(2):63–69

76. Makela SM, Jauhiainen M, Ala-Korpela M et al (2008) HDL2 of heavy alcohol drinkers enhances cholesterol efflux from raw macrophages via phospholipid-rich HDL 2b particles. Alcohol Clin Exp Res 32(6):991–1000

77. Marmillot P, Munoz J, Patel S, Garige M, Rosse RB, Lakshman MR (2007) Long-term ethanol consumption impairs reverse cholesterol transport function of high-density lipoproteins by depleting high-density lipoprotein sphingomyelin both in rats and in humans. Metabolism 56(7):947–953

78. Hoang A, Tefft C, Duffy SJ et al (2008) ABCA1 expression in humans is associated with physical activity and alcohol consumption. Atherosclerosis 197(1):197–203

79. Liinamaa MJ, Hannuksela ML, Kesaniemi YA, Savolainen MJ (1997) Altered transfer of cholesteryl esters and phospholipids in plasma from alcohol abusers. Arterioscler Thromb Vasc Biol 17(11):2940–2947

80. Liinamaa MJ, Kesaniemi YA, Savolainen MJ (1998) Lipoprotein composition influences cholesteryl ester transfer in alcohol abusers. Ann Med 30(3):316–322

81. Kashyap ML, Tavintharan S, Kamanna VS (2003) Optimal therapy of low levels of high density lipoprotein-cholesterol. Am J Cardiovasc Drugs 3(1):53–65

82. van der Gaag MS, van Tol A, Scheek LM et al (1999) Daily moderate alcohol consumption increases serum paraoxonase activity; a diet-controlled, randomised intervention study in middle-aged men. Atherosclerosis 147:405–410

83. Sierksma A, van der Gaag MS, van Tol A, James RW, Hendriks HF (2002) Kinetics of HDL cholesterol and paraoxonase activity in moderate alcohol consumers. Alcohol Clin Exp Res 26(9):1430–1435

84. Rao MN, Marmillot P, Gong M et al (2003) Light, but not heavy alcohol drinking, stimulates paraoxonase by upregulating liver mRNA in rats and humans. Metabolism 52(10):1287–1294

85. Wang X, Huang J, Fan Z et al (2004) Genetic and environmental factors associated with plasma paraoxonase activity in healthy Chinese. Int J Mol Med 13(3):445–450

86. Sierksma A, van der Gaag MS, Kluft C, Hendriks HF (2002) Moderate alcohol consumption reduces plasma C-reactive protein and fibrinogen levels; a randomized, diet-controlled intervention study. Eur J Clin Nutr 56(11):1130–1136

87. Oei HH, van der Meer IM, Hofman A et al (2005) Lipoprotein-associated phospholipase A2 activity is associated with risk of coronary heart disease and ischemic stroke: the Rotterdam Study. Circulation 111(5):570–575

88. Mukamal KJ, Cushman M, Mittleman MA, Tracy RP, Siscovick DS (2004) Alcohol consumption and inflammatory markers in older adults: the Cardiovascular Health Study. Atherosclerosis 173(1):79–87

89. Djousse L, Pankow JS, Arnett DK, Eckfeldt JH, Myers RH, Ellison RC (2004) Apolipoprotein E polymorphism modifies the alcohol-HDL association observed in the National Heart, Lung, and Blood Institute Family Heart Study. Am J Clin Nutr 80(6):1639–1644

90. Hines LM, Stampfer MJ, Ma J et al (2001) Genetic variation in alcohol dehydrogenase and the beneficial effect of moderate

alcohol consumption on myocardial infarction. N Engl J Med 344(8):549–555

91. Hines LM, Hunter DJ, Stampfer MJ et al (2005) Alcohol consumption and high-density lipoprotein levels: the effect of ADH1C genotype, gender and menopausal status. Atherosclerosis 182(2):293–300

92. Corella D, Tucker K, Lahoz C et al (2001) Alcohol drinking determines the effect of the APOE locus on LDL-cholesterol concentrations in men: the Framingham Offspring Study. Am J Clin Nutr 73(4):736–745

93. Kondo I, Berg K, Drayna D, Lawn R (1989) DNA polymorphism at the locus for human cholesteryl ester transfer protein (CETP) is associated with high density lipoprotein cholesterol and apolipoprotein levels. Clin Genet 35(1):49–56

94. Jensen MK, Mukamal KJ, Overvad K, Rimm EB (2008) Alcohol consumption, TaqIB polymorphism of cholesteryl ester transfer protein, high-density lipoprotein cholesterol, and risk of coronary heart disease in men and women. Eur Heart J 29(1):104–112

95. Corbex M, Poirier O, Fumeron F et al (2000) Extensive association analysis between the CETP gene and coronary heart disease phenotypes reveals several putative functional polymorphisms and gene-environment interaction. Genet Epidemiol 19(1):64–80

96. Isaacs A, Sayed-Tabatabaei FA, Njajou OT, Witteman JC, van Duijn CM (2004) The -514 C->T hepatic lipase promoter region polymorphism and plasma lipids: a meta-analysis. J Clin Endocrinol Metab 89(8):3858–3863

97. Fan YM, Lehtimaki T, Rontu R et al (2007) The hepatic lipase gene C-480T polymorphism in the development of early coronary atherosclerosis: the Helsinki Sudden Death Study. Eur J Clin Invest 37(6):472–477

98. Fan YM, Raitakari OT, Kahonen M et al (2009) Hepatic lipase promoter C-480T polymorphism is associated with serum lipids levels, but not subclinical atherosclerosis: the Cardiovascular Risk in Young Finns Study. Clin Genet 76(1):46–53

Effects of Estrogen on HDL Metabolism

Stefania Lamon-Fava

While not very common in premenopausal women, coronary heart disease (CHD) is the leading cause of morbidity and mortality in postmenopausal women [1]. According to the "estrogen hypothesis," the increase in CHD risk with menopause is attributed to the reduced ovarian production of estrogen. In clinical practice, estrogen therapy for the relief of menopausal symptoms started in the 1950s, but it was only in the 1980s that interest on the effect of estrogen on CHD arose. Early observational studies had consistently shown a reduced risk of CHD in postmenopausal women on estrogen therapy, when compared to postmenopausal women not taking estrogen [2]. The reduction in CHD risk with estrogen was particularly evident in young women with early surgical menopause [3]. However, to firmly establish the protective effect of estrogen on CHD risk, randomized clinical trials were carried out. To lower the risk of uterine cancer associated with estrogen use, a combination of estrogen with progestin (hormone therapy, HT) was used in these studies. These trials, including the Heart and Estrogen/progestin Replacement Study (HERS) [4] and the Women' Health Initiative (WHI) [5], have shown no protection or increased risk of CHD with HT use. The lack of protection from CHD in the randomized clinical trials occurred despite HT-induced beneficial changes in intermediate markers of CHD risk, such as reductions in plasma low-density lipoprotein cholesterol (LDL-C) concentrations and increases in plasma high-density lipoprotein cholesterol (HDL-C) concentrations. Recently, reanalysis of the largest randomized intervention trial, the WHI, and of the large observational trial, the Nurses' Health Study, has revealed the significant effect of the time of initiation of HT on CHD outcomes, with initiation of therapy in early menopause associated with reduced CHD risk, and initiation in late menopause associated with increased risk [6, 7]. Therefore, the discrepancy in results between observational and randomized clinical trials may in part be explained by

their different study designs, as HT initiation usually occurred at the time of menopause in the observational studies, but occurred several years after menopause in most randomized studies. Studies using female nonhuman primates as models of the effect of HT on coronary atherosclerosis progression also support the important role of the time of HT initiation, with a reduction in coronary atherosclerosis when HT is initiated at menopause, but a loss of the protective effects when HT is started after a period equivalent to six human postmenopausal years [8]. The causes for the increased risk of CHD with HT in late menopause are unclear, but it has been hypothesized that increased inflammation and thrombogenicity play a role [9, 10].

Estrogen therapy has been shown to significantly affect plasma lipoprotein levels in postmenopausal women. Specifically, estrogen has been shown to significantly reduce plasma LDL-C levels and increase plasma HDL-C levels [11, 12]. In addition, in some studies, estrogen was reported to increase plasma TG levels. When progestin is added to estrogen, a blunting of the estrogen-mediated effect on HDL-C levels usually occurs, and the degree of this opposing effect is dependent on the androgenic potency of the progestin used and its dose [12, 13].

The estrogen-mediated increase in HDL-C levels is mostly due to increases in the HDL subfraction containing only apo A-I (LpAI) and in the large-size HDL subfraction (HDL$_2$) [12, 14, 15]. Two-dimensional gel electrophoresis analysis of HDL subpopulations indicated that estrogen mediates a significant increase in the large α1 and α2 HDL particles [12, 16]. It is generally thought that the LpAI and larger HDL subfractions have stronger antiatherogenic properties than other HDL fractions [17].

Estrogen may be administered orally or transdermally. Both routes of administration achieve premenopausal physiological plasma concentrations of estrogen and result in effective suppression of FSH secretion. However, orally administered estrogen reaches the liver in higher concentrations and, through its first-pass through the liver, is converted to a series of different metabolites, while transdermal estrogen administration slowly delivers estradiol directly into the

S. Lamon-Fava (✉)
Lipid Metabolism Laboratory, Tufts University,
711 Washington Street, Boston, MA 02111, USA
e-mail: stefania.lamon-fava@tufts.edu

---

circulation. Several studies have shown that only the oral administration significantly increases plasma HDL-C levels, while the estrogen transdermal administration causes little or no changes in plasma HDL-C levels [15, 18]. The different rate of conversion to metabolites and the different hepatic concentration of estrogen obtained with the two types of estrogen administration may differentially influence hepatic gene expression and thus HDL metabolism.

Estrogen has been shown to regulate the activity and/or expression of several proteins involved in HDL metabolism. Most of these proteins play an important role in the intra-plasma metabolism of HDL. It has long been known that estrogen lowers the activity of HL [14, 19]. Inhibition of HL leads to the formation of large HDL particles [19]. In addition, the scavenger receptor class B type I (SR-BI), a cell membrane protein involved in cholesterol transport, is regulated by estrogen: in liver cells, SR-BI expression is reduced by estrogen, while in steroidogenic tissues, estrogen causes an increased expression of this protein, thereby facilitating cholesterol uptake by these tissues [20]. There is some indication that cholesteryl ester transfer protein (CETP) may also be affected by estrogen, with higher levels of CETP in premenopausal women than in postmenopausal women, and a significant and positive correlation between CETP and estrogen levels in premenopausal women [21].The estrogen-associated changes in HL and SR-BI would predict to lower the catabolism of HDL, while the increase in CETP would predict to increase HDL catabolism.

Metabolic studies have been carried out to assess the effect of estrogen on the kinetics of apo A-I in HDL, and the general consensus is that estrogen does not affect HDL clearance, but increases apo A-I production (Table 1). In the only study carried out in premenopausal women, Schaefer et al. [22] found that oral administration of 0.1 mg/day ethinyl estradiol was associated with an increase in plasma HDL-C and HDL_2 levels (38 and 150%, respectively), relative to baseline levels. In addition, a 27% increase in apo A-I levels

in HDL was observed with estrogen. The metabolism of HDL was studied by injections of autologous radiolabeled apo A-I HDL at the end of the baseline and estrogen phases: the increase in HDL-C and apo A-I levels in the estrogen phase were accompanied by a 25% increase in apo A-I production, relative to baseline [22].

Walsh et al. [15]. studied the effect of 17β-estradiol, both as oral (2 mg/day) and transdermal (0.1 mg twice weekly) administration, on the kinetics of apo A-I in HDL in eight postmenopausal women. The kinetics of apo A-I were studied using stable isotope methodology by endogenously labeling apolipoproteins with deuterated leucine, administered as a primed-constant infusion over a 14-h period at the end of the placebo and of each treatment phase. Oral estrogen administration was associated with significant increases in the cholesterol and apo A-I content of HDL_2 (40 and 37%, respectively, both $p < 0.05$), relative to placebo [15]. Modest but significant increases in the cholesterol and apo A-I content of HDL_3 (17 and 11%, respectively, $p < 0.05$) were also observed. Relative to placebo, oral estradiol treatment did not affect HDL_2 apo A-I fractional catabolic rate, but was associated with a 36% increase in HDL_2 apo A-I production rate ($p < 0.01$). Also, a modest but significant increase in HDL_3 apo A-I production rate (19%, $p = 0.04$) was observed. Conversely, relative to placebo, treatment with transdermal estradiol had no significant effects on the cholesterol and apo A-I content of HDL_2 and HDL_3, and on apo A-I fractional catabolic rate or production rate. This study clearly indicates that estrogen affects HDL-C levels and apo A-I levels by increasing the production of apo A-I, without affecting the rate of apo A-I clearance.

Brinton [14] studied the effect of oral ethinyl estradiol (0.05 mg/day) in six healthy postmenopausal women. Relative to baseline, estrogen significantly increased plasma levels of HDL-C and apo A-I (36 and 27%, respectively, $p < 0.005$) and plasma levels of LpAI (66%, $p < 0.02$), but not LpAIAII (14%). Apo A-I kinetics was studied by radioactively labeling

Table 1 Studies assessing the effect of hormone therapy on apo A-I metabolism

Author	Subjects	Treatment	Fraction	Apo A-I FCR[a]	Apo A-I PR[a]
Schaefer et al. [22]	Premenopausal, $N=4$	Ethinyl E	HDL	−2%	+25%*
Walsh et al. [15]	Postmenopausal, $N=8$	17β-E, oral	HDL_2	+3%	+36%*
			HDL_3	+10%	+19%*
Walsh et al. [15]	Postmenopausal, $N=8$	17β-E, transdermal	HDL_2	+8%	+7%
			HDL_3	+14%	+4%
Brinton [14]	Postmenopausal, $N=6$	Ethinyl E	LpAI	+7%	+76%*
			LpAIAII	+5%	+22%
Lamon-Fava et al. [23]	Postmenopausal, $N=7$	CEE	HDL	+20%	+47%*
Lamon-Fava et al. [23]	Postmenopausal, $N=8$	CEE+MPA vs. CEE	HDL	−5%	−13%*
Hazzard et al. [24]	Postmenopausal, $N=1$	Ethinyl E	HDL	−42%	−37%
Quintao et al. [25]	Postmenopausal, $N=7$	17β-E	HDL	−45%*	

[a]Percent change from control phase; *FCR* fractional catabolic rate; *PR* production rate
*$p < 0.05$

the autologous HDL fractions containing apo A-I only (LpAI) and the HDL containing both apo A-I and apo A-II (LpAIAII). Subjects received injections of ^{125}I-LpAIAII and ^{131}I-LpAI at baseline and at the end of the estradiol phase. The plasma decay curves of LpAI were similar at baseline and during estrogen (+7%, p=0.2), indicating no significant effect of treatment on apo A-I fractional catabolic rate in this HDL fraction [14]. Similarly, the fractional catabolic rate of LpAIAII was not affected by treatment (+5%, p=0.2). Therefore, the increase in plasma concentration of LpAI was explained by a significant increase in its production (76%, p<0.001), while the production of LpAIAII was modestly and nonsignificantly increased (22%, p=0.2). The activity of the enzymes HL and lipoprotein lipase (LPL) were assessed at the end of each study period. LPL activity was not modified by treatment, while HL activity was significantly reduced (by 66%, p<0.01) by estradiol. Therefore, the reduction in HL activity did not result in a reduced clearance of HDL. Instead, the production of apo A-I in the LpAI fraction of HDL was the main contributor to the HDL-C increase by estrogen.

Our group has assessed the effect of estrogen and progestin on HDL metabolism in postmenopausal women [23]. Eight subjects underwent a placebo-controlled, randomized, crossover study of conjugated equine estrogen (CEE) 0.625 mg/day and CEE plus medroxyprogesterone acetate (MPA) 2.5 mg/day (in one subject, kinetic data during the placebo phase could not be assessed). The kinetic parameters of apo A-I in HDL were assessed at the end of each of three treatment phases. Estrogen significantly increased plasma apo A-I levels by 21%, accompanied by a significant increase in apo A-I production rate (+47%) and a nonsignificant trend for an increase in apo A-I fractional catabolic rate (20%) (Table 2). Therefore, in agreement with the previous studies, oral estrogen administration caused significant increases in plasma HDL-C and apo A-I levels and this effect was due to

an increased synthesis of apo A-I. To assess the independent effect of progestin on apo A-I metabolism, the kinetics of apo A-I during the CEE phase were compared to those during the CEE+MPA phase, The combination of CEE+MPA lowered plasma levels of apo A-I by 9% and this was attributed to the significant 13% reduction in apo A-I production rate, relative to the CEE phase (Table 2). By clearly showing that the addition of a progestin to estrogen in HRT results in a significant drop in apo A-I levels and production rate, this study suggests that the combination treatment may lessen the beneficial effect of estrogen on HDL, and therefore lower the antiatherogenic potential of estrogen. It is likely that the androgenic property of MPA is responsible for the observed reduction in apo A-I PR.

Not all studies assessing the mechanisms by which estrogen replacement increases plasma HDL-C levels have shown an increase in the production rate of apo A-I (Table 1). In two independent studies, estrogen therapy was shown to reduce the clearance of apo A-I in HDL [24, 25].

According to the concept of reverse cholesterol transport, it is conceivable that increasing plasma HDL levels through an increase in apo A-I synthesis will lead to protection from atherosclerosis. Studies in human apo A-I transgenic mice have clearly indicated that overexpression of human apo A-I is associated with the inhibition of vascular lesion formation [26]. Similar findings have been reported in human apo A-I transgenic rabbits [27]. In humans, infusions with reconstituted apo A-I liposome complexes have shown an increase in bile acids and neutral steroids in the feces, compatible with the results in the animal studies [28].

As indicated above, the majority of studies indicate that, in postmenopausal women, treatment with estrogen is associated with an increase in plasma levels of HDL-C and apo A-I due to an increase in the production of apo A-I. Whether this increase in apo A-I synthesis is beneficial in terms of cardiovascular disease prevention is still unclear.

At least three estrogen receptors (ER) have been identified. ERα and ERβ are ligand-activated classic nuclear receptors [29], but a third, membrane-bound receptor belonging to the G protein-coupled receptor family, GPR30, can also bind estrogen and initiate signal transduction [30]. The distribution of these receptors is tissue-dependent. ERα is prevalently expressed in liver and reproductive tissues, but ERα and ERβ are similarly expressed in the vasculature [31]. Less is known about the distribution of GRP30 in the vascular cells. Estrogen receptors affect cell function through both genomic and nongenomic mechanisms. Nongenomic actions are initiated by membrane-bound receptors (either ERs or GRP30), which trigger different signal transduction pathways, including mitogen-activated protein (MAP) kinase, activation of ion channels, and activation of phosphatidylinositol 3-kinase-Akt. The best known example of nongenomic action of estrogen is the activation of NO release from

Table 2 Effects of placebo, conjugated equine estrogen CEE), and medroxyprogesterone acetate (MPA) on plasma concentrations and kinetic parameters of apo A-I in postmenopausal women

Apo A-I	Concentration (mg/dl)	FCR (pools/day)	PR (mg/kg/day)
N=7			
Placebo	126±23	0.202±0.029	11.5±2.9
CEE	150±19	0.240±0.063	15.9±2.9
% change	+21	+20	+47
p value	0.004	0.14	0.04
N=8			
CEE	149±18	0.232±0.062	15.3±3.1
CEE+MPA	136±21	0.221±0.049	13.2±2.0
% change	−9	−3	−13
p value	0.004	0.32	0.02

Values are mean±SD; *FCR* fractional catabolic rate; *PR* production rate

Apo A-I promoter

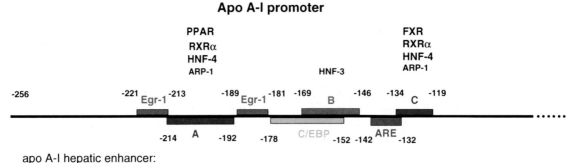

Fig. 1 Apo A-I promoter

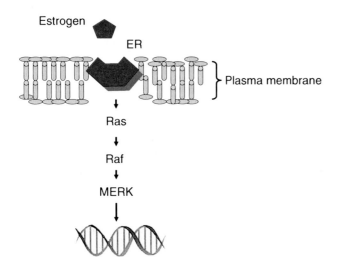

Fig. 2 Gene expression regulation by membrane-bound ERs

endothelial cells [32]. In vitro experiments have been conducted to investigate the effect of estrogen on apo A-I expression. In the human hepatoma cell line HepG2, estrogen was shown to increase both the expression and the secretion of apo A-I [33, 34]. The increased expression was due to increased transcription activation of the apo A-I gene [35]. However, the apo A-I gene does not contain a functional estrogen response element and thus activation of transcription by estrogen is not mediated by a direct interaction of the estrogen receptor with this gene. It has been however demonstrated that estrogen causes an increased expression and binding of two transcription factors, Egr-1 and HNF-3β, to the promoter of the apo A-I gene (Fig. 1) [35]. In HepG2 cells, inhibition of MAPK activity was shown to blunt the increase in apo A-I expression [35]. Therefore, it is concluded that the activation of membrane-bound estrogen receptors and subsequent activation of the MAPK signaling cascade is the molecular mechanism involved in the estrogen activation of apo A-I expression in liver cells (Fig. 2).

References

1. American Heart Association (2008) Heart disease and stroke statistics – 2008 update. American Heart Association, USA
2. Stampfer MJ, Colditz GA (1991) Estrogen replacement therapy and coronary heart disease: a quantitative assessment of epidemiologic evidence. Prev Med 20:47–63
3. Colditz GA, Willett WC, Stampfer MJ, Rosner B, Speizer FE, Hennekens CH (1987) Menopause and the risk of coronary heart disease in women. N Engl J Med 316:1105–1110
4. Hulley SB, Grady D, Bush T, Furberg CD, Herrington DM, Riggs B, Vittinghoff E, for the Heart and Estrogen/progestin Replacement Study (HERS) Research Group (1998) Randomized trial of estrogen plus progestin for secondary prevention of coronary heart disease in postmenopausal women. JAMA 280:605–613
5. Writing Group for the Women's Health Initiative Investigators (2002) Risks and benefits of estrogen plus progestin in healthy postmenopausal women: principal results from the Women's Health Initiative randomized controlled trial. JAMA 288:321–333
6. Rossouw J, Prentice R, Manson JA, Wu L, Barad D, Barnabei V, Marcia K, LaCroix A, Margolis K, Stefanick M (2007) Postmenopausal hormone therapy and risk of cardiovascular disease by age and years since menopause. JAMA 297:1465–1477
7. Grodstein F, Manson JE, Stampfer MJ (2006) Hormone therapy and coronary heart disease: the role of time since menopause and age at hormone initiation. J Womens Health 15:35–44
8. Clarkson TB, Appt SE (2005) Controversies about HRT: lessons from monkey models. Maturitas 51:64–74
9. Smith N, Keckbert S, Lemaitre R, Reiner A, Lumley T, Weiss N (2004) Esterified estrogens and conjugated equine estrogens and the risk of venous thrombosis. JAMA 292:1581–1587
10. Seli E, Guzeloglu-Kayisli O, Cakman H, Kayisli U, Selam B, Arici A (2006) Estradiol increases apoptosis in huma coronary artery endothelial cells by up-regulating Fas and Fas ligand expression. J Clin Endocrinol Metab 91:4995–5001
11. Granfone A, Campos H, McNamara JR, Schaefer MM, Lamon-Fava S, Ordovas JM, Schaefer EJ (1992) Effects of estrogen replacement on plasma lipoproteins and apolipoproteins in postmenopausal dyslipidemic women. Metabolism 41:1193–1198
12. Lamon-Fava S, Postfai B, Asztalos BF, Horvath KV, Dallal G, Schaefer EJ (2004) Effects of estrogen and medroxyprogesterone acetate on subpopulations of triglyceride-rich lipoproteins and high-density lipoproteins. Metabolism 52:1330–1336
13. The writing group for the PEPI Trial (1995) Effects of estrogen or estrogen/progestin regimens on heart disease risk factors in

postmenopausal women. The Postmenopausal Estrogen/Progestin Interventions (PEPI) Trial. JAMA 273:199–208

14. Brinton EA (1996) Oral estrogen replacement therapy in postmenopausal women selectively raises levels and production rates of lipoprotein AI and lowers hepatic lipase activity without lowering the catabolic rate. Arterioscler Thromb Vasc Biol 16:431–440

15. Walsh BW, Li H, Sacks FM (1994) Effects of postmenopausal hormone replacement with oral and transdermal estrogen on high density lipoprotein metabolism. J Lipid Res 35:2083–2093

16. Lamon-Fava S, Herrington DM, Reboussin BA, Sherman M, Horvath KV, Schaefer EJ, Asztalos BF (2009) Changes in remnant and high-density lipoproteins associated with hormone therapy and progression of coronary artery disease in postmenopausal women. Atherosclerosis 205(1):325–330

17. Barbaras R, Puchois P, Fruchart JC, Ailhaud G (1987) Cholesterol efflux from culture adipose tissue cells is mediated by LpAI particles but not by LpAIAII particles. Biochem Biophys Res Comm 1:63–70

18. Vrablik M, Fait T, Kovar J, Poledne R, Ceska R (2008) Oral but not transdermal estrogen replacement therapy changes the composition of plasma lipoproteins. Metabolism 57:1086–1092

19. Applebaum-Bowden D, McLean P, Steinmetz A, Fontana D, Matthys C, Warnick GR, Cheung MC, Albers JJ, Hazzard WR (1989) Lipoprotein, apolipoprotein, and lipolytic enzyme changes following estrogen administration in postmenopausal women. J Lipid Res 30:1895–1906

20. Landschulz KT, Pathak RK, Rigotti AKM, Hobbs HH (1996) Regulation of scavenger receptor, class B, type 1, a high density lipoprotein receptor, in liver and steroidogenic tissues of the rat. J Clin Invest 98:984–995

21. Zhang C, Zhuang Y, Qiang H, Liu X, Xu R, Wu Y (2001) Relationship between endogenous estrogen concentrations and serum cholesteryl ester transfer protein concentrations in Chinese women. Clin Chim Acta 314:77–83

22. Schaefer EJ, Foster DM, Zech LA, Lindgren FT, Brewer HBJ, Levy RI (1983) The effects of estrogen administration on plasma lipoprotein metabolism in premenopausal women. J Clin Endocrinol Metab 57:262–267

23. Lamon-Fava S, Postfai B, Diffenderfer M, deLuca C, O'Connor J Jr, Welty FK, Dolnikowski GG, Barrett P, Schaefer EJ (2006) Role of the estrogen and progestin in hormonal replacement therapy on apolipoprotein A-I kinetics in postmenopausal women. Arterioscler Thromb Vasc Biol 26:385–391

24. Hazzard WR, Haffner S, Kushwaha R, Applebaum-Bowden D, Foster DM (1984) Preliminary report: kinetic studies on the modulation of high-density lipoprotein, apolipoprotein, and subfraction metabolism by sex steroids in a postmenopausal woman. Metabolism 33:779–784

25. Quintao E, Nakandakare E, Oliveira HCF, Rocha J, Garcia RC, de Melo N (1991) Oral estradiol-117beta raises the level of plasma high-density lipoprotein in menopausal women by slowing down its clearance rate. Acta Endocrinol (Copenh) 125:657–661

26. Rubin E, Krauss R, Spangler E, Verstuyft J, Clift S (1991) Inhibition of early atherogenesis in transgenic mice by human apolipoprotien A-I. Nature 353:265–267

27. Duverger N, Kruth H, Emmanuel F, Caillaud J, Viglietta C, Castro GR, Tailleux A, Fievet C, Fruchart JC, Houdebine L, Denefle P (1996) Inhibition of atherosclerosis development in cholesterol-fed human apolipoprotein A-I-transgenic rabbits. Circulation 94: 713–717

28. Eriksson M, Carlson LA, Miettinen T, Angelin B (1999) Stimulation of fecal steroid excretion after infusion of recombinant proapolipoprotein A-I. Potential reverse cholesterol transport in humans. Circulation 100:594–598

29. Kuiper GG, Enmark E, Pelto-Huikko M, Nilsson S, Gustafsson J-A (1996) Cloning of a novel receptor expressed in rat prostate and ovary. Proc Natl Acad Sci USA 93:5925–5930

30. Thomas P, Pang Y, Filardo EJ, Dong J (2005) Identity of an estrogen membrane receptor coupled to a G protein in human breast cancer cells. Endocrinology 146:624–632

31. Mendelsohn M, Karas R (1999) The protective effects of estrogen on the cardiovascular system. N Engl J Med 340:1801–1811

32. Stirone C, Boroujerdi A, Duckles SP, Krause DN (2005) Estrogen receptor activation of phosphoinositide-3 kinase, akt, and nitric oxide signaling in cerebral blood vessels: rapid and long-term effects. Mol Pharmacol 67:105–113

33. Tam S, Archer T, Deeley R (1985) Effects of estrogen on apolipoprotein secretion by the human hepatocarcinoma cell line Hep G2. J Biol Chem 260:1670–1675

34. Lamon-Fava S (2000) Genistein activates apolipoprotein A-I gene expression in the human hepatoma cell line Hep G2. J Nutr 130:2489–2492

35. Lamon-Fava S, Micherone D (2004) Regulation of apo A-I gene expression: mechanism of action of estrogen and genistein. J Lipid Res 45:106–112

Effects of Niacin on HDL Metabolism

Stefania Lamon-Fava

The cholesterol-lowering effects of nicotinic acid, or niacin, were discovered by Altschul et al. [1] more than 50 years ago. Since then, nicotinic acid has been shown to be very effective in reducing the risk of coronary heart disease (CHD). The Coronary Drug Project was the first randomized clinical trial to show a significant reduction in recurrent non-fatal myocardial infarctions over a follow-up of 6.5 years in 3,908 men with a prior CHD who had been randomized to 3 g/day of immediate-release nicotinic acid, relative to pla-cebo [2]. Subsequently, other studies, including the CLAS (Cholesterol-Lowering Atherosclerosis Study) [3], FATS (Familial Atherosclerosis Treatment Study) [4], HATS (HDL-Atherosclerosis Treatment Study) [5], and ARBITER 2 (Arterial Biology for the Investigation of the Treatment Effects of Reducing cholesterol) [6] studies, have shown that nicotinic acid in combination with other lipid-lowering med-ications significantly lowers CHD risk or coronary artery disease progression.

Niacin is the most potent HDL-C-raising medication currently available. In addition to increasing HDL-C levels, niacin decreases plasma TG and LDL-C levels [2, 7, 8]. Niacin is also one of the few lipid-modifying medications capable of reducing plasma levels of another atherogenic lipoprotein, lipoprotein(a) [Lp(a)] [9]. However, the use of niacin in the treatment of plasma lipid abnormalities and the reduction of CHD risk has been limited by significant side effects, such as flushing. The extended-release formulation of niacin is preferred over the immediate-release formulation for its greater tolerability. Treatment with extended-release niacin has been shown to lower plasma TG levels by 20–50%, LDL-C by 0–15%, and Lp(a) by 25–30%, and to increase plasma HDL-C levels by 20–40% [7, 10]. Even though the clinical benefits of niacin treatment are well established, the effects of niacin on plasma lipoprotein metabolism have not been clearly defined.

S. Lamon-Fava (✉)
Lipid Metabolism Laboratory, Tufts University,
711 Washington Street, Boston, MA 02111, USA
e-mail: stefania.lamon-fava@tufts.edu

In 2003, three groups independently identified a specific receptor for nicotinic acid, named GPR109A (also known as HM74A in humans and PUMA-G in mice) [11–13]. GPR109A is a member of the G protein-coupled receptors in cell mem-branes, and is expressed in adipose tissue, spleen, and immune cells but not in liver, intestine, kidney, or muscle [11, 13–15]. Animal studies have indicated that this receptor is involved in the nicotinic acid-mediated reduction in adipocyte lipolysis and release of free fatty acids (FFA) [12] (Fig. 1). It has been hypothesized that the reduction in plasma TG levels follow-ing niacin administration is mediated by the niacin-induced inhibition of FFA release from adipose tissue, which may lead to reduced substrate availability for TG synthesis and secretion by hepatic cells [16]. However, in humans, the inhi-bition of FFA release by niacin is short-termed and is fol-lowed by a significant rebound in plasma FFA levels less than 4 h after administration [17], while the reduction in TG levels is sustained over 24 h. Previously, Wang et al. [18] have reported that the production of TG in very low-density lipo-protein (VLDL) was lowered by niacin in normolipidemic women, but this reduction was not fully explained by the effect of niacin on FFA levels. In vitro experiments have also suggested that niacin inhibits the activity of diglycerol acyl-transferase-2 (DGAT-2), an enzyme involved in TG synthesis in hepatic cells [19]. Altogether, these experiments suggest that the primary effect of niacin on VLDL is a reduction in hepatic VLDL production. However, two studies aimed at understanding the mechanism of action of niacin on apo B-containing lipoprotein metabolism have been carried out in subjects with elevated TG levels and have come to the conclu-sion that niacin increases the clearance of VLDL particles. In one hypertriglyceridemic subject, clearance of autologous ^{125}I-labeled VLDL was faster after niacin treatment, relative to the absence of niacin treatment, suggesting that mecha-nisms other than a reduction in TG-rich lipoprotein synthesis may contribute to lowering of plasma TG levels. In another study, conducted by our group in five subjects with dyslipi-demia, extended-release niacin lowered plasma TG and VLDL apo B levels, relative to placebo, and these reductions were accompanied by faster VLDL apo B clearance [10].

E.J. Schaefer (ed.), *High Density Lipoproteins, Dyslipidemia, and Coronary Heart Disease,*
DOI 10.1007/978-1-4419-1059-2_18, © Springer Science+Business Media, LLC 2010

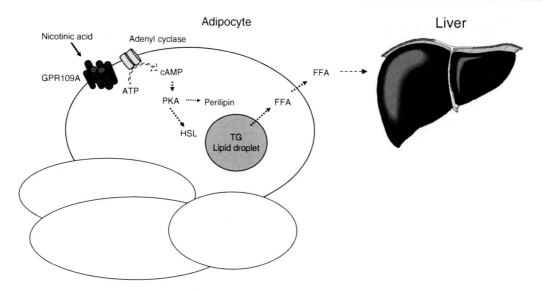

Fig. 1 Effect of nicotinic acid-mediated activation of the nicotinic acid receptor on adipocytes. *Dotted lines* indicate inhibition. *PKA* protein kinase A; *HSL* hormone sensitive lipase. Reprinted from Lamon-Fava S, et al. Extended-release niacin alters the metabolism of plasma apolipoprotein (Apo) A-1 and ApoB containing lipoproteins. Arterioscler Thromb Vasc Biol 2008; 28:1672–1678

Niacin is the most effective medication currently available for raising HDL-C levels. Specifically, niacin has been shown to selectively increase the HDL subfraction containing only apo A-I (LpAI), with little effect on the HDL subfraction containing both apo A-I and apo A-II (LpAIAII) [20, 21]. LpAI is thought to be more atheroprotective than LpAIAII [22]. An increase in large HDL particles and a reduction in small HDL particles with niacin were observed by nuclear magnetic resonance spectroscopy [23]. HDL subfractions were assessed by two-dimensional gel electrophoresis in the HATS study, where subjects with CHD were randomized to placebo or a combination of niacin/simvastatin, and plasma levels of the large α1 HDL particles were significantly increased by 115% in subjects treated with niacin/simvastatin, relative to placebo [24]. Additionally, the increase in the α1 HDL subpopulation was significantly and inversely correlated with the progression of coronary atherosclerosis during the trial [24]. This association indicates that the changes in HDL caused by niacin are beneficial: either the increased particle number or the change in HDL composition make HDL more efficient in the reverse cholesterol transport.

To date, three studies have attempted to elucidate the effect of niacin on HDL metabolism by studying the kinetics of apo A-I and apo A-II in HDL. Two of these studies were conducted in young, normocholesterolemic subjects [25, 26], while the third was conducted in dyslipidemic subjects [10]. In the first study, Blum et al. [25] found that, in two young normolipidemic subjects, immediate-release niacin (1 g three times daily) increased HDL-C levels (from 36 to 44 mg/dL) and the ratio of cholesterol/protein in HDL (from 0.32 to 0.37). After injection of autologous ^{125}I-HDL, treatment with nicotinic acid was associated with slower plasma

Table 1 Effects of placebo and extended-release niacin on plasma lipid concentrations in five dyslipidemic subjects

	Placebo (mg/dL)	Niacin (mg/dL)	Percent change	p value
TC	224±39	199±29	−10	0.14
TG	382±1.35	259±1.59	−21	0.04
LDL-C	117±38	115±16	+3	0.59
HDL-C	30±6	43±9	+44	0.001

Values are mean±SD

radioactivity decay, indicating slower apo A-I clearance. In the second study, Shepherd et al. [26] studied the effect of immediate-release niacin (1 g three times daily) on HDL metabolism in five young healthy subjects. Niacin significantly increased plasma HDL-C (from 52 to 64 mg/dL, $p < 0.05$) and apo A-I (135 mg/dL vs. 145 mg/dL, $p < 0.05$) levels, but significantly reduced plasma apo A-II levels (29 mg/dL vs. 25 mg/dL, $p < 0.05$) [26]. Subjects underwent injections with autologous HDL labeled with ^{131}I-apo A-I and ^{125}I-apo A-II before and after treatment with niacin: measurement of plasma radioactivity decay indicated a slower catabolism and reduced synthesis of apo A-II with nicotinic acid but no effect on apo A-I kinetic parameters [26].

In the third study, five men with dyslipidemia (TG ≥ 150 mg/dL, LDL-C ≥ 130 mg/dL, and HDL-C ≤ 40 mg/dL) underwent a placebo-controlled, randomized, crossover study of the effect of extended-release niacin (2 g/day) on the kinetics of apo A-I and apo A-II in HDL [10]. Subjects with elevated TG and low HDL-C levels are the ideal targets of treatment with nicotinic acid. Relative to placebo, a significant reduction in plasma TG levels (−21%) and a significant increase in plasma HDL-C levels (+44%) were observed (Table 1). The metabolism of HDL was studied by endogenous labeling of apolipoproteins with deuterated leucine, administered as a primed-constant infusion over a period of 15 h at the end of the placebo and the niacin phases. Niacin significantly increased plasma apo A-I concentrations by 15% and apo A-I production rate by 24%, without affecting apo A-I fractional catabolic rate (Table 2). On the other hand, apo A-II plasma levels and kinetic parameters were not significantly affected by niacin (Table 2). These results suggest that, in dyslipidemic subjects, niacin increases plasma apo A-I levels by increasing its synthesis and secretion. These findings are in contrast with those in the two previous human metabolic studies [25, 26]. The discrepancy between studies may be explained by differences in the characteristics of the study subjects and in study design: subjects with abnormal plasma TG and HDL-C levels may respond differently to niacin compared to young, healthy, and normolipidemic subjects. In addition, in the study by Lamon-Fava et al. [10], apolipoproteins were endogenously labeled with a stable isotope, a method which has the advantages of labeling nascent particles and conserving the structure, metabolism, and binding characteristics of lipoproteins [27].

In vitro experiments using the human hepatoma cell line HepG2 have shown that niacin increases the apo A-I concentration in the media (47%) by reducing its hepatic re-uptake (17%) without affecting apo A-I gene expression [28]. Recently, it was shown that this effect is mediated by the inhibition of the expression of ATP synthase β chain, a protein involved in apo A-I uptake in liver cells [29]. These experiments indicate that the modulation of apo A-I levels by niacin may involve the catabolism and not the production of apo A-I in liver cells and support the findings from the earlier human metabolic studies. However, it is not clear if these mechanisms of apo A-I regulation may be effective in dyslipidemic subjects.

It should be pointed out that, in the study of five dyslipidemic subjects, the observed increase in plasma apo A-I levels (+15%) was less than the increase in plasma HDL-C levels (+44%) [10]. Therefore, only part of the increase in HDL-C levels could be explained by the effect of niacin on

apo A-I production. The additional effect of niacin on HDL-C levels is consistent with remodeling of HDL, leading to the formation of larger, cholesterol-enriched HDL particles [23, 24] (Fig. 2). In fact, a significant increase in the large α1 and α2 HDL particles was observed in these subjects in the niacin phase, relative to placebo (Table 3) [10]. The formation of larger, cholesterol-enriched HDL may be mediated by an inhibition of cholesteryl ester transfer protein (CETP) activity. This enzyme plays an important role in HDL metabolism by mediating the exchange of TG in VLDL and LDL with cholesteryl ester (CE) in HDL. In a recent study conducted in mice carrying the apo E3 Leiden mutation without (E3L) or with (E3L/CETP) the human CETP gene, it was observed that while the E3L mice responded to niacin treatment with a reduction in TG levels, only the E3L/CETP mice responded to niacin treatment with a reduction in TG levels and an increase in HDL-C levels [30]. The increase in HDL-C levels with niacin in the E3L/CETP mouse was accompanied by an increase in the residence time of apo A-I. In addition, a reduction in the hepatic CETP mRNA levels and in CETP

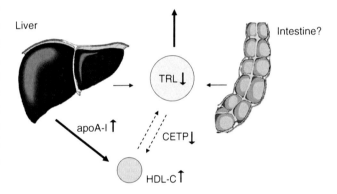

Fig. 2 Niacin may increase HDL-C levels by increasing the synthesis of apo A-I by liver cells (and potentially intestinal cells), and by reducing the activity of CETP. Reprinted from Lamon-Fava S, et al. Extented-release niacin alters the metabolism of plasma apolipoprotein (Apo) A-1 and ApoB- containing lipoproteins. Arterioscler Thromb Vasc Biol 2008; 28:1672–1678

Table 2 Effects of placebo and extended-release niacin on plasma concentrations and kinetic parameters of apo A-I and apo A-II in HDL in five dyslipidemic subjects

	Placebo	Niacin	Percent change	p value
Apo A-I				
C (mg/dL)	103 ± 11	118 ± 5	+15	0.001
FCR (pools/day)	0.205 ± 0.03	0.217 ± 0.03	+7	0.47
PR (mg/kg/day)	9.5 ± 1.5	11.5 ± 1.0	+24	0.04
Apo A-II				
C (mg/dL)	25 ± 3	26 ± 4	+6	0.47
FCR (pools/day)	0.135 ± 0.02	0.127 ± 0.2	−5	0.79
PR (mg/kg/day)	1.48 ± 0.11	1.46 ± 0.23	−1	0.99

Values are mean ± SD

C concentration; *FCR* fractional catabolic rate; *PR* production rate

Table 3 Effects of placebo and extended-release on apo A-I-containing HDL subpopulation concentrations in five dyslipidemic subjects

	Placebo	Niacin	Percent change	p value
Preβ$_1$	18.1 ± 5.5	16.3 ± 5.4	−7	0.32
Preβ$_2$	2.7 ± 1.1	3.0 ± 1.0	+18	0.10
α$_1$	7.1 ± 3.5	14.1 ± 5.9	+122	0.006
α$_2$	27.0 ± 5.6	33.5 ± 2.2	+27	0.02
α$_3$	25.4 ± 5.9	22.5 ± 6.9	−12	0.27
α$_4$	11.8 ± 1.7	10.2 ± 2.0	−12	0.28
Preα$_1$	2.4 ± 2.1	7.8 ± 5.1	+338	0.02
Preα$_2$	4.1 ± 1.0	6.8 ± 2.1	+66	0.02
Preα$_3$	2.9 ± 0.9	2.8 ± 0.7	+1	0.99
Preα$_4$	1.5 ± 0.6	1.3 ± 0.4	−7	0.85

Values are mean ± SD; HDL subpopulations expressed as mg/dL of apo A-I

plasma levels was observed with niacin in E3L/CETP mice. A reduction in CETP activity may indeed lead to an increase in the cholesterol content of HDL and to larger HDL particles [31]. In addition, since niacin significantly lowers plasma levels of VLDL, which serve as substrate for the TG/CE exchange, it is likely that niacin causes a further reduction in CETP activity.

In conclusion, despite the large body of evidence supporting the efficacy of niacin in favorably affecting plasma lipid levels and in reducing CHD risk, there is a paucity of data on the mechanisms by which niacin exerts these effects. Understanding the mechanism of action of niacin on lipoprotein metabolism will help in developing other medications with similar beneficial effects but greater tolerability. The effects of niacin on lipoprotein metabolism need to be further studied in patients with hyperlipidemia or dyslipidemia, who are the ideal subjects for this treatment. In addition, the molecular basis for the effect of nicotinic acid on lipoprotein metabolism is not known. It is important to identify the molecular targets of niacin in the liver because this tissue is a major regulator of lipoprotein metabolism and does not express the nicotinic acid receptor GPR109A.

References

1. Altschul R, Hoffer A, Stephen JD (1955) Influence of nicotinic acid on serum cholesterol in man. Arch Biochem 54:558–559
2. The Coronary Drug Project Research Group (1975) Clofibrate and niacin in coronary heart disease. JAMA 231:360–381
3. Blankenhorn DH, Nessim SA, Johnson RL, Sanmarco ME, Azen SP, Cashin-Hemphill L (1987) Beneficial effects of combined colestipol/niacin therapy on coronary atherosclerosis and coronary venous bypass grafts. JAMA 257:3233–3240
4. Brown G, Albers JJ, Fisher L, Schaefer SM, Lin JT, Kaplan C, Zhao XQ, Bisson BD, Fitzpatrick VF, Dodge HT (1990) Regression of coronary artery disease as a result of intensive lipid-lowering therapy in men with high levels of apolipoprotein B. N Engl J Med 323:1289–1298
5. Brown B, Zhao X, Chait A, Fisher L, Cheung M, Morse J, Dowdy A, Marino E, Bolson E, Alaupovic P, Frohlich J, Albers J (2001) Simvastatin and niacin, antioxidant vitamins, or the combination for the prevention of coronary disease. N Engl J Med 345:1583–1592
6. Taylor AJ, Sullenberger LE, Lee HJ, Lee J, Grace KA (2004) Arterial Biology for the Investigation of the Treatment Effects of Reducing Cholesterol (ARBITER) 2: a double-blind, placebo-controlled study of extended-release niacin on atherosclerosis progression in secondary prevention patients treated with statins. Circulation 110:3512–3517
7. Capuzzi DM, Guyton JR, Morgan J, Goldberg AC, Kreisberg RA, Brusco OA, Brody J (1998) Efficacy and safety of an extended-release niacin (Niaspan): a long-term study. Am J Cardiol 82:74U–81U
8. Knopp RH, Ginsberg J, Albers JJ, Hoff C, Ogilvie JT, Warnick GR, Burrows E, Retzlaff B, Poole M (1985) Contrasting effects of unmodified and time-release forms of niacin on lipoproteins in hyperlipidemic subjects: clues to mechanism of action of niacin. Metabolism 34:642–650
9. Carlson LA, Hamsten A, Asplund A (1989) Pronounced lowering of serum levels of lipoprotein Lp(a) in hyperlipidemic subjects treated with nicotinic acid. J Intern Med 226(271):276
10. Lamon-Fava S, Diffenderfer M, Barrett PH, Buchsbaum A, Nyaku M, Horvath KV, Asztalos BF, Otokozawa S, Ai M, Matthan N, Lichtenstein AH, Dolnikowski GG, Schaefer EJ (2008) Extended-release niacin alters the metabolism of plasma apolipoprotein (apo) A-I and apoB-containing lipoproteins. Arterioscler Thromb Vasc Biol 28:1672–1678
11. Wise A, Foord SM, Fraser NJ, Barnes AA, Elshourbagy N, Eiler M, Ignar DM, Murdock PR, Steplewski K, Green A et al (2003) Molecular identification of high and low affinity receptors for nicotinic acid. J Biol Chem 278:9869–9874
12. Tunaru S, Kero J, Schaub A, Wufka C, Blaukat A, Pfeffer K, Offermanns S (2003) PUMA-G and HM74 are receptors for nicotinic acid and mediate its anti-lipolytic effect. Nat Med 9:352–355
13. Soga T, Kamohara M, Takasaki J, Matsumoto S-H, Saito T, Ohishi T, Hiyama H, Matsuo A, Matsushime H, Furuichi K (2003) Molecular identification of nicotinic acid receptor. Biochem Biophys Res Commn 303:364–369
14. Lorenzen A, Stannek C, Lang H, Andrianov V, Kalvinsh I, Schwabe U (2001) Characterization of a G-protein-coupled receptor for nicotinic acid. Mol Pharmacol 59:349–357
15. Lorenzen A, Stannek C, Burmeister A, Kalvinsh I, Schwabe U (2002) G protein-coupled receptor for nicotinic acid in mouse macrophages. Biochem Pharmacol 64:645–648
16. Carlson LA, Oro L (1962) The effect of nicotinic acid on the plasma free fatty acids. Acta Med Scand 172:641–645
17. Vega GL, Cater NB, Meguro S, Grundy SM (2005) Influence of extended-release nicotinic acid on nonesterified fatty acid flux in the metabolic syndrome with atherogenic dyslipidemia. Am J Cardiol 95:1309–1313
18. Wang W, Basinger A, Neese RA, Shane B, Myong S-A, Christiansen M, Hellerstein MK (2001) Effect of nicotinic acid administration on hepatic very low-density lipoprotein-triglyceride production. Am J Physiol Endocrinol Metab 43:E540–E547
19. Ganji SH, Tavintharan S, Zhu D, Xing Y, Kamanna VS, Kashyap ML (2004) Niacin noncompetitively inhibits DGAT2 but not DGAT1 activity in HepG2 cells. J Lipid Res 45:1835–1845
20. Atmeh RF, Shepherd J, Packard CJ (1983) Subpopulations of apo A-I in human HDLs. Their metabolic properties and response to drug therapy. Biochim Biophys Acta 751:175–188
21. Sakai T, Kamanna VS, Kashyap ML (2001) Niacin, but not gemfibrozil, selectively increases LpAI, a cardioprotective subfraction of HDL, in patients with low HDL cholesterol. Arterioscler Thromb Vasc Biol 21:1783–1789
22. Barbaras R, Puchois P, Fruchart JC, Ailhaud G (1987) Cholesterol efflux from culture adipose tissue cells is mediated by LpAI particles but not by LpAIAII particles. Biochem Biophys Res Comm 1:63–70
23. Kuvin JT, Dave DM, Sliney KA, Mooney P, Patel AR, Kimmelstiel CD, Karas R (2006) Effects of extended-release niacin on lipoprotein particle size, distribution, and inflammatory markers in patients with coronary artery disease. Am J Cardiol 98:743–745
24. Asztalos BF, Batista M, Horvath KV, Cox CE, Dallal G, Morse JS, Brown GB, Schaefer EJ (2003) Change in alpha1 HDL concentration predicts progression in coronary artery stenosis. Arterioscler Thromb Vasc Biol 23:847–852
25. Blum CB, Levy RI, Eisenberg S, Hall M III, Goebel RH, Berman M (1977) High density lipoprotein metabolism in man. J Clin Invest 60:795–807
26. Shepherd J, Packard CJ, Patsch JR, Gotto AM, Taunton OD (1979) Effects of nicotinic acid therapy on plasma high density lipoprotein subfraction distribution and composition and on apolipoprotein A metabolism. J Clin Invest 63:858–867

27. Marsh J, Welty FK, Schaefer EJ (2000) Stable isotope turnover of apolipoproteins of high-density lipoproteins in humans. Curr Opin Lipidol 11:261–266

28. Jin FY, Kamanna VS, Kashyap ML (1997) Niacin decreases removal of high-density lipoprotein apolipoprotein A-I but not cholesterol ester by Hep G2 cells. Arterioscler Thromb Vasc Biol 17:2020–2028

29. Zhang L-H, Kamanna VS, Zhang MC, Kashyap ML (2008) Niacin inhibits surface expression of ATP synthase beta chain in HepG2 cells; implications for raising HDL. J Lipid Res 49:1195–1201

30. van der Hoorn JWA, de Haan W, Berbee JF, Havekes LM, Jukema JW, Rensen PC, Princen HM (2008) Niacin increases HDL by reducing hepatic expression and plasma levels of cholesteryl ester transfer protein in apoE*Leiden.CETP mice. Arterioscler Thromb Vasc Biol 28:2016–2022

31. Asztalos BF, Horvath KV, Kajinami K, Nartsupha C, Cox CE, Batista M, Schaefer EJ, Inazu A, Mabuchi H (2004) Apolipoprotein composition of HDL in cholesteryl ester transfer protein deficiency. J Lipid Res 45:448–455

Effects of Statins on HDL Metabolism

Stefania Lamon-Fava

Primary and secondary prevention studies have clearly documented a reduction in coronary heart disease (CHD) risk with statins [1]. Statins, a family of cholesterol-lowering medications, inhibit the endogenous synthesis of cholesterol by competitively blocking the activity of 3-hydroxy-3-methylglutaryl coenzyme A (HMG CoA) reductase, a step-limiting enzyme in the synthesis of cholesterol (Fig. 1). In liver cells, the inhibition of cholesterol synthesis by statins activates the sterol regulatory element-binding protein (SREBP), a transcription factor that acts as a sensor of intracellular cholesterol, triggering an increase in the expression of the low-density lipoprotein (LDL) receptor [2]. Thus, the primary effect of statins is to reduce plasma concentrations of atherogenic LDL through an increase in LDL clearance [3–6]. In addition, statins are very effective in reducing plasma triglyceride (TG) levels. Statins are also known to modestly increase plasma levels of high-density lipoproteins (HDL) [7]. Randomized clinical trials have shown that statins variably increase plasma HDL-C levels by 1–13% [7]. Atorvastatin and rosuvastatin are the most effective statins in lowering LDL-C levels, but differ on their effect on HDL-C levels: in studies comparing the effect of different statins on HDL-C levels, atorvastatin increased this parameter less than other statins, while rosuvastatin had the greatest raising effect [7–10]. Generally, while statins have been documented to lower plasma LDL-C levels in a dose-dependent manner, no true dose–response effect of different statins on HDL-C levels has been observed (Fig. 2) [11], with a few exceptions. For example, high-dose atorvastatin has been shown to reverse the increase in HDL-C levels observed at lower doses [6, 12]. In the Statin Therapies for Elevated Lipid Levels Compared Across Doses to Rosuvastatin (STELLAR) study, doses of 10, 20, 40, and 80 mg/day of atorvastatin in 605 hypercholesterolemic patients resulted in HDL cholesterol increases

of 5.7, 4.8, 4.4, and 2.1%, respectively [12]. On the other hand, in the same study, a trend toward a dose-dependent increase in HDL-C levels was observed with rosuvastatin [12]. Statins also increase apo A-I levels, but the effect on apo A-I is more modest than that on HDL-C levels, resulting in a shift toward larger, more cholesterol-enriched, HDL particles [11]. It has been suggested that this effect is mediated by a reduction in the activity of cholesteryl ester transfer protein (CETP), which mediates the exchange of TG in TG-rich lipoproteins for cholesteryl esters in HDL [13]. This reduction in CETP activity during statin therapy may be explained by the significant reduction in TG-rich lipoproteins and LDL, which serve as substrate for CETP, but also by reduced expression of the CETP gene [14].

The clinical significance of the increase in HDL-C levels effected by statins is not well defined, but analyses performed in the Scandinavian Simvastatin Survival Study (4S) and the GREek Atorvastatin and Coronary heart disease Evaluation (GREACE) study have shown that the change in plasma HDL-C levels during treatment with statins was a significant predictor of CHD outcome even after controlling for the LDL-C lowering effect [15, 16].

Several metabolic studies have been conducted to assess the effect of statins on the production and clearance of apo A-I in HDL (Table 1). An earlier study by Ginsberg et al. [17], published only as an abstract, showed an increase in HDL-C levels in seven hypoalphalipoproteinemia subjects after treatment with lovastatin. In this study, the increase in HDL-C was associated with a significant 18% increase in apo A-I production rate (PR) [17]. In a study conducted in six normolipidemic subjects treated with pravastatin 40 mg/day, nonsignificant increases in both HDL-C and apo A-I levels were observed, associated with a 16% increase in apo A-I PR and a slight increase (5%) in apo A-I fractional catabolic rate (FCR) [18]. Currently, six independent groups have assessed the effect of atorvastatin on HDL metabolism, and have concluded that this statin does not affect significantly the kinetics of apo A-I in HDL. Watts et al. [3] studied the effects of atorvastatin 40 mg/day on the kinetics of apo A-I in HDL in a randomized, placebo-controlled, double-blind

S. Lamon-Fava (✉)
Lipid Metabolism Laboratory, Tufts University,
711 Washington Street, Boston, MA 02111, USA
e-mail: stefania.lamon-fava@tufts.edu

E.J. Schaefer (ed.), *High Density Lipoproteins, Dyslipidemia, and Coronary Heart Disease*,
DOI 10.1007/978-1-4419-1059-2_19, © Springer Science+Business Media, LLC 2010

study of 11 men with the metabolic syndrome. There was no significant effect of atorvastatin on plasma HDL-C (+1%) and apo A-I concentrations (−1%) after 5 weeks of atorvastatin, relative to placebo. In addition, no significant changes in apo A-I PR and FCR were observed. However, study subjects experienced a significant reduction in CETP activity during the atorvastatin phase relative to placebo [3]. Bilz et al. [19] studied eight subjects with elevated TG levels and normal or elevated LDL-C levels in an open-label study. The kinetics of apo A-I were studied at baseline and at the end of 8 weeks of atorvastatin 80 mg/day. Atorvastatin treatment resulted in a significant 18% increase in plasma HDL-C levels and a nonsignificant 4% increase in plasma apo A-I levels, compared to baseline [19]. No changes in apo A-I PR or FCR were observed between atorvastatin and baseline in

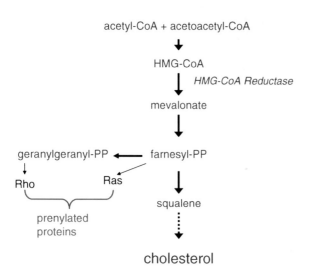

Fig. 1 *Cholesterol biosynthesis pathway*. Statins are competitive inhibitors of HMG-CoA reductase and thus inhibit the endogenous synthesis of cholesterol. Inhibition of cholesterol synthesis also leads to reduced formation of intermediates such as geranylgeranyl-diphosphate and farnesyl-diphosphate, which play a role in posttranslational modification of proteins

this study, suggesting that the effect of atorvastatin on the cholesterol content of HDL is independent of apo A-I kinetics [19]. Mauger et al. [20] compared the kinetics of apo A-I during treatment with 40 mg/day atorvastatin and during 80 mg/day simvastatin in a randomized, double-blind, crossover study of seven hypercholesterolemic subjects. Plasma HDL-C levels were similar at the end of the atorvastatin and simvastatin treatment phases, but plasma apo A-I levels were 8.1% lower ($P < 0.05$) during atorvastatin than during simvastatin treatment. The apo A-I reduction in apo A-I levels was associated with a significant 14.5% reduction in apo A-I PR during atorvastatin, relative to simvastatin. Due to the lack of a placebo or baseline phase in this study, it is not possible to state whether the observed effects were a result of an increase in apo A-I PR during simvastatin or its reduction during atorvastatin. The effects of atorvastatin on apo A-I kinetics were also studied in seven patients (four men and three women) with type 2 diabetes mellitus and mixed dyslipidemia [21]. Subjects were studied at the end of the placebo lead-in phase and at the end of 8 weeks of treatment with atorvastatin 40 mg/day, in a nonrandomized fashion. Treatment with atorvastatin was not associated with significant changes in HDL-C levels or apo A-I concentrations and kinetic parameters [21]. Also, in 12 obese subjects with dyslipidemia, treatment with atorvastatin 40 mg/day was not associated with significant changes in plasma HDL-C or apo A-I levels and A-I metabolism, relative to 12 subjects receiving placebo [22]. We have conducted a randomized, double-blind, placebo-controlled, crossover study to assess the effect of a low-dose (20 mg/day) and a high-dose (80 mg/day) of atorvastatin on the kinetics of apo A-I in HDL in nine subjects (five men and four women) with dyslipidemia [6]. Plasma HDL-C and apo A-I levels were not significantly affected by the two doses of atorvastatin when measured in the fasted state. However, in the fed state, HDL-C levels were significantly increased by low-dose atorvastatin (+14%), relative to placebo, and significantly lowered by

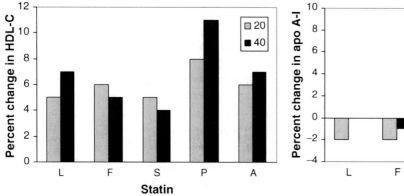

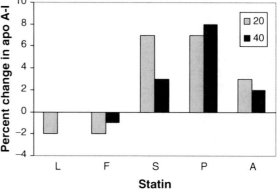

Fig. 2 *Dose-effect of statins*. Effect of 20 and 40 mg/day of different statins on plasma HDL-C levels (*left panel*) and apo A-I (*right panel*) levels. *L* lovastatin; *F* fluvastatin; *S* simvastatin; *P* pravastatin; *A* atorvastatin (see reference 11)

Table 1 Published studies on the effect of statins on the metabolism of apo A-I in HDL

Reference	Subjects	Statin	Outcome HDL-C (% Δ)	Apo A-I (% Δ)	Effect on apo A-I kinetics
Ginsberg et al. [17]	Hypoalphalipoproteinemia, $N=7$	Lovastatin			PR: +18%*
Schaefer et al. [18]	Normocholesterolemic, $N=6$	Pravastatin 40 mg	+13	+12	PR: +16%; FCR: +5%
Watts et al. [3]	Metabolic syndrome, $N=11$	Atorvastatin 40 mg	+1	−1	PR: −1%; FCR: 0%
Bilz et al. [19]	Mixed hyperlipidemic, $N=8$	Atorvastatin 80 mg	+18*	+4	PR: 0%; FCR: −7%
Mauger et al. [20]	Hypercholesterolemic, $N=7$	Atorvastatin 40 mg vs. simvastatin 80 mg	−1	−8*	PR: −15%*; FCR: −6%
Bach-Ngohou et al. [21]	T2DM with mixed hyperlipidemia, $N=7$	Atorvastatin 40 mg	+15	+2	PR: −9%; FCR: −13%
Chan et al. [22]	Obese, $N=2$	Atorvastatin 40 mg	+4	+3	PR: 0%; FCR: +4%
Lamon-Fava et al. [6]	Combined dyslipidemia, $N=9$	Atorvastatin 20 mg	+14*,[a]	0[a]	PR: −1%; FCR: −2%
		Atorvastatin 80 mg	+6[a]	−5[a]	PR: −5%; FCR: −1%
Ooi et al. [24]	Metabolic syndrome, $N=12$	Rosuvastatin 10 mg	+4	+4	PR: −7%; FCR: −10%*
		Rosuvastatin 40 mg	+10*	+2	PR: −17%*; FCR: −18%*
Verges et al. [25]	T2DM with dyslipidemia, $N=8$	Rosuvastatin 20 mg	+5	0	PR: −21%*; FCR: −22%*

[a]Non-fasting
*$P<0.05$

high-dose atorvastatin (−6%), relative to low-dose atorvastatin [6]. In agreement with the other studies on the effect of atorvastatin on apo A-I metabolism, we did not observe a significant effect of this statin on plasma apo A-I levels or on apo A-I kinetics (Table 1) [6]. This study confirmed previous reports of a blunting effect of atorvastatin on HDL-C at the highest dose of 80 mg/day. However, we observed only a nonsignificant trend toward a reduction in apo A-I PR at the 80 mg/day dose, as compared to placebo (−5%, $P=0.18$) [6]. This may indicate that the observed reduction in apo A-I at the highest atorvastatin dose may be mediated, at least in part, by very modest reductions in apo A-I PR. In the absence of significant changes in apo A-I concentrations, atorvastatin induced a significant shift in HDL subpopulation profile, with an increase in the concentration of the large α1 particles and a significant reduction in the small α3 particles [6], which is consistent with the inhibition of CETP activity [23]. Recently, Ooi et al. [24] studied the effect of low-dose (10 mg/day) and high-dose (40 mg/day) rosuvastatin on HDL-C levels and apo A-I kinetics in 12 subjects with metabolic syndrome using a randomized, double-bind, placebo-controlled crossover study design. Low-dose rosuvastatin caused modest and nonsignificant elevations in plasma HDL-C and apo A-I levels, and a significant reduction in apo A-I FCR (−10%) without changes in apo A-I PR [24]. However, high-dose rosuvastatin was effective in significantly increasing plasma levels of HDL-C but not apo A-I, and in significantly reducing both the clearance and the production of apo A-I in HDL. In this study, both doses of rosuvastatin effectively reduced CETP mass and activity. In addition, the high-dose rosuvastatin significantly increased HDL particle size, and this increase was significantly associated with the reduction in plasma TG levels, thus supporting

the role of the statin-related reduction in CETP activity in the remodeling of HDL. The results of this study support previous findings of a dose-dependent increase in HDL-C levels with rosuvastatin [12]. Verges et al. [25] studied the effect of 20 mg/day rosuvastatin in eight patients with type 2 diabetes and associated dyslipidemia (TG > 150 mg/dl and HDL-C < 40 mg/dl) using a randomized, double-blind, placebo-controlled, crossover design. Plasma HDL-C and apo A-I levels were not significantly affected by rosuvastatin. However, consistent with the findings of Ooi et al. [24], it was shown that rosuvastatin 20 mg significantly reduced both the FCR and PR of apo A-I [25]. It was also shown that rosuvastatin treatment restored apo A-I FCR and PR to values observed in a group of healthy subjects [25].

A few observations emerge from the review of these studies on the effect of different statins on the kinetics of apo A-I in HDL: (1) in agreement with previous studies conducted in large group of subjects, the increase in plasma HDL-C levels is usually greater than that in apo A-I levels; (2) the effect on plasma apo A-I concentrations is modest; (3) different statins seem to modulate apo A-I metabolism in different ways. The lack of agreement on the effect of statins on HDL metabolism may be explained by the different type of patients selected for the different studies, and sample size. It is also possible that different statins affect HDL metabolism differently, with atorvastatin having no effect, but rosuvastatin reducing both the production and the clearance of apo A-I. It is not clear that the hydrophilic (pravastatin, rosuvastatin) or hydrophobic (lovastatin, atorvastatin) characteristics of each statin play a role in their effect on HDL metabolism.

It should be pointed out that, in spite of the blunting effect on HDL cholesterol levels exerted by high-dose atorvastatin, randomized prospective trials have clearly documented a greater reduction in CHD events with this dose treatment as compared with either lower doses of atorvastatin or other lower-potency statins. In the Pravastatin or Atorvastatin Evaluation and Infection Therapy (PROVE-IT) trial, a comparison between atorvastatin 80 mg/day and pravastatin 40 mg/day showed greater plasma LDL-C reductions and CHD primary endpoints hazard ratio reductions with atorvastatin over a mean period of 2 years [26]. Also, in the Treating to New Targets (TNT) trial, in which regimens of 10 and 80 mg/day atorvastatin were compared for the secondary prevention of CHD, a 22% reduction in relative risk of cardiovascular events was reported with the higher dose [27]. In the Incremental Decrease in Endpoints through Aggressive Lipid lowering (IDEAL) study, while 80 mg/day atorvastatin had a similar effect as 20 mg/day simvastatin on the combined primary endpoint of coronary death, acute myocardial infarction and cardiac arrest in a secondary CHD prevention setting, atorvastatin was more effective that simvastatin in preventing reoccurrence of nonfatal myocardial infarction [28].

In agreement with the observed increase in apo A-I PR in the early studies by Ginsberg et al. [17] and Schaefer et al. [18], experiments conducted in the human hepatoma cell line HepG2 have shown an increase in the expression of the apo A-I gene with statins. Pitavastatin, a potent lipophilic statin, was shown to increase apo A-I mRNA levels in HepG2, in a dose- and time-dependent manner [29]. The increase in apo A-I gene expression was mediated by an activation of the apo A-I promoter and required the −256 to −128 region of the promoter, which contains the peroxisome proliferator activated receptor α (PPARα) element. In fact, it was demonstrated that pitavastatin increased the expression of PPARα. Addition of mevalonate to the culture media completely abolished the effect of pitavastatin on apo A-I expression and on PPARα activation, suggesting that inhibition of HMG-CoA reductase is responsible for the effect of statins on apo A-I expression. This could possibly be mediated by metabolites downstream of the HMG-CoA inhibition (Fig. 1): in fact, coincubation with geranylgeranyl-PP, bur not farnesyl-PP, completely abolished the effect on PPARα, similar to the effect of mevalonate. It was therefore concluded that geranylgeranylation (or prenylation, a posttranslational modification of proteins) of Rho GTP-binding proteins, which leads to translocation of Rho to the membrane, inhibits PPARα [29]. Statins, by inhibiting the formation of downstream products in the cholesterol biosynthesis pathway, inhibit the prenylation of proteins and thus affect gene expression. Atorvastatin has been shown to activate apo A-I expression in HepG2 cells much less efficiently than pitavastatin [30]. However, rosuvastatin was shown to increase apo A-I expression in HepG2 cells in a manner similar to pitavastatin [31]. Since the only two studies assessing the in vivo effects of rosuvastatin on apo A-I kinetics have shown a reduction in

apo A-I PR [24, 25], it is difficult to interpret the relevance of these results obtained in HepG2 cells.

In conclusion, the raising effect on HDL-C and apo A-I levels by statins may be compound-specific. The metabolism of HDL may be affected by statins through an inhibition of CETP activity and subsequent reduction of HDL clearance. The effect of statins on apo A-I synthesis is less clear.

References

1. Gotto AM (2005) Review of primary and secondary prevention trials with lovastatin, pravastatin, and simvastatin. Am J Cardiol 96: 34F–38F
2. Brown MS, Goldstein JL (1997) The SREBP pathway regulation of cholesterol metabolism by proteolysis of a membrane-bound transcription factor. Cell 89:331–340
3. Watts GF, Barrett P, Ji J, Serone AP, Chan DC, Croft KD, Loehrer F, Johnson AG (2003) Differential regulation of lipoprotein kinetics by atorvastatin and fenofibrate in subjects with the metabolic syndrome. Diabetes 52:803–811
4. Parhofer K, Barrett P, Dunn J, Schonfeld G (1993) Effect of pravastatin on metabolic parameters of apolipoprotein B in patients with mixed hyperlipoproteinemia. Clin Investig 71:939–946
5. Aguilar-Salinas CA, Barrett PH, Pulai J, Zhu X, Schonfeld G (1997) A familial combined hyperlipidemic kindred with impaired apolipoprotein B catabolism. Kinetics of apolipoprotein B during placebo and pravastatin therapy. Arterioscler Thromb Vasc Biol 17:72–82
6. Lamon-Fava S, Diffenderfer M, Barrett PH, Buchsbaum A, Matthan N, Lichtenstein AH, Dolnikowski GG, Horvath KV, Asztalos BF, Zago V, Schaefer EJ (2007) Effects of different doses of atorvastatin on human apolipoprotein B-100, B-48, and A-I metabolism. J Lipid Res 48:1746–1753
7. Asztalos BF, Schaefer EJ (2006) The effects of statins on high-density lipoproteins. Curr Atheroscler Rep 8:41–49
8. Ballantyne C, Blazing M, Hunningake D, Yuan Z, DeLucca P, Ramsey K, Hustad C, Palmisano J (2003) Effect on high-density lipoprotein cholesterol of maximum doses of simvastatin and atorvastatin in patients with hypercholesterolemia: results of the Comparative HDL Efficacy and Safety Study (CHESS). Am Heart J 146:862–869
9. Crouse JR, Frohlich J, Ose L, Mercuri M, Tobert JA (1999) Effects of high doses of simvastatin and atorvastatin on high-density lipoprotein cholesterol and apolipoprotein A-I. Am J Cardiol 83:1476–1477
10. Leiter LA, Rosenson RS, Stein E; POLARIS study investigators (2007) Efficacy and safety of rosuvastatin 40 mg versus atorvastatin 80 mg in high-risk patients with hypercholesteolemia: results of the POLARIS study. Atherosclerosis 194:e154–e164
11. Asztalos BF, Horvath KV, McNamara JR, Roheim PS, Rubistein JJ, Schaefer EJ (2002) Comparing the effects of five different statins on the HDL subpopulation profiles of coronary heart disease patients. Atherosclerosis 164:361–369
12. Jones PH, Davidson MH, Stein EA, Bays HF, McKenney JM, Miller E, Cain VA, Blasetto JW; STELLAR Study Group (2003) Comparison of the efficacy and safety of rosuvastatin versus atorvastatin, simvastatin, and pravastatin across doses (STELLAR Trial). Am J Cardiol 92:152–160
13. Guerin M, Lassel TS, Le Goff W, Farnier M, Chapman J (2000) Action of atorvastatin in combined hyperlipidemia: preferential reduction of cholesteryl ester transfer from HDL to VLDL1 particles. Arterioscler Thromb Vasc Biol 20:189–197
14. de Haan W, van der Hoogt CC, Westerterp M, Hoekstra M, Dallinga-Thie G, Princen HM, Romijn JA, Jukema JW, Havekes LM,

Rensen PC (2008) Atorvastatin increases HDL cholesterol by reducing CETP expression in cholesterol-fed APOE*3-Leiden. CETP mice. Atherosclerosis 197:57–63

15. Pedersen TR, Olsson AG, Faergeman O, Kjekshus J, Wedel H, Berg K, Wilhelmsen L, Haghfelt T, Thorgeirsson G, Pyorala K, Miettinen T, Christophersen B, Tobert J, Musliner T, Cook T; Scandinavian Simvastatin Study Group (1998) Lipoprotein changes and reduction in the incidence of major coronary heart disease events in the Scandinavian Simvastatin Survival Study (4S). Circulation 97:1453–1460

16. Athyros V, Mikhailidis D, Papageorgiou A, Symeonidis A, Mercouris B, Pehlivanidis A, Boukoukos V, Elisaf M; GREACE Collaborative Group (2004) Effect of atorvastatin on high density lipoprotein-cholesterol and its relationship with coronary events: a subgroup analysis of the GREek Atorvastatin and Coronary-heart-disease Evaluation (GREACE) Study. Curr Med Res Opin 20:627–637

17. Ginsberg HN, Ngai C, Ramakrishnan R (1991) Lovastatin increases apolipoprotein A-I levels in subjects with isolated reductions in high-density lipoproteins. Circulation 84:II–140

18. Schaefer JR, Schweer H, Ikewaki K, Stracke H, Seyberth HJ, Kaffarnik H, Maisch B, Steinmetz A (1999) Metabolic basis of high-density lipoproteins and apolipoprotein A-I increase by HMG-CoA reductase inhibition in healthy subjects and a patient with coronary artery disease. Atherosclerosis 144:177–184

19. Bilz S, Wagner S, Schmitz M, Bedynek A, Keller U, Demant T (2004) Effects of atorvastatin versus fenofibrate on apo B-100 and apo A-I kinetics in mixed hyperlipidemia. J Lipid Res 45:174–185

20. Mauger J-F, Couture P, Paradis M-E, Lamarche B (2005) Comparison of the impact of atorvastatin and simvastatin on apo A-I kinetics in men. Atherosclerosis 178:157–163

21. Bach-Ngohou K, Ouguerram K, Frenais R, Maugere P, Ripolles-Piquer B, Zair Y, Krempf M, Bard JM (2005) Influence of atorvastatin on apolipoprotein E and A-I kinetics in patients with type 2 diabetes. J Pharmacol Exp Ther 315:363–369

22. Chan D, Watts GF, Nguyen MN, Barrett P (2006) Factorial study of the effect of n-3 fatty acid supplementation and atorvastatin on the kinetics of HDL apolipoproteins A-I and A-II in men with abdominal obesity. Am J Clin Nutr 84:37–43

23. Asztalos BF, Horvath KV, McNamara JR, Roheim PS, Rubistein JJ, Schaefer EJ (2002) Effects of atorvastatin on the HDL subpopulation profile of coronary heart disease patients. J Lipid Res 43:1701–1707

24. Ooi EMM, Watts GF, Nestel PJ, Sviridov D, Hoang A, Barrett PH (2008) Dose-dependent regulation of high-density lipoprotein metabolism with rosuvastatin in the metabolic syndrome. J Clin Endocrinol Metab 93:430–437

25. Verges B, Florentin E, Baillot-Rudoni S, Petit J-M, Brindisi MC, de Barros J-P Pais, Lagrost L, Gambert P, Duvillard L (2009) Rosuvastatin 20 mg restores normal HDL-apoA-I kinetics in type 2 diabetes. J Lipid Res 50:1209–1215

26. Cannon CP, Braunwald E, McCabe CH, Rader DJ, Rouleau JL, Belder R, Joyal SV, Hill KA, Pfeffer MA, Skene AM (2004) Intensive versus moderate lipid lowering with statins after acute coronary syndromes. N Engl J Med 350:1495–1504

27. LaRosa JC, Grundy SM, Waters DD, Shear C, Barter P, Fruchart JC, Gotto AM, Greten H, Kastelein JJ, Shepherd J, Wenger NK; Treating to New Targets (TNT) Investigators (2005) Intensive lipid lowering with atorvastatin in patients with stable coronary disease. N Engl J Med 352:1425–1435

28. Pedersen TR, Faergeman O, Kastelein JJP, Olsson AG, Tikkanen MJ, Holme I, Larsen ML, Bendiksen FS, Lindhal C, Szarek M, Tsai J; Incremental Decrease in End points through Aggressive Lipid lowering study group (2005) High-doses atorvastatin vs usual-dose simvastatin for the secondary prevention after myocardial infarction. The IDEAL study: a randomized controlled trial. JAMA 294:2437–2445

29. Martin G, Duez H, Blanquart C, Berezowski V, Poulain P, Fruchart JC, Najib-Fruchart J, Glineur C, Staels B (2001) Statin-induced inhibition of the Rho-signaling pathway activates PPARalpha and induces HDL apo A-I. J Clin Invest 107:1423–1432

30. Maejima T, Yamazaki H, Aoki T, Tamaki T, Sato F, Kitahara M, Saito Y (2004) Effect of pitavastatin on apolipoprotein A-I production in HepG2 cells. Biochem Biophys Res Commun 324:835–839

31. Qin S, Koga T, Ganji SH, Kamanna VS, Kashyap ML (2008) Rosuvastatin selectively stimulates apolipoprotein A-I but not apolipoprotein A-II synthesis in HepG2 cells. Metabolism 57:973–979

Therapeutic Regulation of High-Density Lipoprotein Transport in the Metabolic Syndrome

Dick C. Chan, P.H.R. Barrett, and Gerald F. Watts

Abbreviations

Apo	Apolipoprotein
CETP	Cholesteryl ester transfer protein
CVD	Cardiovascular disease
HDL	High-density lipoprotein
FCR	Fractional catabolic rate
IDL	Intermediate-density lipoprotein
LDL	Low-density lipoprotein
LPL	Lipoprotein lipase
MetS	Metabolic syndrome
PPAR	Peroxisome proliferator-activated receptor
PR	Production rate
RCT	Reverse cholesterol transport
TRL	Triglyceride-rich lipoprotein
VLDL	Very low-density lipoprotein

Introduction

Visceral obesity, insulin resistance, dyslipidaemia, hypertension and a pro-inflammatory/thrombotic state collectively define the metabolic syndrome (MetS) [1]. Individuals with MetS have a significant increase in cardiovascular morbidity and mortality [2]. Disturbances in high density lipoprotein (HDL) metabolism, reflected by decreased levels of HDL cholesterol, is particularly common in MetS and one of the major factors contributing to vascular risk [3]. Raising HDL-cholesterol is therefore a captivating notion for coronary disease prevention [4].

HDL plays an important role in transporting cholesterol from peripheral tissues directly back to the liver or indirectly via intermediate density lipoprotein (IDL) and low density

G.F. Watts (✉)
Metabolic Research Centre, School of Medicine and Pharmacology, University of Western Australia, GPO Box X2213, Perth 6847, WA, Australia
e-mail: gerald.watts@uwa.edu.au

lipoprotein (LDL) particles, in a process popularly referred to as reverse cholesterol transport (RCT) [5]. In human plasma, apoA-I and apoA-II are the major apolipoproteins of HDL. According to apolipoprotein composition, HDLs can also be classified into lipoprotein (Lp) A-I particles, containing apoA-I without apoA-II, and LpA-I:A-II particles, containing both apoA-I and apoA-II. Compelling evidence supports the anti-atherogenic role of apoA-I in preventing CVD [6], with less consistent data available for apoA-II [7, 8]. However, HDL metabolism is complex and abnormal plasma concentrations can result from alterations in the rates of production and/or catabolism of the various HDL particles. Static measures of either lipid or lipoprotein concentrations do not provide information on the underlying pathogenic mechanisms. Tracer studies, whether utilising radioactive or stable isotopes, provide novel insight that furthers understanding of metabolic disorders and effects of treatments. This chapter focuses on the dysregulation and therapeutic regulation of HDL transport in MetS from studies chiefly carried out in vivo with stable isotope tracers.

Principles of Tracer Methods

Tracer studies are employed to infer information about a substance in a system. The term "tracee" is defined as the substance of interest, for example apoA-I, to be traced kinetically. A "tracer" is a labelled substance introduced into the "system" to infer information about the kinetics of the tracee. For example, stable isotopically labelled amino acids (typically ^{13}C-leucine or D$_3$-leucine) can be administered intravenously as a bolus or primed infusion with serial blood sampling over several hours/days to study the turnover of VLDL, IDL and LDL-apoB, as well as HDL apoA-I. For the purpose of lipoprotein studies, the system should be maintained in a steady state, where the rates of input and output for a given tracee are equal and time-invariant. Enrichment data are generated by gas-chromatography mass-spectrometry (GCMS) analysis after separation of the relevant apolipoproteins. The data are then subjected to multicompartmental analysis to assess the

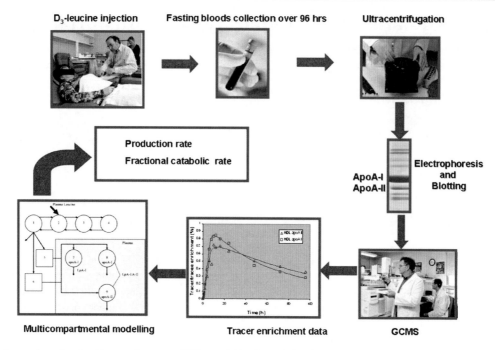

Fig. 1 Steps and procedures involved in carrying out an HDL-apoA kinetic study in a human subject

fractional turnover and conversion rates of lipoproteins, from which absolute transport rates are calculated (Fig. 1). Full methodological details of the aforementioned techniques are provided in several of our publications [9, 10].

HDL Tracer Kinetics in Metabolic Syndrome

Oversecretion of very-low density lipoprotein (VLDL)-apoB is a cardinal feature of MetS [11]. This abnormality is also associated with delayed clearance of IDL and LDL [12]. Recent stable-isotopic studies also found that Mets subjects have markedly increased fractional catabolic rate (FCR) of apoA-I and, to a lesser extent, increased apoA-I production, accounting for a net lowering of plasma HDL-apoA-I concentrations [13, 14]. The hypercatabolism of HDL-apoA-I in these subjects is reflected by both accelerated catabolism of HDL LpA-I and LpA-I:A-II particles [15]. Although plasma concentration of apoA-I is partly determined by its production rate [16], the hypercatabolism of apoA-I may have a more dominant effect on HDL concentration in subjects with MetS. Figure 2 illustrates the kinetic defects of apoB-100 and apoA-I metabolism in MetS.

The underlying mechanisms regulating HDL-apoA-I catabolism are not fully understood. Animal and human kinetic studies have previously shown that enhanced HDL-apoA-I clearance is a function of triglyceride enrichment of HDL and on the activity of hepatic lipase (HL) [17]. In insulin

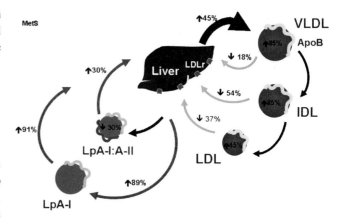

Fig. 2 Kinetic defects in apoA and apoB transport in the metabolic syndrome

resistance, hepatic overproduction of VLDL together with decreased lipoprotein lipase (LPL) activity results in expansion in the pool of triglyceride-rich lipoproteins (TRLs) enhances cholesteryl ester transfer protein (CETP)-mediated exchange of neutral lipids and results in the formation of unstable triglyceride-enriched HDL particles that are rapidly removed from the plasma via the action of HL [11]. Consistent with this, hypertriglyceridemia, as driven by over-secretion of VLDL-apoB, was found to be highly associated with hypercatabolism of HDL-apoA-I [18] (Fig. 3a). Another important association of hypertriglyceridemia is increased apoC-III. Elevated plasma apoC-III was also found to be a predictor of hypercatabolism of HDL-apoA-I in subjects with

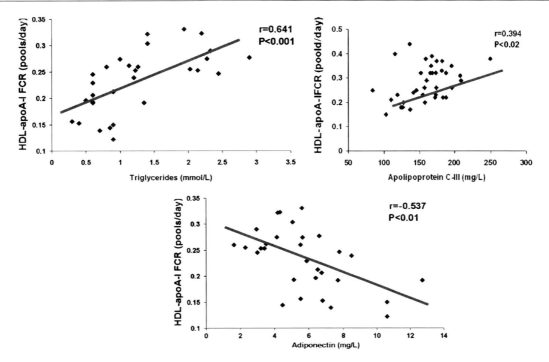

Fig. 3 Association between HDL-apoA-I fractional catabolic rate and plasma triglyceride, apoC-III, and adiponectin concentrations

central obesity [19]. Given the functional role of apoC-III in inhibiting hydrolysis of triglycerides, it is conceivable that accumulation of apoC-III in plasma will favour the formation of unstable triglyceride-rich HDL particles, thereby increasing the FCR of HDL-apoA-I (Fig. 3b). Recent reports also highlight the importance of liver fat content in the regulation of TRL metabolism. High liver fat content is associated with hepatic oversecretion of triglyceride-rich $VLDL_1$ particles, as well as with postprandial lipemia [20, 21]. Accumulation of liver fat therefore impacts indirectly on HDL metabolism by increasing HDL-apoA-I FCR.

Adiponectin is an adipocytokine that has been known to be closely related to obesity and insulin resistance in MetS [22]. Low plasma adiponectin levels have been shown in humans to be correlated with hypertriglyceridemia and low HDL cholesterol. Recent kinetic data also found that low plasma adiponectin levels predicted elevated plasma VLDL-apoB concentration, and that this was chiefly due to impaired catabolism of VLDL-apoB [23]. In addition, low plasma adiponectin levels are also associated with enhanced HL activity in vivo. Adiponectin may therefore have a dual effect on the VLDL-triglyceride pool and HL, both of which may influence HDL-apoA-I catabolism. Verges et al. found that plasma adiponectin concentration was negatively correlated with HDL-apoA-I FCR in a heterogeneous group including type 2 diabetic subjects [24]. However, a recent study could only confirm the predictive role of adiponectin on HDL-apoA-I FCR in non-obese subjects [18] (Fig. 3c). This suggests that that in non-diabetic

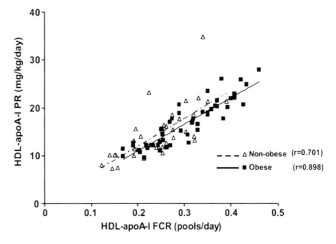

Fig. 4 Direct association between production rate and fractional catabolic rate of HDL-apoA-I

obese men, the impact of adiponectin on HDL metabolism might have been masked by other factors, such as body fat distribution.

It is also important to note that HDL-apoA-I PR, as opposed to HDL-apoA-I FCR, was significantly associated with plasma apoA-I concentration in MetS. That plasma apoA-I concentration is associated with its production rate is therefore possibly secondary to the increased catabolism of HDL-apoA-I, a "balancing feedback" mechanism that drives hepatic apoA-I production attempting to maintain apoA-I concentration (Fig. 4). However, this hypothesis needs further investigation.

Intervention Studies on HDL Kinetics in Metabolic Syndrome

As reviewed elsewhere [25], regulation of hypertriglyceridemia and low HDL levels with lifestyle modifications and pharmacotherapy is an established recommendation for subjects with MetS. The putative mechanisms of action of these agents on HDL metabolism as applied to MetS are summarized in Table 1. Only the kinetics effects of weight loss, fish oils, statins and fibrates on HDL metabolism in MetS will be reviewed. Readers should refer to the studies on the effects of phytosterol supplementation, PPAR-γ agonists, niacins and CETP inhibitors published elsewhere for further details [26–29].

Weight Loss

Several studies have shown that modest weight reduction through dieting in obese subjects is associated with improvement in a wide spectrum of cardiovascular risk factors, including dyslipidaemia. In a placebo-controlled study of obese men with MetS, weight loss employing a standard low-fat, low-caloric diet decreased both the catabolic and production rates of HDL-apoA-I, thereby not altering plasma HDL-apoA-I nor HDL-cholesterol concentrations [30]. The catabolic changes in HDL with weight loss could relate to reduction in the plasma VLDL triglyceride pool available for exchange with HDL. The decrease in HDL catabolism was found to be associated with the rise in adiponectin, consistent with the aforementioned role of adiponectin in HDL catabolism. A "balancing feedback" mechanism probably accounts for the tight correlation between changes in catabolism and production of HDL-apoA-I following weight loss. It is also worthy to note that weigh loss also decreased plasma apoB concentration by enhancing the catabolism of LDL-apoB and reducing the secretion of VLDL-apoB. That HDL kinetic

changes were associated with increased catabolism of apoB-containing lipoproteins explaining the favourable effect on apoB/apoA-I ratio and cardiovascular benefits of weight loss. In the same study, weight loss also decreased the production rate of HDL-apoA-II and, to a lesser extent, decreased apoA-II fractional catabolic rate, accounting for a net lowering of plasma HDL-apoA-II concentrations [31]. However, the cardiometabolic significance of this effect on HDL-apoA-II metabolism remains to be further investigated.

Fish Oil Supplementation

Fish oils are a rich source of n–3 fatty acids, eicosapentaenoic acid and docosahexaenoic acid. Increasing evidence suggests that fish oil consumption protects against atherosclerotic heart disease [32]. Modification of lipid and lipoprotein metabolism by fish oils may also confer anti-atherogenic benefits. Frenais et al. reported that in five diabetic patients, HDL-apoA-I FCR and production rate were significantly decreased after treatment with n–3 fatty acid supplementation [33]. The concentration of HDL apoA-I was not significantly changed. In another study of obesity, 6-week supplementation with fish oil capsules (4 g/day) decreased the catabolism of HDL apoA-I and apoA-II [34]. As with weight loss, this was coupled with a significant decrease in the corresponding production rates, accounting for the lack of treatment effect on plasma apoA-I and apoA-II concentrations, another example of "balancing feedback". The reduction in HDL catabolism was related to the decrease in plasma triglycerides, which in turn stabilizes HDL particles; that is, the HDL particles become larger, retain more cholesterol and are less susceptible to catabolism by hepatic and renal pathways. Notwithstanding their many other favourable CVS properties, the offset of fish oils on RCT remains unknown.

Table 1 Kinetic effects of lifestyle and drug interventions on HDL-apoA-I and apoA-II metabolism in the metabolic syndrome

Intervention	HDL-apoA-I			HDL-apoA-II		
	Concentration	FCR	PR	Concentration	FCR	PR
Weight loss	↔	↓	↓	↓	↓	↓↓
Fish oils	↔	↓	↓	↔	↔	↔
Plant sterols	↔	↔	↔	N/A	N/A	N/A
Statins	↔ or ↑	↔ or ↓	↔ or ↓	↔	↔	↔
PPAR-α agonists	↑	↑	↑↑	↑	↑	↑↑
PPAR-γ agonists	↔	↔	↔	N/A	N/A	N/A
Niacins[a]	↑	↔	↑	↔	↔	↔
CETP inhibitor	↑	↓	↔	↑	↓	↔

"↔" denotes no effect; "↓" denotes decreased; "↑" denotes increased
N/A not available; FCR fractional catabolic rate; PR production rate
[a]Combined hyperlipidaemic subject

Peroxisome Proliferator-Activated Receptor-α Agonists

Fibrates are PPAR-α ligands that have been shown to significantly decrease the progression of coronary atherosclerosis and cardiovascular events in MetS and type 2 diabetes [35]. The benefit of fibrates in clinical endpoint trials may be partly related to the correction of lipid and lipoprotein metabolism, in particular HDL metabolism. The effects of fenofibrate on HDL metabolism have been examined in MetS. Fenofibrate increased plasma concentration of apoA-I chiefly by enhancing the production of apoA-I. Fenofibrate also increased the production of both LpA-I:A-II and apoA-II, accounting for significant increases of their corresponding plasma concentrations [36]. As shown in Fig. 5, fenofibrate also reduced the concentrations of apoB-containing lipoproteins by increasing their catabolic rates. The mechanisms of action of fibrates on HDL metabolism are consistent with experimental data showing that the activation of PPAR-α stimulates apoA-I and apoA-II expression [37]. Importantly, the catabolism of apoA-I was also accelerated by fenofibrate implying overall enhancement in RCT. In a recent study, Millar et al. found that activation of PPAR-α with LY518674 (a potent and selective PPAR-α agonist) significantly increased the production of HDL-apoA-I and apoA-II [38]. However, this was coupled with a significant increase in the corresponding fractional catabolic rates, accounting for the lack of treatment effect on plasma apoA-I and apoA-II concentrations. The effects of these changes in HDL metabolism may have a net beneficial impact on RCT, but this requires further investigation.

Statins

Several clinical end-point trials have demonstrated that statins can decrease cardiovascular events in patients with impaired glucose tolerance, type 2 diabetes mellitus and the metabolic syndrome [39, 40]. Inhibition of de novo cholesterol synthesis by statins is well recognized to upregulate LDL receptor activity in vitro. Consistent with this, the FCR of apoB in the VLDL, IDL and LDL fractions increased with statin treatment. However, statins do not appreciably elevate plasma HDL-cholesterol concentrations. The significant increases reported are probably consequent on a triglyceride-lowering effect. By decreasing plasma triglyceride levels and the associated compositional changes in HDL, statins may potentially alter the kinetics of HDL particles. Several studies have examined the effect of statins on HDL apoA-I

metabolism in subjects with the metabolic syndrome, including obese and type 2 diabetes [14, 34, 41, 42]. However, most have consistently failed to demonstrate significant changes in the production and catabolic rates of HDL-apoA-I. It is possible that increase in the residence time of larger HDL particles in plasma could potentially be counterbalanced by increased uptake of the particles by hepatic HDL receptors, but this speculation requires investigation. However, rosuvastatin, a more potent statin shown to have a greater HDL-cholesterol-raising effect than other statins, decreased the catabolism of HDL-apoA-I in type 2 diabetes [43]. The decrease in HDL-apoA-I FCR was correlated with the reduction of plasma triglyceride and HDL-triglyceride. In another study of MetS, treatment with rosuvastatin dose-dependently increased plasma HDL and LpA-I concentrations chiefly by decreasing LpA-I particle catabolism [44]. Rosuvastatin also resulted in a dose-dependent increase in HDL particle size, but did not change the concentration nor kinetics of LpA-I:A-II. These findings suggest a diverging impact of different statins on HDL metabolism.

Conclusions

Decreased apoA-I and HDL-cholesterol concentrations are both strong predictors of coronary events in MetS. Tracer kinetic studies have contributed significantly to our understanding of HDL metabolism in these subjects. Accelerated catabolism of HDL-apoA-I and apoA-II is largely associated with dysregulation of VLDL-apoB metabolism (i.e. elevated plasma triglyceride and apoC-III concentration and overproduction of VLDL-apoB), and to a less extent low adiponectin concentration. In MetS, interventions (e.g. weight loss and fish oils) that decrease plasma triglycerides and/or VLDL-apoB secretion lower the fractional catabolism of HDL. A balancing feedback mechanism results in a fall in apoA-I production, with no net change in HDL concentrations, however. This appears to be a short-term phenomenon, and a net increase in RCT or apoA/apoB ratio is possible with longer periods of intervention. PPAR-α agonists are the only agents that increase apoA-I production in MetS and potentially enhance RCT. The differential effect of rosuvastatin and fenofibrate on HDL metabolism provides a good rationale for their use as combination therapy (Fig. 5), but the impact on CVS outcomes needs investigation. The significance of lifestyle and pharmacological interventions on HDL metabolism must be viewed in light of their favourable therapeutic alterations in apoB metabolic pathways. New clinical methods are also needed for investigating cellular and in vivo cholesterol transport.

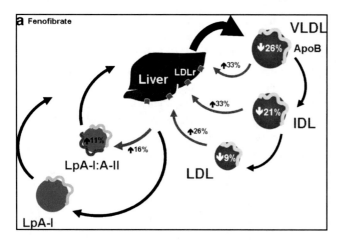
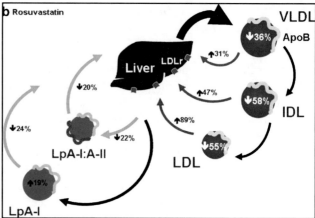

Fig. 5 Kinetic effects of fenofibrate and rosuvastatin on apoA and apoB-100 in the metabolic syndrome

References

1. Expert Panel on Detection, Evaluation, and Treatment of High Blood Cholesterol in Adults (2001) Executive Summary of the Third Report of the National Cholesterol Education Program (NCEP) Expert Panel on Detection, Evaluation, and Treatment of High Blood Cholesterol in Adults (Adult Treatment Panel III). JAMA 285:2486–2497

2. Isomaa B, Almgren P, Tuomi T et al (2001) Cardiovascular morbidity and mortality associated with the metabolic syndrome. Diabetes Care 24:683–689

3. Castelli WP, Garrison RJ, Wilson PW et al (1986) Incidence of coronary heart disease and lipoprotein cholesterol levels. The Framingham Study. JAMA 256:2835–2838

4. Singh IM, Shishehbor MH, Ansell BJ (2007) High-density lipoprotein as a therapeutic target: a systematic review. JAMA 298:786–798

5. Lewis GF, Rader DJ (2005) New insights into the regulation of HDL metabolism and reverse cholesterol transport. Circ Res 96:1221–1232

6. van der Steeg WA, Holme I, Boekholdt SM et al (2008) High-density lipoprotein cholesterol, high-density lipoprotein particle size, and apolipoprotein A-I: significance for cardiovascular risk: the IDEAL and EPIC-Norfolk studies. J Am Coll Cardiol 51:634–642

7. Birjmohun RS, Dallinga-Thie GM, Kuivenhoven JA et al (2007) Apolipoprotein A-II is inversely associated with risk of future coronary artery disease. Circulation 116:2029–2035

8. Blanco-Vaca F, Escolà-Gil JC, Martín-Campos JM, Julve J (2001) Role of apoA-II in lipid metabolism and atherosclerosis: advances in the study of an enigmatic protein. J Lipid Res 42:1727–1739

9. Barrett PHR, Chan DC, Watts GF (2006) Design and analysis of lipoprotein tracer kinetics studies in humans. J Lipid Res 47:1607–1619

10. Chan DC, Wats GF (2004) Lipoprotein transport in the metabolic syndrome. Part I. Methodological aspects of stable isotope kinetics studies. Clin Sci 107:221–232

11. Adiels M, Olofsson SO, Taskinen MR, Boren J (2008) Overproduction of very low-density lipoproteins is the hallmark of the dyslipidemia in the metabolic syndrome. Arterioscler Thromb Vasc Biol 28:1225–1236

12. Chan DC, Watts GF, Redgrave TG, Mori TA, Barrett PHR (2002) Apolipoprotein B-100 kinetics in visceral obesity: associations with plasma apolipoprotein C-III concentration. Metabolism 29:1041–1046

13. Chan DC, Barrett PH, Watts GF (2006) Recent studies of lipoprotein kinetics in the metabolic syndrome and related disorders. Curr Opin Lipidol 17:28–36

14. Watts GF, Barrett PH, Ji J et al (2003) Differential regulation of lipoprotein kinetics by atorvastatin and fenofibrate in subjects with the metabolic syndrome. Diabetes 52:803–811

15. Ji J, Watts GF, Johnson AG et al (2006) High-density lipoprotein (HDL) transport in the metabolic syndrome: application of a new model for HDL particle kinetics. J Clin Endocrinol Metab 91:973–979

16. Ooi EM, Watts GF, Farvid MS, Chan DC, Allen MC, Zilko SR, Barrett PH (2005) High-density lipoprotein apolipoprotein A-I kinetics in obesity. Obes Res 13:1008–1016

17. Rashid S, Watanabe T, Sakaue T, Lewis GF (2003) Mechanisms of HDL lowering in insulin resistant, hypertriglyceridemic states: the combined effect of HDL triglyceride enrichment and elevated hepatic lipase activity. Clin Biochem 36:421–429

18. Chan DC, Barrett PHR, Ooi EMM, Ji J, Chan DT, Watts GF (2009) Very low density lipoprotein metabolism and plasma adiponectin as predictors of high-density lipoprotein apolipoprotein A-I kinetics in obese and nonobese men. J Clin Endocrinol Metab 94:989–997

19. Chan DC, Nguyen MN, Watts GF, Barrett PH (2008) Plasma apolipoprotein C-III transport in centrally obese men: associations with very low-density lipoprotein apolipoprotein B and high-density lipoprotein apolipoprotein A-I metabolism. J Clin Endocrinol Metab 93:557–564

20. Adiels M, Taskinen MR, Packard C et al (2006) Overproduction of large VLDL particles is driven by increased liver fat content in man. Diabetologia 49:755–765

21. Matikainen N, Manttari S, Westerbacka J et al (2007) Postprandial lipemia associates with liver fat content. J Clin Endocrinol Metab 92:3052–3059

22. Matsuzawa Y, Funahashi T, Kihara S, Shimomura I (2004) Adiponectin and metabolic syndrome. Arterioscler Thromb Vasc Biol 24:29–33

23. Ng TWK, Watts GF, Farvid MS, Chan DC, Barrett PHR (2005) Adipocytokines and VLDL metabolism: independent regulatory effects of adiponectin, insulin resistance, and fat compartments on VLDL apolipoprotein B-100 kinetics? Diabetes 54:795–802

24. Verges B, Petit JM, Duvillard L et al (2006) Adiponectin is an important determinant of apoA-I catabolism. Arterioscler Thromb Vasc Biol 26:1364–1369

25. Rader DJ (2007) Mechanisms of disease: HDL metabolism as a target for novel therapies. Nat Clin Pract Cardiovasc Med 4:102–109

26. Ooi EM, Watts GF, Barrett PH et al (2007) Dietary plant sterols supplementation does not alter lipoprotein kinetics in men with the metabolic syndrome. Asia Pac J Clin Nutr 16:624–631

27. Nagashima K, Lopez C, Donovan D et al (2005) Effects of the PPAR gamma agonist pioglitazone on lipoprotein metabolism in patients with type 2 diabetes mellitus. J Clin Invest 115:1323–1332

28. Lamon-Fava S, Diffenderfer MR, Barrett PHR et al (2008) Extended-release niacin alters the metabolism of plasma apolipo-protein (apo) A-I and ApoB-containing lipoproteins. Arterioscler Thromb Vasc Biol 28:1672–1678

29. Brousseau ME, Diffenderfer MR, Millar JS et al (2005) Effects of cholesteryl ester transfer protein inhibition on high-density lipopro-tein subspecies, apolipoprotein A-I metabolism, and fecal sterol excretion. Arterioscler Thromb Vasc Biol 25:1057–1064

30. Ng TWK, Watts GF, Barrett PH et al (2007) Effect of weight loss on LDL and HDL kinetics in the metabolic syndrome: associations with changes in plasma retinol-binding protein-4 and adiponectin levels. Diabetes Care 30:2945–2950

31. Ng TWK, Chan DC, Barrett PHR, Watts GF (2009) Effect of weight loss on HDL-apoA-II kinetics in the metabolic syndrome. Clin Sci (Lond) 118(1):79–85

32. Mori TA, Beilin LJ (2001) Long-chain omega 3 fatty acids, blood lipids and cardiovascular risk reduction. Curr Opin Lipidol 12:11–17

33. Frenais R, Ouguerram K, Maugeais C et al (2001) Effect of dietary omega-3 fatty acids on high-density lipoprotein apolipoprotein AI kinetics in type II diabetes mellitus. Atherosclerosis 157: 131–135

34. Chan DC, Watts GF, Nguyen MN, Barrett PH (2006) Factorial study of the effect of n-3 fatty acid supplementation and atorvasta-tin on the kinetics of HDL apolipoproteins A-I and A-II in men with abdominal obesity. Am J Clin Nutr 84:37–43

35. Robins SJ (2001) PPARα ligands and clinical trials: cardiovascular risk reduction with fibrates. J Cardiovasc Risk 8:195–201

36. Chan DC, Watts GF, Ooi EMM et al (2009) Regulatory effects of fenofibrate and atorvastatin on lipoprotein A-I and lipoprotein A-I:A-II kinetics in the metabolic syndrome. Diabetes Care 32(11):2111–2113

37. Staels B, Dallongeville J, Auwerx J, Schoonjans K, Leitersdorf E, Fruchart JC (1998) Mechanism of action of fibrates on lipid and lipoprotein metabolism. Circulation 98:2088–2093

38. Millar JS, Duffy D, Gadi R et al (2009) Potent and selective PPAR-α agonist LY518674 upregulates both ApoA-I production and catabo-lism in human subjects with the metabolic syndrome. Arterioscler Thromb Vasc Biol 29:140–146

39. Goldberg RB, Mellies MJ, Sacks FM, Moyé LA, Howard BV, Howard WJ, Davis BR, Cole TG, Pfeffer MA, Braunwald E (1998) Cardiovascular events and their reduction with pravastatin in dia-betic and glucose-intolerant myocardial infarction survivors with average cholesterol levels: subgroup analyses in the cholesterol and recurrent events (CARE) trial. The Care Investigators. Circulation 98:2513–2519

40. Nissen SE, Nicholls SJ, Sipahi I et al (2006) Effect of very high-intensity statin therapy on regression of coronary atherosclerosis: the ASTEROID trial. JAMA 295:1556–1565

41. Bilz S, Wagner S, Schmitz M, Bedynek A, Keller U, Demant T (2004) Effects of atorvastatin versus fenofibrate on apoB-100 and apoA-I kinetics in mixed hyperlipidemia. J Lipid Res 45:174–185

42. Bach-Ngohou K, Ouguerram K, Frenais R et al (2005) Influence of atorvastatin on apolipoprotein e and AI kinetics in patients with type 2 diabetes. J Pharmacol Exp Ther 315:363–369

43. Vergès B, Florentin E, Baillot-Rudoni S, Petit JM et al (2009) Rosuvastatin 20 mg restores normal HDL-apoA-I kinetics in type 2 diabetes. J Lipid Res 50:1209–1215

44. Ooi EMM, Watts GF, Nestel PJ et al (2008) Dose-dependent regula-tion of high-density lipoprotein metabolism with rosuvastatin in the metabolic syndrome. J Clin Endocrinol Metab 93:430–437

Effects of Cholesterol Ester Transfer Protein Inhibition on HDL Metabolism

Ernst J. Schaefer

Introduction

Early studies in the laboratories of Donald Zilversmit and Philip Barter documented in rabbits that cholesteryl ester (CE) could readily exchange between lipoproteins, especially from high-density lipoproteins (HDLs) to triglyceride-rich lipoproteins (TRLs). Moreover, it was learned that this transfer was facilitated by cholesteryl ester transfer protein or CETP. In the postprandial state there is an influx of TRL from the intestine. These lipoproteins rapidly undergo lipolysis via the action of lipoprotein lipase (activated by apolipoprotein C-II) in the capillary bed, and their cores become depleted in triglyceride (see Fig. 1a–e). After lipolysis TRL pick up CE from HDL in exchange for triglyceride (TG) (see Fig. 2 for proposed shuttle mechanism) [1]. During this process, intestinal chylomicrons become cholesterol enriched chylomicron remnants and hepatic very-low-density lipoproteins (VLDLs) become intermediate-density lipoproteins (IDLs) and finally low-density lipoproteins (LDLs).

The transfer of cholesteryl ester from HDL to TRL in exchange for triglyceride is mediated by CETP, a 60-angstrom long tunnel capable of holding four lipid molecules, and plugged by an amphipathic phosphatidylcholine at each end [1]. The two tunnel openings are large enough to allow lipid access, which is aided by a flexible helix and a mobile flap. The curvature of the concave surface of CETP matches the radius of curvature of HDL particles, and potential conformational changes occur to accomodate larger lipoprotein particles. Point mutations blocking the middle of the tunnel abolish lipid-transfer activities [1]. See Fig. 3a, b for models of the crystal structure of CETP. Chylomicron remnants enriched in cholesteryl ester also contain apolipoprotein (apo) B-48, and apoE are removed from the plasma by liver receptors that recognize apoE. LDLs are removed by many cells via LDL receptors which recognize apoB-100. Chylomicron remnants, IDLs,

and LDLs are all atherogenic particles. Zilversmit proposed that the postprandial state was an atherogenic situation.

Inazu, Mabuchi, and colleagues from Kanazawa, Japan described a kindred with familial CETP deficiency. These patients had very high HDL cholesterol levels, normal or low LDL cholesterol, and no evidence of heart disease [2]. Dr. Mabuchi has provided a chapter on human CETP deficiency for this book, and it has been documented that the HDL from patients with CETP deficiency are substantially larger than normal, and they are enriched in apoA-I, apoA-II, and apoE, in contrast to large alpha-1 HDL from normal subjects, which contains only apoA-I [3]. However, the HDL particles from these subjects have been shown to be as effective as control HDL in serving as an acceptor of both ATP-binding cassette protein A1 (ABCA-I)-mediated cellular cholesterol efflux from J774 macrophages or scavenger receptor B1 (SR-B1)-mediated cholesterol efflux from Fu5AH hepatoma cells [4]. The discovery of familial CETP deficiency led to the documentation that such kindreds had defects in the CETP gene [2]. It was also recognized that mice and rats lack CETP activity, and are very resistant to diet-induced atherosclerosis, while hamsters, rabbits, nonhuman primates, and humans all have CETP, and are sensitive to diet-induced atherosclerosis.

CETP Genetic Variation and CHD Risk

Moreover, the common genetic variant Taq1B at the CETP locus has been associated with increased HDL cholesterol, decreased CETP mass, and decreased risk of CHD in the Framingham Offspring Study [5] and decreased recurrent CHD risk in the Veteran Affairs HDL Intervention Trial [6]. In addition, a specific mutation (I405V) conferring decreased CETP mass and increased HDL has been associated with enhanced longevity in an Ashkenazi Jewish population [7]. However, other investigators have reported that CETP deficiency and common variants in the CETP gene, which raise HDL cholesterol, are not beneficial in terms of CHD risk reduction [8–10]. Japanese investigators have noted that in several kindred affected with combined CETP and hepatic lipase deficiency

E.J. Schaefer (✉)
Lipid Metabolism Laboratory, Tufts University, 711 Washington Street, Boston, MA, 02111, USA
e-mail: ernst.schaefer@tufts.edu

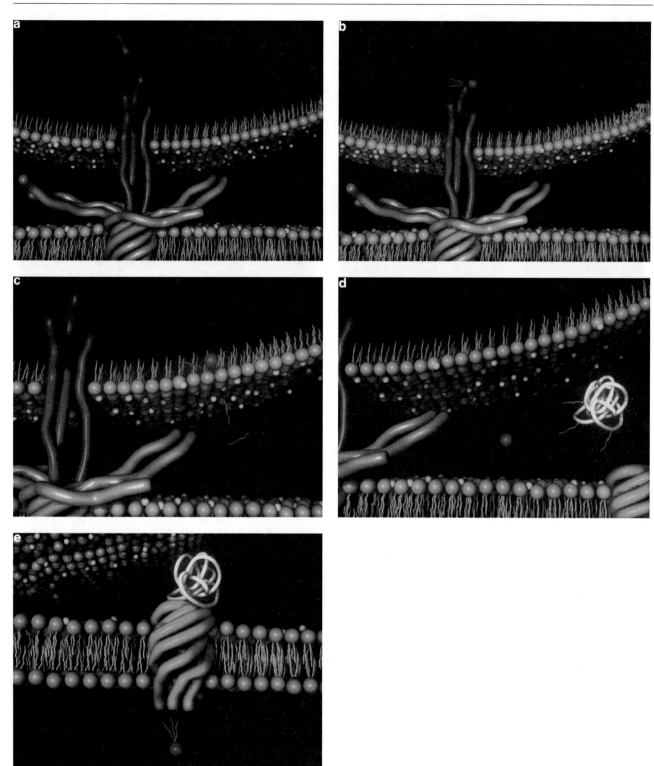

Fig. 1 The hydrolysis of lipoprotein triglyceride is shown by the action of lipoprotein lipase. In (**a**) a triglyceride-rich lipoprotein (either a chylomicron or a very low density lipoprotein, is sitting on top of a lipoprotein lipase stalk (*orange*) attached to an endothelial cell wall by heparin sulfate (*yellow*). The lipoprotein lipase has punctured the surface layer of the particle which consists of phospholipids with two fatty acids attached (*blue*) and free cholesterol (*green*), and is about to interact with a triglyceride molecule with three fatty acids attached (*purple*). In (**b**) the triglyceride molecule is resting on the tip of the lipoprotein lipase stalk. In (**c**) the fatty acids have been separated from the spherical glycerol backbone and leave the particle and go into the plasma space. In (**d**) the fatty acids bind to albumin (*yellow*) while the glycerol is rapidly cleared from plasma. In (**e**) albumin with the fatty acid attached binds to fatty acid binding protein (*green*) on the cell surface surface. The fatty acids cross into the cell and are reformed into triglyceride (*purple*) for energy storage. Created by Mr. Martin Jacob. Courtesy of Boston Heart Lab Corporation, Framingham, MA, USA

there is excess CHD risk [8]. In the Copenhagen Heart Study, CETP gene variants were associated with excess CHD risk in women [9]. In an analysis of 812 men treated with a statin had excess risk of total mortality over 10 years if they carried the Taq1B variant at the CETP gene locus [10]. Finally, Cambridge University investigators have carried out a review of 46 studies involving 113,833 individuals with data on 27,196 CHD cases and concluded that three genetic variants (Taq1B, I405V, and −692C>A) were associated with modest reductions in CHD risk, which was commensurate with the degree to which their HDL cholesterol levels were raised as compared to control populations [11]. The overall data suggest that genetic variation at the CETP locus causing higher HDL cholesterol levels in associated with CHD risk reduction [11].

The Development of CETP Inhibitors

Vaccine

A vaccine containing CETP has been developed and tested in rabbits on an atherogenic diet. Use of the vaccine resulted in antibodies against CETP, CETP inhibition, increases in HDL, and reductions in aortic atherosclerosis lesions in the rabbits [12].

Dalcetrapib

The discovery of CETP deficiency and its association with elevated HDL cholesterol, led pharmaceutical companies such as Japan Tobacco, Pfizer, and Merck to develop CETP inhibitors. It was documented that the CETP inhibitor JTT-705, developed by Japan Tobacco, protected against diet-induced atherosclerosis in rabbits fed an atherogenic diet [13]. The chemical structure of dalcetrapib is shown in Fig. 4. Moreover, this agent was tested in humans and was found to be effective in raising HDL cholesterol by about 30% whether given as monotherapy or together with pravastatin [14, 15]. This agent has also been shown to decrease the cholesteryl ester content

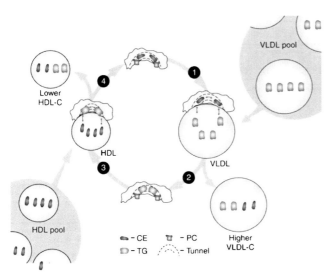

Fig. 2 The proposed shuttle mechanism for the transfer of cholesteryl ester (CE) from high density lipoproteins (HDL) to triglyceride-rich lipoproteins (TRL, in this case very low density lipoproteins or VLDL) in exchange for triglyceride (TG) via cholesteryl ester transfer protein (CETP) is shown. The CETP sits on the surface of HDL and picks up CE while donating TG, then it shuttles to VLDL or chylomicron remnants to donate CE and pick up TG. The figure is derived and modified from reference 1. PC is phosphatidylcholine, the major phospholipid on the surface of HDL, and is also a component of CETP. The ideal TRL particles to participate in this process are those that have undergone lipolysis and have room in their cores to pick up CE, while the ideal HDL particles to participate in this process are large alpha migrating HDL that are rich in CE. This process is thought to be enhanced in metabolic syndrome, diabetes, and hypertriglyceridemia where circulating levels of TRL are elevated

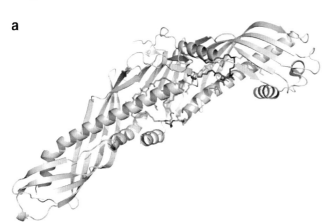

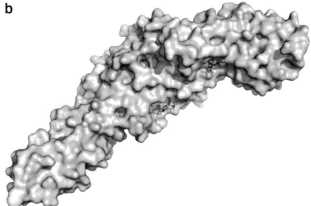

Fig. 3 (a) The ribbon model of the crystal structure of cholesteryl ester transfer protein (CETP) is shown with water and four bound lipid molecules. (b) The surface of the CETP crystal structure model is shown with two of the four bound lipid molecules still being visible and presumably available for transfer (as modified from Qiu X, Mistry A, Ammirati MJ, Chrunyk BA, et al. Crystal structure of cholesteryl ester transfer protein reveals a long tunnel and four bound lipid molecules. Nat Struct Mol Biol 2007;14:106–113)

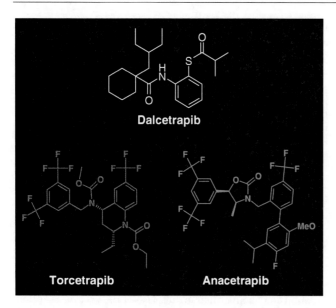

Fig. 4 The structures of the cholesteryl ester transfer protein inhibitors dalcetrapib (*top*), torcetrapib (*lower left*), and anacetrapib (*lower right*) are shown, indicating that dalcetrapib is structurally very different than the other two CETP inhibitors, and may be more of a CETP modulator than an inhibitor

of atherogenic remnant-like lipoprotein particles [16]. Moreover, this agent was found to be well tolerated and does not raise blood pressure. Subsequently, this agent was licensed to the pharmaceutical company Roche and has been named dalcetrapib.

Dalcetrapib was then tested in 838 subjects as either monotherapy or together with pravastatin and effective HDL cholesterol raising of about 30% was documented with no effect on blood pressure. The incidence of adverse events was similar in subjects on 300 and 600 mg/day as compared to placebo, but was slightly higher than placebo at the 900 mg/day dose [17]. In vitro studies indicated that torcetrapib, but not dalcetrapib increased aldosterone synthesis and mRNA levels in in vitro cell culture studies [17]. This agent is currently being studied in three clinical trials. The largest of these, known as dal-OUTCOMES is a phase III trial in which approximately 16,000 patients hospitalized for acute coronary syndrome are being randomized to dalcetrapib versus placebo [18, 19]. The second study, known as dal-VESSEL, is a phase II trial in which approximately 500 patients with CHD or CHD risk equivalent status are being randomized to dalcetrapib versus placebo and having endothelial function assessed [18, 19]. In the third study, known as dal-PLAQUE, approximately 100 patients are being placed on dalcetrapib and having their plaques evaluated by positron emission tomography, computed tomography angiography, and magnetic resonance imaging [18, 19]. The results of the large phase III study will be pivotal for the further clinical development of CETP inhibitors.

Torcetrapib

The pharmaceutical company Pfizer developed another CETP inhibitor known as torcetrapib, and its chemical structure is shown in Fig. 4 [20]. This agent was shown to raise HDL cholesterol by about 50% or more, and to lower LDL cholesterol by a modest amount, especially when given together with atorvastatin [21–23]. Moreover, this agent was shown to increase the size of both LDL and HDL particles [21, 24]. In careful metabolic studies in humans, torcetrapib – whether given alone or together with atorvastatin – the increases in HDL cholesterol, and apolipoprotein (apo) A-I and apoA-II were associated with significantly delayed fractional catabolism, with no effect on synthesis [24, 25]. Torcetrapib dramatically increased the levels of large protective alpha-1 HDL particles, but had no effect on fecal cholesterol excretion [24]. It has also been reported in rabbits that torcetrapib increases HDL cholesteryl ester by delaying its fractional clearance [26]. Studies in human have also documented that torcetrapib significantly enhances the clearance of apoB-100 and apoE in TRL [27, 28]. Torcetrapib has reported to decrease the atherogenicity of postprandial lipoproteins in patients with type IIb hyperlipidemia, as well as to correct the abnormalities noted in HDL subfractions in these patients [29, 30]. The serum of patients treated with torcetrapib is able to provide normal cellular cholesterol efflux via ABCA1 and SR-B1 mediated mechanisms, as has been reported for dalcetrapib [31, 32]. Similar to dalcetrapib, torcetrapib has been shown to decrease diet-induced atherosclerosis in rabbits [33].

However, a major concern however has been that torcetrapib has been reported to form a "nonproductive" complex with CETP and HDL [20]. In addition, recently torcetrapib has been reported to induce the production of aldosterone and cortisol by an intracellular calcium-mediated mechanism that is independent of its inhibition of cholesteryl ester transfer protein [34]. Such findings may explain the lack of benefit of torcetrapib at a dose of 60 mg/day in addition to atorvastatin therapy in clinical trials. This agent was tested in multiple clinical trials (15,067 CHD and high risk patient clinical endpoint study, intravascular ultrasound study in 1,188 CHD patients, and carotid intimal medial thicjness studies in 904 patients with familial hypercholesterolemia and 752 patients with dyslipidemia) [35–39]. In these trials, the use of torcetrapib was associated with no significant benefit on clinical endpoints, coronary atherosclerosis or carotid intimal medial thickness. Moreover, the large clinical endpoint trial was terminated prematurely because of excess cardiovascular endpoints (hazards ratio 1.25, $p=0.001$), with 464 events versus 373 events (CHD death, nonfatal myocardial infarction, stroke, and hospitalization for unstable angina) in the torcetrapib group versus placebo [32]. Moreover, there was also excess total mortality (93 vs. 59 deaths, with 6 vs. 0 fatal strokes, 9 vs. 0 fatal infections, and 24 vs. 14 cancer deaths) in the torcetrapib group versus the placebo group [35]. In all trials, torcetrapib use was associated with increased blood pressure, lowering of serum potassium, and increases in serum aldosterone levels [35–39]. However, post hoc analysis has indicated that those patients who received torcetrapib and had the highest on-trial HDL cholesterol levels appeared to get the most benefit on terms of CHD risk reduction in the endpoint trial and less progression or regression of coronary atherosclerosis in the intravascular ultrasound study [35, 37].

Anacetrapib

A third pharmaceutical company Merck has also developed a CETP inhibitor named anacetrapib. Its chemical structure is shown in Fig. 4. This agent has not been shown to increase blood pressure or to inhibit or induce CYP3A activity [40, 41]. Moreover, anacetrapib at doses of 10, 40, 150, and 300 mg/day in a total of 589 patients with hypercholesterolemia or mixed dyslipidemia has been reported to increase HDL cholesterol 44, 86, 139, and 133%, respectively, while reducing LDL cholesterol by 16, 27, 40, and 39%, respectively [42]. Similar effects were observed when the drug was added to atorvastatin [42]. Moreover, the drug was well tolerated, and the adverse event profile was similar to that observed in the placebo group [42]. It should also be noted that anacetrapib significantly lowers levels of lipoprotein(a).

Conclusions

Of the three CETP inhibitors that have been brought to clinical trials, one, namely torcetrapib, has been abandoned because of off-target effects, specifically raising aldosterone and blood pressure, and lowering potassium levels, along with adverse clinical outcomes. This agent has also been shown to increase cortisol levels in cells, which may account for the excess mortality from fatal infections observed in the endpoint trial, as well as the excess total mortality [34, 35]. The other two CETP inhibitors, dalcetrapib and anacetrapib, do not appear to have these off-target effects, and both significantly increase HDL cholesterol levels, and can be given together with statin therapy [15, 16, 41, 42]. The beneficial effect of CETP inhibition in my view is that cholesteryl ester transfer to TRL is prevented, resulting in a delay in the fractional clearance of large HDL particles, and enhanced fractional clearance of atherogenic remnant lipoprotein particles of both liver and intestinal origin [24, 25, 27, 28]. By enhancing the clearance of these latter particles, the ability of apo(a) to attach to apoB-100 TRL is decreased, and Lp(a)

is probably more readily cleared from the circulation [43]. However, Lp(a) metabolism before and after CETP inhibition requires more investigation. In addition, the natural inhibitor of CETP is apoC-I, and CETP is not stimulated by dietary cholesterol in the presence of a high-fat diet in animals [44, 45]. These latter observations require further study as well. CETP inhibitors can reduce the risk of CHD by lowering the amount of cholesteryl ester on atherogenic lipoprotein remnant particles of both intestinal and liver origin, and increase the amount of cholesteryl ester on large protective HDL particles [17, 46–49]. There is currently controversy as to whether CETP inhibitors without off-target effects will be beneficial [50]. The outcome of the large phase III trial currently underway with dalcetrapib is critical for the future development of CETP inhibitors.

References

1. Qiu X, Mistry A, Ammirati MJ, Chrunyk BA et al (2007) Crystal structure of cholesteryl ester transfer protein reveals a long tunnel and four bound lipid molecules. Nat Struct Mol Biol 14:106–113
2. Inazu A, Brown ML, Hesler CB, Agellon LB, Koizumi J, Takata K, Maruhama Y, Mabuchi H, Tall AR (1990) Increased high density lipoprotein levels caused by a common cholesteryl-transfer protein gene mutation. N Engl J Med 323:1234–1238
3. Asztalos BF, Horvath KV, Kajinami K, Nartsupha C, Cox CE, Batista M, Schaefer EJ, Inazu A, Mabuchi H (2004) Apolipoprotein composition of HDL in cholesteryl ester transfer protein deficiency. J Lipid Res 45:448–455
4. Miwa K, Inazu A, Kawashiri M, Nohara A, Higashikata T, Kobayashi J, Koizumi J, Nakajima K, Nakano T, Niimi M, Mabuchi H, Yamaqishi M (2009) Cholesterol efflux from J774 macrophages and Fu5AH hepatoma cells to serum is preserved in CETP-deficient patients. Clin Chim Acta 402:19–24
5. Ordovas JM, Cupples LA, Corella D, Otvos JD, Osgood D, Martinez A, Lahoz C, Coltell O, Wilson PW, Schaefer EJ (2000) Association of cholesteryl ester transfer protein – TaqIB polymorphism with variations in lipoprotein subclasses and coronary heart disease risk. The Framingham Study. Arterioscler Thromb Vasc Biol 20:1323–1329
6. Brousseau ME, O'Connor JJ, Ordovas JM, Collins D, Otvos JD, Massov T, McNamara JR, Rubins HB, Robins SJ, Schaefer EJ (2002) Cholesteryl ester transfer protein TaqI B2B2 genotype is associated with higher HDL cholesterol levels and lower risk of coronary heart disease endpoints in men with HDL deficiency. Veterans Affairs HDL Cholesterol Intervention Trial. Arterioscler Thromb Vasc Biol 22:1148–1154
7. Barzilai N, Atzmon G, Schechter C, Schaefer EJ, Cupples AL, Lipton R, Cheng S, Shuldiner AR (2003) Unique lipoprotein phenotype and genotype associated with exceptional longevity. JAMA 290:2030–2040
8. Hirano K, Yamashita S, Matsuzawa Y (2000) Pros and cons of inhibiting cholesteryl ester transfer protein. Curr Opin Lipidol 11:589–596
9. Agerholm-Larsen B, Nordestgaard BG, Steffensen R, Jensen G, Tybjaeg-Hansen A (2000) Elevated HDL cholesterol is a risk factor for ischemic heart disease in white women when caused by a common mutation in the cholesteryl ester transfer protein gene. Circulation 101:1907–1912

10. Regieli JJ, Jukema JW, Grobbee DE, Kastelein JJ, Kuivenhoven JA, Zwinderman AH, van der Graaf Y, Bots ML, Doevendans PA (2008) CETP genotype predicts increased mortality in statin-treated men with proven cardiovascular disease: an adverse pharmacogenetic interaction. Eur Heart J 22:2792–2799

11. Thompson A, Di Angelantonio E, Sarwar N, Erquo S, Saleheen D, Dullaart RP, Keavney B, Ye Z, Danesh J (2008) Association of cholesteryl ester transfer protein genotypes with CETP mass and activity, lipid levels and coronary heart disease. JAMA 299:2377–2388

12. Rittershaus CW, Miller DP, Thomas LJ, Picard MD, Honan CM, Emmett CD et al (2000) Vaccine-induced antibodies inhibit CETP activity in vivo and reduce aortic atherosclerosis in a rabbit model of atherosclerosis. Arterioscler Thromb Vasc Biol 20:2106–2112

13. Okamoto H, Yonemori F, Wakitani K, Minowa T, Maeda K, Shinkai A (2000) A cholesteryl ester transfer protein inhibitor attenuated atherosclerosis in rabbits. Nature 406:203–207

14. de Grooth GJ, Kuivenhoven JA, Stalenhoef AF, de Graaf J, Zwinderman AH, Posma JL, Van Tol A, Kastelein JJ (2002) Efficacy and safety of a novel cholesteryl ester transfer protein inhibitor, JTT-705, in humans: a randomized phase II dose response study. Circulation 105:2159–2165

15. Kuivenhoven JA, de Grooth GJ, Kawamura H, Klerkx AH, Wilhelm F, Trip MD, Kastelein JJ (2005) Effectiveness of of inhibition of cholesteryl ester transfer protein by JTT-705 in combination with pravastatin in type II dyslipidemia. Am J Cardiol 95:1085–1088

16. Stein EA, Stroes ES, Steiner G, Buckley BM, Capponoi AM, Burgess T, Niesor EJ, Kallend D, Kastelein JJ (2009) Safety and tolerability of dalcetrapib. Am J Cardiol 104:82–91

17. Okamoto H, Miyai A, Sasase T, Furukawa N, Matsushita M, Nakano T, Nakajima K (2006) Cholesteryl ester transfer protein promotes the formation of cholesterol-rich remnant like lipoprotein particles in human plasma. Clin Chim Acta 372:15–21

18. Davidson MH, Ballantyne CM, Chapman MJ (2009) HDL controversy: what have we learned from the clinical trials? Medscape CME June 19

19. http://www.clinicaltrials.gov

20. Clark RW, Ruggieri RB, Cunningham D, Bamberger MJ (2006) Description of the torcetrapib series of cholesteryl ester protein inhibitors, including mechanism of action. J Lipid Res 47:537–552

21. Brousseau ME, Schaefer EJ, Wolfe ML, Bloedan LT, Digenio AG, Clark RW, Mancuso JP, Rader DJ (2004) Effects of an inhibitor of cholesteryl ester transfer protein on HDL cholesterol. N Engl J Med 350:1505–1515

22. Clark RW, Surfin TA, Ruggeri RB, Willauer AT, Sugarman ED, Magnus-Aritey G, Cosgrove PG, Sand TM, Wester RT, Williams JA, Perlman ME, Bamberger MF (2004) Raising high-density lipoproteins in humans through inhibition of cholesteryl ester transfer protein: an initial multidose study of torcetrapib. Arterioscler Thromb Vasc Biol 24:490–497

23. Davidson MH, McKenney JM, Shear CL, Revkin JH (2006) Efficacy and safety of torcetrapib, a novel cholesteryl ester transfer protein inhibitor, in individuals with below average high density lipoprotein cholesterol levels. J Am Coll Cardiol 48:1782–1790

24. Brousseau ME, Diffenderfer MR, Millar JS, Nartsupha C, Asztalos BF, Welty FK, Wolfe ML, Rudling M, Bjorkham I, Angelin B, Mancuso JP, Digenio AG, Rader DJ, Schaefer EJ (2005) Effects of cholesteryl ester transfer protein inhibition on high-density lipoprotein subspecies, apolipoprotein A-I metabolism, and fecal sterol excretion. Arterioscler Thromb Vasc Biol 25:1057–1064

25. Brousseau ME, Millar JS, Diffenderfer MR, Nartsupha C, Asztalos BF, Wolfe ML, Mancuso JP, Digenio AG, Rader DJ, Schaefer EJ (2009) Effects of cholesteryl ester transfer protein inhibition on apolipoprotein (apo) A-II-containing HDL subspecies and apoA-II metabolism. J Lipid Res 50:1456–1462

26. Kee P, Cantazza D, Rye KA, Barrett PH, Morehouse LA, Barter PJ (2006) Effect of inhibiting cholesteryl ester protein on the kinetics of high-density lipoprotein cholesteryl ester transport in plasma. In vivo studies in rabbits. Arterioscler Vasc Thromb Biol 26:884–890

27. Millar JS, Brousseau ME, Diffenderfer MR, Barrett PH, Welty FK, Faruqi A, Wolfe ML, Nartsupha C, Digenio AG, Mancuso JP, Dolnokowski GG, Schaefer EJ, Rader DJ (2006) Effects of the cholesteryl ester transfer protein inhibitor torcetrapib on apolipoprotein B100 metabolism. Arterioscler Thromb Vasc Biol 26:1350–1356

28. Millar JS, Brousseau ME, Diffenderfer MR, Barrett PH, Welty FK, Cohn JS, Wilson A, Wolfe ME, Schaefer PM, Nartsupha C, Schaefer PM, Digenio AG, Mancuso JP, Dolnikowski GG, Schaefer EJ, Rader DJ (2008) Effects of the cholesteryl ester transfer protein inhibitor torcetrapib on VLDL apolipoprotein E metabolism. J Lipid Res 49:543–549

29. Guerin M, Le Goff W, Duchene E, Julia Z, Nguyen T, Thuren T, Shear CL, Chapman MJ (2008) Inhibition of CETP by torcetrapib attenuates the atherogenicity of postprandial TG-rich lipoproteins in type IIB hyperlipidemia. Arterioscler Thromb Vasc Biol 28:148–154

30. Catalano G, Julia Z, Friedal E, Vedie B, Fiurnier N, Le Goff W, Chapman MJ (2009) Torcetrapib differentially modulates the biological activities of HDL2 and HDL3 particles in the reverse cholesterol transport pathway. Arterioscler Thromb Vasc Biol 29:268–275

31. Masson D, Jiang XC, Lagrost L, Tall A (2009) The role of plasma lipid transfer proteins in lipoprotein metabolism and atherogenesis. J Lipid Res 50:S201–S206

32. Rader DJ, Alexander ET, Weibel GL, Bilheimer J, Rothblat GH (2009) The role of reverse cholesterol transport in animals and humans in relationship to atherosclerosis. J Lipid Res 50:S189–S194

33. Morehouse LA, Sugarman ED, Bourassa PA, Sand TM, Zimetti F, Gao F, Rothblat GH, Milici AJ (2007) Inhibition of CETP activity by torcetrapib reduces susceptibility to diet-induced atherosclerosis in New Zealand White rabbits. J Lipid Res 48:1263–1272

34. Hu X, Dietz JD, Xia C, Knight DR, Loging WT, Smith AH, Yuan H, Perry DA, Keider J (2009) Torcetrapib induces aldosterone and cortisol production by an intracellular calcium-mediated mechanism independently of cholesteryl ester transfer protein inhibition. Endocrinology 150:2211–2219

35. Barter PJ, Caulfield M, Eriksson M, Grundy SM, Kastelein JJ, Komajda M et al (2007) Effects of torcetrapib in patients at high risk for coronary events. N Engl J Med 357:2109–2122

36. Nissen SE, Tardif JC, Nicholls SJ, Revkin JH, Shear CL, Duggan WT, Ruzyllo W, Bachinsky WB, Lasala GP, Tuzcu EM; ILLUSTRATE Investigators (2007) Effects of torcetrapib on progression of coronary atherosclerosis. N Engl J Med 356:1304–1316

37. Nicholls SJ, Tuzcu EM, Brennan DM, Tardif JC, Nissen SE (2008) Cholesteryl ester transfer protein inhibition, high density lipoprotein raising, and progression of coronary atherosclerosis: insights from ILUSTRATE (Investigation of Lipid Level Management Using Coronary Ultrasound to Assess Reduction of Atherosclerosis by CETP Inhibition and HDL Elevation). Circulation 118:2 506–2514

38. Kastelein JJ, van Leuven SI, Burgess L, Evan GW, Kuivenhoven JA, Barter PJ, Revkin JH, Grobbee DE, Riley WA, Shear CL, Bots ML; RADIANCE 1 Investigators (2007) Effect of torcetrapib on carotid atherosclerosis in familial hypercholesterolemia. N Eng J Med 356:1620–1630

39. Bots ML, Visseren FL, Evans GW, Riley WA, Revkin JH, Tegeler CH, Shear CL, Duggan WT, Vicari RM, Grobbee DE, Kastelein JJ; RADIANCE 2 Investigators (2007) Torcetrapib and carotid intima-media thickness in mixed dyslipidemia (RADIANCE 2 study): a randomized, double-blind trial. Lancet 370:107–108

40. Krishna R, Bergman AJ, Jin B, Garg A, Roadcap B, Chiou R, Dru J, Cote J, Laethem T, Wang RW, Didolkar V, Vets E, Gottesdiener K, Wagner J (2009) Assessment of the CYP3A-mediated drug interaction potential of anacetrapib, a potent cholesteryl ester transfer protein (CETP) inhibitor, in healthy volunteers. J Clin Pharm 49:80–87

41. Krishna R, Anderson MS, Bergman AJ, Jin B, Fallon M, Cote J, Rosko K, Chavez-Eng C, Lutz R, Bloomfield DM, Guiterrez M, Doherty J, Biebersdorf F, Chodakewitz J, Gottesdiener KM, Wagner J (2007) Effect of the cholesteryl ester transfer protein inhibitor, anacetrapib, on lipoproteins in patients with dyslipidemia and on 24-h ambulatory blood pressure in healthy individuals:two double-blinded randomized placebo-controlled phase 1 trials. Lancet 370:1907

42. Bloomfield D, Carlson GL, Sapre A, Tribble D, McKenney JM, Littlejohn TW 3rd, Sisk CM, Mitchel Y, Pasternak RC (2009) Efficacy and safety of the cholesteryl ester transfer protein inhibitor anacetrapib as monotherapy and coadministered with atorvastatin in dyslipidemic patients. Am Heart J 157:352–360

43. Jenner JL, Seman LJ, Millar JS, Lamon-Fava S, Welty FK, Dolnikowski GG, Marcovina SM, Lichtenstein AH, Barrett PHR, deLuca C, Schaefer EJ (2005) The metabolism of apolipoproteins (a) and B-100 within plasma lipoprotein(a) in human beings. Metabolism 54:361–369

44. Dumont L, Gauthier T, de Barros JP, Laplanche H, Blache D, Ducuroy P, Fruchart J, Fruchart JC, Gambert P, Masson D, Lagrost L (2005) Molecular mechanism of the blockade of plasma cholesteryl ester protein by its physiologic inhibitor apolipoprotein CI. J Biol Chem 280:38108–38116

45. Cheema SK, Agarwal-Mawal A, Murray CM, Tucker S (2005) Lack of stimulation of cholesteryl ester transfer protein by cholesterol in the presence of a high fat diet. J Lipid Res 46:2356–2366

46. Asztalos BF, Cupples LA, Demissie S, Horvath K, Cox CE, Batista MC, Schaefer EJ (2004) High-density lipoprotein subpopulation profile and coronary heart disease prevalence in male participants in the Framingham Offspring Study. Arterioscler Thromb Vasc Biol 24:2181–2187

47. Asztalos BF, Collins D, Cupples LA, Demissie S, Horvath KV, Bloomfield HE, Robins SJ, Schaefer EJ (2005) Value of high density lipoprotein (HDL) subpopulations in predicting recurrent cardiovascular events in the Veterans Affairs HDL Intervention Trial. Arterioscler Thromb Vasc Biol 25:2185–2191

48. Asztalos BF, Batista M, Horvath KV, Cox CE, Dallal GE, Morse JS, Brown GB, Schaefer EJ (2003) Change in alpha 1 HDL concentration predicts progression in coronary artery stenosis. Arterioscler Thromb Vasc Biol 23:847–852

49. McNamara JR, Shah PK, Nakajima K, Cupples LA, Wilson PWF, Ordovas JM, Schaefer EJ (2001) Remnant-like particle (RLP) cholesterol is an independent cardiovascular disease risk factor in women: results from the Framingham Heart Study. Atherosclerosis 154:229–236

50. Zhao L, Jin W, Rader D, Packard C, Feuerstein G (2009) A translational medicine perspective of the development of torcetrapib:does the failure of torcetrapib development cast a shadow on the future development of lipid modifying agents, HDL elevation strategy, or CETP as a viable molecular target for atherosclerosis? A case study of the use of biomarkers and translational medicine in atherosclerosis drug discovery and development. Biochem Pharmacol 78:315–325

HDL Infusion Therapy

H. Bryan Brewer

Over the last three decades, clinical trials utilizing statins to reduce LDL in high risk patients have resulted in a 30–40% reduction in clinical events [1–6]. However, despite a significant reduction in LDL, many patients continue to have clinical events. The residual risk present in statin treated high risk patients has resulted in the search for additional therapeutic approaches to reduce clinical events. Epidemiological studies have identified HDL cholesterol (HDL-C) as an independent risk factor for cardiovascular disease [7, 8]. In addition, low HDL-C levels are often present in high risk patients [9], and analyses of clinical trials of statin therapy have indicated that the baseline level of HDL-C is an important determinant of the clinical benefit associated with statin treatment [1, 4, 5]. As a result, focus has now turned to increasing HDL as a potential approach to reduce the residual cardiovascular risk in statin treated patients.

Several lines of evidence suggest that increasing HDL will reduce cardiovascular events. Initial studies with infusions of HDL in cholesterol fed rabbits [10] and increasing HDL-C by overexpression of the apoA-I gene in transgenic mice resulted in decreased aortic atherosclerosis [11, 12]. Overexpression of the LCAT gene in cholesterol fed transgenic rabbits was associated with a significant increase in HDL-C and dramatic reduction in aortic atherosclerosis [13]. An initial clinical trial with niacin which increases HDL-C resulted in a reduction of myocardial infarctions as well as long-term mortality [14]. The combination of niacin and statin therapy in patients with coronary atherosclerosis in the FATS trial resulted in an angiographically documented decrease in coronary artery plaque size and reduced clinical events [15]. In the ARBITER 2 and 3 trials, statin therapy was associated with a decrease in the progression of carotid intimal-medial thickness (CIMT), while the addition of niacin to the patients receiving statin therapy resulted in an increased HDL-C and regression of the CIMT [16, 17].

The clinical importance of the 3–14% increase in HDL-C associated with statin therapy has also been reviewed in four clinical trials using intravascular ultrasound (IVUS) to quantitate coronary atherosclerosis. In this analysis, the increase in HDL-C independent of the reduction of LDL-C was correlated with the reduction in atherosclerosis [18]. Aggressive LDL reduction to the 60 mg/dl range was associated with regression of coronary atherosclerosis. On the basis of the analysis of these four clinical trials, a reduction of LDL to <87.5 mg/dl and a 7.5% increase in HDL-C resulted in the regression of atherosclerosis [18]. A meta-analysis of statin trials targeted to lower LDL as well as trials using a combination of LDL lowering and HDL raising therapies supported the thesis that statins were associated with a decrease in the progression of coronary artery atherosclerosis; however, that concomitant LDL reduction and an increase in HDL-C were required for regression of vascular disease [15].

Recently, significant progress has been made in our understanding of the potential mechanisms by which HDL may reduce atherosclerosis. For the last four decades, the key mechanism proposed for the HDL mediated reduction in atherosclerosis was reverse cholesterol transport [19]. A process by which HDL removes excess cholesterol from the cholesterol loaded peripheral cell and transports the cholesterol back to the liver, where the excess cholesterol may be removed from the body. Until recently, the mechanism by which HDL removes cholesterol from peripheral cells was poorly understood. The discovery of the molecular defect in the ABCA1 transporter as the genetic defect in Tangier disease [20–26] and the identification of the role of the ABCG1 transporter in cholesterol efflux [27, 28] have provided a dual mechanism for cellular cholesterol efflux (Fig. 1). The ligands for the ABCA1 and ABCG1 transporters are lipid poor apoA-I/preβ-HDL and mature αHDL, respectively [29–31]. An improved understanding of the mechanisms involved in cholesterol efflux and additional new knowledge on the receptors, enzymes, and transfer proteins involved in lipid transport has resulted in an updated model of cellular cholesterol efflux and reverse cholesterol transport from the cholesterol loaded peripheral cell to the liver (Fig. 1). Increased levels of intracellular cholesterol in peripheral

H.B. Brewer (✉)
Lipoprotein and Atherosclerosis Research, Cardiovascular Research Institute, MedStar Research Institute, Washington Hospital Center, Suite 4B-1, 110 Irving Street, Washington, DC 20010, USA
e-mail: Bryan.Brewer@MedStar.net

E.J. Schaefer (ed.), *High Density Lipoproteins, Dyslipidemia, and Coronary Heart Disease*,
DOI 10.1007/978-1-4419-1059-2_22, © Springer Science+Business Media, LLC 2010

173

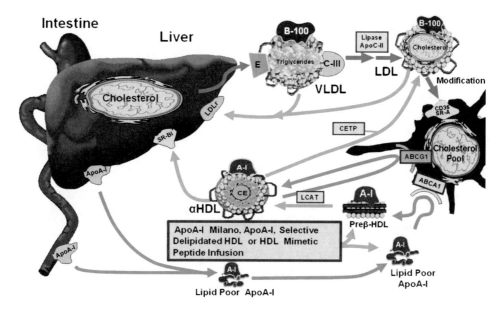

Fig. 1 Schematic model of cholesterol efflux and reverse cholesterol transport. Lipid lipid poor/preβ-HDL and αHDL facilitate cholesterol efflux by the ABCA1 and ABCG1 transporter pathways, respectively. HDL cholesterol is transported back to the liver by both transfer of cholesteryl esters to the apoB containing lipoproteins by the cholesterol ester transfer protein (CETP) with ultimate hepatic uptake via the LDL receptor or directly following interaction with the hepatic SR-BI receptor. Acute HDL infusion therapy dramatically increases cholesterol efflux by increasing the ligand for the ABCA1 transporter, lipid poor/preβ-HDL

macrophages result in an increased level of expression of the ABCA1 transporter. Newly synthesized lipid poor apoA-I from the liver and intestine bind to the ABCA1 transporter and mediate cholesterol efflux resulting in an increase in cholesterol within preβ-HDL [32]. The cholesterol is esterified by the LCAT enzyme and preβ-HDL is converted to αHDL. Efflux from peripheral cells to αHDL is mediated by ABCG1. The cholesterol in HDL is transported back to the liver directly by binding to the SR-BI receptor or following transfer to the apoB containing lipoproteins by the cholesterol ester exchange protein (CETP), thus completing the reverse cholesterol transport cycle. An initial human study which involved the infusion of a reconstituted proapoA-I/lipid complex increased both plasma HDL-C and fecal sterol excretion consistent with the concept that apoA-I mediates reverse cholesterol transport [33].

In addition to reverse cholesterol transport, HDL has been proposed to protect against the development of cardiovascular disease by several other mechanisms. HDL has been shown to be an effective anti-inflammatory agent in both in vitro studies as well as animal models [34–36]. A pivotal mechanism involved in the anti-inflammatory function of HDL is the reduction of both the protein as well as RNA of endothelial cell adhesion molecules. HDL has also been shown to protect LDL from oxidation [37, 38], increase NO levels [39, 40], and transport a number of potentially important biologically active molecules [41].

ApoA-I Infusions

A major stimulus in the interest of incorporating increasing HDL in therapeutic programs to reduce clinical cardiovascular events in high risk patients was the initial results of a clinical trial of HDL infusion therapy with apoA-I Milano. ApoA-I Milano was discovered in a small village in Italy in patients with high triglycerides and low HDL but no increased risk of cardiovascular disease [42]. ApoA-I Milano is a mutant A-I apolipoprotein with a single amino acid substitution of a cysteine residue for arginine at position 173 resulting in an apolipoprotein that can form dimmers [43]. Employing radiolabeled HDL kinetic studies, the low plasma HDL levels in apoA-I Milano heterozygotes were shown to be due to increased catabolism of the monomeric apoA-I Milano protein [44]. The lack of increased risk of cardiovascular disease in kindreds with low HDL resulted in the initiation of a clinical trial to determine the effect of apoA-I Milano infusions on coronary artery atherosclerosis quantitated by IVUS in acute coronary artery syndrome (ACS) patients [45]. In this trial, IVUS results were obtained during an initial clinically indicated cardiac catherization, and following 5 weekly control infusions or reconstituted apoA-I Milano/phospholipid infusions in 11 control patients and 36 treated patients (21, 15 mg/kg; 15, 45 mg/kg), respectively. In the combined 36 patients who received apoA-I Milano infusions, the total atheroma volume and the 10 mm most

Table 1 Comparison of the changes in IVUS Parameters in ApoA-I Milano and selective HDL delipidation acute HDL infusion trials

Variable (mean ± SD)	ApoA-I Milano (n = 36)	Selective HDL delipidation (n = 14)
Change in total atheroma volume (mm³)	−14.10 ± 0.50	−12.18 ± 36.75
Change in % atheroma volume (plaque burden)	−1.1 ± 3.2	−1.0 ± 4.0
Change in 10 mm³ most disease segment (mm³)	−7.20 ± 12.60	−6.24 ± 17.95

diseased segment decreased by −14.10 ± 39.5 mm³ and −7.20 ± 12.60 mm³ when compared to the atherosclerosis quantitated at baseline (Table 1). It is important to note that each control and infused patient serves as his/her own control with the atherosclerosis quantitated at baseline compared to the atherosclerosis ascertained at the end of 5 weeks of standard care in patients with control infusions and following the 5 weekly apoA-I Milano infusions in the treated patients. The observed results were unexpected since it was anticipated that it would take months or even years to obtain significant regression in patients with established coronary artery atherosclerosis.

The reduction in IVUS quantitated plaque volume in patients who received apoA-I Milano infusions suggested that acute HDL infusion therapy in ACS patients might be associated with decreased clinical cardiovascular events.

In 2004, at the time the apoA-I Milano infusion study was completed, a great deal of speculation surrounded the potential mechanism(s) for such a dramatic reduction in coronary atherosclerosis. The elucidation of the genetic defect in Tangier disease provided the unique opportunity to discover the ABCA1 transporter, the major pathway for cellular cholesterol efflux and lipid poor apoA-I/preβ-HDL as the ligand for the ABCA1 transporter. This data provided a major insight into the potential mechanism for the atheroprotective results obtained with the apoA-I Milano infusions. In normal plasma lipid poor apoA-I/preβ-HDL is only approximately 3–5% of the total plasma HDL. The reconstituted apoA-I Milano/phospholipid complex is a lipid poor apoA-I/preβ-HDL like particle and infusion of this recombined complex dramatically expanded the pool size of the ligand for the ABCA1 transporter facilitating both cholesterol efflux as well as increasing the anti-inflammatory potential of plasma HDL. An increased plasma capacity for both cholesterol efflux as well as reduced vascular inflammation provide potential mechanisms for the dramatic effects of apoA-I Milano infusions on coronary atherosclerosis.

The elucidation of the ABCA1-apoA-I/preβ-HDL pathway for reducing coronary atherosclerosis resulted in the quest for additional approaches to obtain lipid poor apoA-I/preβ-HDL for infusions in high risk ACS patients. The development of a plasma method for selective HDL delipidation

with the conversion of αHDL to lipid poor apoA-I/preβ-HDL without any other change in the plasma apoB lipoproteins provided a unique convenient source of autologous lipid poor apoA-I/preβ-HDL for infusions [46]. During this process plasma is removed, and passed through an LS PDS-2 delipidation device which removes selectively cholesterol from HDL converting αHDL into lipid poor apoA-I/preβ-HDL. The selective HDL delipidated plasma is then reinfused back into the patient.

Data on the initial clinical safety and efficacy of selective HDL delipidated plasma was determined in hyperlipidemic African Green monkeys [46]. Plasma from control monkeys was selectively delipidated and infused weekly for 12 weeks into five hyperlipidemic monkeys for a total of 123 infusions. Complete lipoprotein and clinical chemistry profiles obtained throughout the course of the study were unremarkable and the infusions were well tolerated. Changes in aortic atherosclerotic lesions were evaluated by comparison of IVUS quantitated aortic plaques obtained at baseline and following the completion of the 12 weekly infusions. A comparison of aortic plaques at baseline and posttreatment revealed a 6.9% decrease (p = 0.03) in total atheroma volume associated with infusions of selective HDL delipidated plasma. Detailed HDL kinetic studies were also performed to determine the metabolic fate of the infused lipid poor apoA-I/preβ-HDL. The lipid poor apoA-I/preβ-HDL had a plasma residence time of 8 ± 6 h and was converted to the large mature αHDL with a residence time of 13–14 h. The results of the monkey infusion study established that the metabolic pathway for infused lipid poor apoA-I/preβ-HDL was similar to the maturation of normal preβ-HDL to αHDL and that infused lipid poor apoA-I/preβ-HDL was associated with decreased aortic atherosclerosis in this primate model.

Following completion of the monkey selective HDL delipidated plasma infusion study, a human clinical trial employing this novel autologous selective HDL delipidated plasma methodology was initiated in ACS patients [47]. This first-in-man trial involved baseline quantitation of atherosclerosis in a nontargeted coronary artery (20–50% luminal obstruction) during a clinically indicated coronary artery catherization in patients with ACS. The patients were randomized to receive either 7 weekly infusion of autologous selective HDL delipidated plasma (15 mg/kg apoA-I) or undelipidated plasma. Plasma was removed and either stored for control subjects or delipidated using the LS PDS-2 delipidation devise, and the control or delipidated plasma was reinfused back into the patient. Following completion of the seven infusions, a second cardiac catherization was performed, and the change in coronary artery atherosclerosis in the same selected vessel was determined. Fourteen control and 14 treated patients participated in the clinical trial. Twenty-six of the 28 subjects (92.1%) complete the entire protocol. The plasma collection, delipidation, and reinfusion procedures were well tolerated except for occasional transient hypotension during the plasma collection. The exploratory analyses of the IVUS data obtained at baseline and following completion of the 7 weekly infusions revealed a 2.8 ± 21.3 mm^3 and -12.18 ± 36.75 mm^3 changes in absolute atheroma volume in control and selective HDL delipidated plasma treated patients respectively. The percent change in atheroma volume was $-1.0 \pm 4\%$ for selective HDL delipidated plasma infused patients and $0.0 \pm 4\%$ in control infused patients. Although the small sample size precluded definitive statistical analysis of the reduction of atheroma volume observed in the treated patients, the results are consistent with the conclusion that infusion of selective HDL delipidated plasma may represent a new therapeutic approach to decrease plaque burden in ACS patients.

An additional HDL infusion clinical trial, the ERASE Trial (Effect of rHDL on Atherosclerosis-Safety and Efficacy), was performed in patients using a reconstituted normal apoA-I/lipid complex [48]. The trial enrolled ACS patients at the time of a clinically indicated cardiac catherization followed by 4 weekly infusions of either saline control or an apoA-I/lipid complex (40 or 80 mg/kg). A total of 54 control and 105 apoA-I/lipid complex treated (40 mg/kg) ACS patients completed the 4 week infusion study. The 12 patient receiving the apoA-I/lipid complex at a dose of 80 mg/kg were terminated during the course of the trial because of liver function test abnormalities. In this relatively short study, the change in total atheroma volume determined at baseline and following completion of the infusions in saline control subjects and the 40 mg/kg apoA-I/lipid complex treated group was -1.6% ($p=0.04$) and -3.4% ($p<0.001$) respectively ($p=0.48$ between placebo and treated groups). The percent change in atheroma volume was -1.1% for apoA-I/lipid complex treated patients ($p<0.001$ vs. baseline) and -0.1% for control placebo patients ($p=0.07$ vs. baseline). In addition, both an improved coronary score based on quantitative coronary angiography and plaque characterization indexes obtained by IVUS were significantly different between the placebo and apoA-I/lipid complex treated group supporting the conclusion that HDL infusions in ACS patients reduce coronary atherosclerosis.

It is of interest to compare the IVUS results of the currently available HDL infusion trials (Table 1), in which each patient serves as his or her own control with paired comparisons performed between the baseline and end-of-study quantitation of atheroma burden. The reduction of absolute atheroma volume and plaque in the 10 mm most diseased segment were similar in the apoA-I Milano and selective HDL delipidation trials (Table 1). The reduction in total atheroma volume with the infusion of reconstitue apoA-I in the shorter ERASE trail was statistically significant but less than the other two trials, however the data for the 10 mm most disease segment was not reported.

It is also of interest to compare the results of the changes in atherosclerosis obtained with weekly infusions of reconstituted HDL in the apoA-I Milano and selective HDL delipidation trials with IVUS atherosclerosis data obtained following 18 months of high-dose statin therapy. The rapid reduction in atherosclerosis obtained with the HDL infusion trials is in contrast to the results obtained in the REVERSAL (Reversal of Atherosclerosis with Aggressive Lipid Lowering) Trial in 502 ACS patients [49]. At the end of the 18 month trial, the total atheroma volume and 10 mm most diseased segment in the high dose statin arm (80 mg atorvastatin) were -0.04 mm^3 and -4.2 mm^3, respectively. Thus, the reductions in atherosclerosis quantitated by IVUS in the HDL infusion trials following 5–7 weeks of therapy were nearly doubled that achieved with high dose statin therapy for 18 months.

These combined results add support to the concept that increasing poorly lipidated apoA-I/preβ-HDL by acute HDL infusions in ACS patients may result in a rapid reduction in atheroma burden with stabilization of the plaque and potential decreased future clinical events.

HDL Mimetic Peptides

The infusion of apoA-I as a therapeutic approach to the treatment of high risk cardiovascular patients presents a challenge due to the requirements for the synthesis of the 243 amino acid apoA-I protein and the large quantity of protein required for each infusion. As a result, there has been an expanding interest in the development of synthetic HDL mimetic peptides. Following the determination of the amino acid sequence of apoA-I [50], a number of studies were undertaken to develop apoA-I mimetic peptides. These shorter peptides may have only a minimal similarity in amino acid sequence to apoA-I; however, they maintain the characteristic amphipathic helix present in apoA-I and the other apolipoproteins [51–54]. A number of the synthetic amphipathic peptides were modification of the 18pA and 37pA model hydrophobic peptides which contained amphipathic helices characteristic of apoA-I [54].

Several synthetic apoA-I mimetic peptides are currently under development. ETC 642 is a 22 amino acid amphipathic peptide modified to optimize the ability of the peptide to increase LCAT activity similar to apoA-I [55]. In culture studies, ETC 642 facilitated cholesterol efflux from cholesterol loaded THP-1 cells. In these studies, saturation of cholesterol efflux was observed; however, at the protein concentration, tested ETC 642 did not exhibit saturation. In contrast to apoA-I (lipid free) and rHDL, ETC 642 mediated cholesterol efflux from Tangier disease fibroblasts was both ABCA1 dependent (lipidated peptide) and ABCA1 independent (lipid free peptide).

In addition, ETC 642 was able to efflux cholesterol from formaldehyde fixed cells which occurred by an energy-independent passive process. Additional animal as well as clinical studies are underway to further evaluate the potential efficacy of ETC 642 to reduce atherosclerosis.

D-4F is an 18 amino acid peptide which contains D-amino acids which are resistant to degradation by intestinal proteases facilitating oral administration of the peptide. D-4F contains four phenylalanine substitutions in the 18A peptide [56]. A pivotal feature of D-4F is its anti-inflammatory property [56–59]. HDL isolated from mice treated with D-4F have greater anti-inflammatory properties than control HDL when assayed by the ability of HDL to inhibit LDL-induced monocyte chemotactic activity in a human endothelial cell coculture in vitro system. D-4F also binds fatty acid hyperoxides and proinflammatory oxidized phospholipids. Oral administration of D-4F in LDLr and apoE knockout mice reduced aortic atherosclerosis with no change in the plasma lipoproteins. In addition, D-4F was able to reduce the inflammatory response of influenza A infected mice [60] and human type II pneumocytes in culture [61]. A human clinical trial using a dose escalating single oral administration of D-4F has been reported [62]. The single dose of D-4F was well tolerated, and the HDL isolated from the participants at the two highest doses was anti-inflammatory relative to placebo HDL when tested in the endothelial cell culture assay system.

NIH 5A is a 37 amino acid bi-helical peptide modeled after the 37pA peptide [63]. One helical domain is highly hydrophobic, and the second helix was modified to reduce the hydrophobicity and to selectively increase the efflux from the ABCA1 pathway with minimal non-ABCA1 mediated efflux. NIH-5A did not significantly efflux cholesterol from cholesterol loaded Tangier disease fibroblasts or formaldehyde treated fixed cells [63–65]. Aortic atherosclerosis was significantly decreased following 6 weeks of 3× week injections of NIH 5A in apoE knockout mice. NIH-5A administration was anti-inflammatory with a significant reduction in CD11B expression in PMA activated monocytes [64].

LSI-518P contains 38 amino acids with two amphipathic helices. LSI-518P efficiently increased selectively ABCA1 mediated cholesterol efflux with no significant non-ABCA1 mediated efflux or efflux from SR-BI expressing cells, formaldehyde fixed cells, or cholesterol loaded Tangier disease fibroblasts [66]. In preclinical animal models, LSI-518P increased plasma HDL-C, and decreased aortic atherosclerosis in apoE knockout mice. In addition, LSI-518P inhibited expression of PMA induced CD11B in human monocytes, and inhibited VCAM-1 adhesion molecule expression of human cardiac endothelial cells in culture. Thus, LSI-518P was similar to apoA-I in its ability to facilitate cholesterol efflux from cholesterol loaded cells in vitro, increase plasma HDL-C, decrease atherosclerosis in the apoE-KO animal model, and decrease inflammation.

An initial report on ATI-5261, a small amphipathic helical peptide, indicated that this amphipathic peptide was able to efflux cholesterol from the ABCA1 pathway in vitro and decrease aortic atherosclerosis in the apoE-KO mouse model [67].

Summary

The recurrent clinical events in high risk ACS patients are a challenge to the cardiovascular physician. Acute HDL therapy with HDL infusions may provide an approach to decrease clinical events in ACS patients. To date, HDL infusion therapy utilizing either reconstituted apoA-I Milano/phospholipid complexes, selective HDL delipidated plasma, or reconstituted normal apoA-I/phospholipid complexes has been shown to decrease coronary atherosclerotic plaques in IVUS imaging trials in ACS patients. HDL mimetic peptides based on the amphipathic structure of apoA-I have been shown in preclinical studies to increase plasma HDL-C and decrease aortic atherosclerosis in mouse model systems. This growing body of evidence suggests that acute HDL therapy using HDL infusions may provide a new exciting therapeutic approach to decrease vascular disease. Future clinical trials will ultimately be required to definitively establish if acute HDL therapy with HDL infusions with either apoA-I or HDL mimetic peptides will result in a rapid decrease in coronary atheroma burden and decreased clinical events in high risk ACS patients.

References

1. Scandinavian Simvastatin Survival Study Group (1994) Randomized trial of cholesterol lowering in 4444 patients with coronary heart disease: the Scandinavian Simvastatin Survival Study (4S). Lancet 344:1383–1389
2. Shepherd J, Cobbe SM, Ford I et al (1995) Prevention of coronary heart disease with pravastatin in men with hypercholesterolemia. N Engl J Med 333:1350–1351
3. Sacks FM, Pfeffer MA, Moye LA et al (1996) The effect of pravastatin on coronary events after myocardial infarction in patients with average cholesterol levels. N Engl J Med 335:1001–1009
4. Downs JR, Clearfield M, Weis S et al (1998) Primary prevention of acute coronary events with lovastatin in men and women with average cholesterol levels: results of AFCAPS/TexCAPS. Air Force/Texas Coronary Atherosclerosis Prevention Study. JAMA 279:1615–1622
5. Heart Protection Study Collaborative Group (2002) MRC/BHF Heart Protection Study of cholesterol lowering with simvastatin in 20,536 high-risk individuals: a randomized placebo-controlled trial. Lancet 360:7–22
6. Baigent C, Keech A, Kearney PM et al (2005) Efficicay and safety of cholesterol lowering treatment:prospective meta-analysis of data from 90,056 participants in 14 randomized trials of statins. Lancet 366:1267–1278

7. Castelli WP, Anderson K, Wilson PW et al (1992) Lipids and risk of coronary heart disease: The Framingham Study. Ann Epidemiol 2:23–28

8. Gordon DJ, Rifkind BM (1989) High-density lipoprotein: the clinical implications of recent studies. N Engl J Med 321:1311–1316

9. Barter P, Gotto AM, LaRosa JC et al; Treating to New Targets Investigators (2007) HDL cholesterol, very low levels of LDL cholesterol, and cardiovascular events. N Engl J Med 357:1301–1310

10. Badimon JJ, Badimon L, Fuster V (1990) Regression of atherosclerotic lesions by high density lipoprotein plasma fraction in the cholesterol-fed rabbit. J Clin Invest 85:1234–1241

11. Rubin EM, Krauss RM, Spangler EA et al (1991) Inhibition of early atherogenesis in transgenic mice by human apolipoprotein AI. Nature 353:265–267

12. Plump AS, Scott CJ, Breslow JL (1994) Human apolipoprotein A-I gene expression increases high density lipoprotein and suppresses atherosclerosis in the apolipoprotein E-deficient mouse. Proc Natl Acad Sci USA 91:9607–9611

13. Hoeg JM, Santamarina-Fojo S, Bérard AM et al (1996) Overexpression of lecithin:cholesterol acyltransferase in transgenic rabbits prevents diet-induced atherosclerosis. Proc Natl Acad Sci USA 93:11448–11453

14. Canner PL, Berge KG, Wenger NK et al (1986) Fifteen year mortality in Coronary Drug Project patients: long-term benefit with niacin. J Am Coll Cardiol 8:1245–1255

15. Brown BG, Stukovsky KH, Zhao XQ (2006) Simultaneous low-density lipoprotein-C lowering and high-density lipoprotein-C elevation for optimum cardiovascular disease prevention with various drug classes, and their combinations: a meta-analysis of 23 randomized lipid trials. Curr Opin Lipidol 17:631–636

16. Taylor AJ, Sullenberger LE, Lee HJ et al (2004) Arterial Biology for the Investigation of the Treatment Effects of Reducing Cholesterol (ARBITER) 2: a double-blind, placebo-controlled study of extended-release niacin on atherosclerosis progression in secondary prevention patients treated with statins. Circulation 8:1245–1255

17. Taylor A, Lee H, Sullenberger LE (2006) The effect of 24 months of combination statin and extended-release niacin on carotid intima-media thickness: ARBITER 3. Curr Med Res Opin 22:2243–2250

18. Nicholls SJ, Tuzcu EM, Sipahi I et al (2007) Statins, high-density lipoprotein cholesterol, and regression of coronary atherosclerosis. JAMA 297:499–508

19. Glomset JA (1968) The plasma lecithin:cholesterol acyltransferase reaction. J Lipid Res 9:155–167

20. Brooks-Wilson A, Marcil M, Clee SM et al (1999) Mutations in ABC1 in Tangier disease and familial high-density lipoprotein deficiency. Nat Genet 22:336–345

21. Bodzioch M, Orso E, Klucken J et al (1999) The gene encoding ATP-binding cassette transporter 1 is mutated in Tangier disease. Nat Genet 22:347–351

22. Rust S, Rosier M, Funke H et al (1999) Tangier disease is caused by mutations in the ATP binding cassette transporter 1 (ABC1) gene. Nat Genet 22:352–355

23. Remaley AT, Rust S, Rosier M et al (1999) Human ATP-binding cassette transporter 1 (ABC1): genomic organization and identification of the genetic defect in the original Tangier disease kindred. Proc Natl Acad Sci USA 96:12685–12690

24. Brousseau ME, Schaefer EJ, Dupuis J et al (2000) Novel mutations in the gene encoding ATP-binding cassette 1 in four tangier disease kindreds. J Lipid Res 41:433–441

25. Lawn RM, Wade DP, Garvin MR et al (1999) The Tangier disease gene product ABC1 controls the cellular apolipoprotein-mediated lipid removal pathway. J Clin Invest 104:R25–R31

26. Santamarina-Fojo S, Peterson K, Knapper C et al (2000) Complete genomic sequence of the human ABCA1 gene: analysis of the human and mouse ATP-binding cassette A promoter. Proc Natl Acad Sci USA 97:7987–7992

27. Wang N, Lan D, Chen W et al (2004) ATP-binding cassette transporters G1 and G4 mediate cellular cholesterol efflux to high-density lipoproteins. Proc Natl Acad Sci USA 31: 9774–9779

28. Kennedy MA, Barrera GC, Nakamura K et al (2005) ABCG1 has a critical role in mediating cholesterol efflux to HDL and preventing cellular lipid accumulation. Cell Metab 1:121–131

29. Oram JF, Vaughan AM (2000) ABCA1-mediated transport of cellular cholesterol and phospholipids to HDL apolipoproteins. Curr Opin Lipidol 11:253–260

30. Remaley AT, Stonik JA, Demosky SJ et al (2001) Apolipoprotein specificity for lipid efflux by the human ABCA1 transporter. Biochem Biophys Res Commun 280:818–823

31. Yancey PG, Bortnick AE, Kellner-Weibel G et al (2003) Importance of different pathways of cellular cholesterol efflux. Arterioscler Thomb Vasc Biol 23:712–719

32. Castro GR, Fielding CJ (1988) Early incorporation of cell-derived cholesterol into pre-beta-migrating high-density lipoprotein. Biochemistry 27:25–29

33. Eriksson M, Carlson LA, Miettinen TA, Angelin B (1999) Stimulation of fecal steroid excretion after infusion of recombinant proapolipoprotein A-I. Potential reverse cholesterol transport in humans. Circulation 100:594–598

34. Dimayuga P, Zhu J, Oguchi S et al (1999) Reconstituted HDL containing human apolipoprotein A-1 reduces VCAM-1 expression and neointima formation following periadventitial cuff-induced carotid injury in apoE null mice. Biochem Biophys Res Commun 264:465–468

35. Barter PJ, Baker PW, Rye KA (2002) Effect of high-density lipoproteins on the expression of adhesion molecules in endothelial cells. Curr Opin Lipidol 13:285–288

36. Nicholls SJ, Cutri B, Worthley SG et al (2005) Impact of short-term administration of high-density lipoproteins and atorvastatin on atherosclerosis in rabbits. Arterioscler Thromb Vasc Biol 25: 2416–2421

37. Mackness MI, Arrol S, Abbott C et al (1993) Protection of low-density lipoprotein against oxidative modification by high-density lipoprotein associated paraoxonase. Atherosclerosis 104:129–135

38. Marathe GK, Zimmerman GA, McIntyre TM (2002) Platelet-activating factor acetylhydrolase, and not paraoxonase-1, is the oxidized phospholipid hydrolase of high density lipoprotein particles. J Biol Chem 278:3937–3947

39. Mineo C, Deguchi H, Griffin JH et al (2006) Endothelial and anti-thrombotic actions of HDL. Circ Res 98:1352–1364

40. Mineo C, Shaul PW (2007) Role of high-density lipoprotein and scavenger receptor B type I in the promotion of endothelial repair. Trends Cardiovasc Med 17:156–161

41. Vaisar T, Pennathur S, Green PS et al (2007) Shotgun proteomics implicates protease inhibition and complement activation in the antiinflammatory properties of HDL. J Clin Invest 117:746–756

42. Franceschini G, Sirtori CR, Capurso A 2nd, Weisgraber KH, Mahley RW (1980) A-IMilano apoprotein. Decreased high density lipoprotein cholesterol levels with significant lipoprotein modifications and without clinical atherosclerosis in an Italian family. J Clin Invest 66:892–900

43. Weisgraber KH, Bersot TP, Mahley RW, Franceschini G, Sirtori CR (1980) A-Imilano apoprotein. Isolation and characterization of a cysteine-containing variant of the A-I apoprotein from human high density lipoproteins. J Clin Invest 66:901–907

44. Roma P, Gregg RE, Meng MS et al (1993) In vivo metabolism of a mutant form of apolipoprotein A-I, apoA-IMilano, associated with familial hypoalphalipoproteinemia. J Clin Invest 91:1445–1452

45. Nissen SE, Tsunoda T, Tuzcu EM et al (2003) Effect of recombinant ApoA-I Milano on coronary atherosclerosis in patients with acute coronary syndromes: a randomized controlled trial. JAMA 290:2292–2300

46. Sacks FM, Rudel LL, Conner A et al (2009) Selective delipidation of plasma HDL enhances reverse cholesterol transport in vivo. J Lipid Res 50:894–907

47. Waksman R, Kent K, Pichard G et al (2008) A first-in-man, randomized, placebo-controlled study to evaluate the safety and feasibility of autologous delipidated high density lipoprotein plasma infusions in patients with acute coronary syndrome. Circulation 118:S371

48. Tardif JC, Grégoire J, L'Allier PL et al; Effect of rHDL on Atherosclerosis-Safety and Efficacy (ERASE) Investigators (2007) Effects of reconstituted high-density lipoprotein infusions on coronary atherosclerosis: a randomized controlled trial. JAMA 297:1675–1682

49. Nissen SE, Tuzcu EM, Schoenhagen P et al; REVERSAL Investigators (2004) Effect of intensive compared with moderate lipid-lowering therapy on progression of coronary atherosclerosis: a randomized controlled trial. JAMA 291:1071–1080

50. Brewer HB Jr, Fairwell T, LaRue A et al (1978) The amino acid sequence of human apoA-I, an apolipoprotein isolated from high density lipoproteins. Biochem Biophys Res Commun 80:623–630

51. Assmann G, Brewer HB Jr (1974) A molecular model of high density lipoproteins. Proc Natl Acad Sci USA 71:1534–1538

52. Segrest JP, Jackson RL, Morrisett JD et al (1974) A molecular theory of lipid-protein interactions in the plasma lipoproteins. FEBS Lett 38:247–258

53. Segrest JP, Jones MK, De Loof H et al (1992) The amphipathic helix in the exchangeable apolipoproteins: a review of secondary structure and function. J Lipid Res 33:141–166

54. Epand RM, Gawish A, Iqbal M et al (1987) Studies of synthetic peptide analogs of the amphipathic helix. Effect of charge distribution, hydrophobicity, and secondary structure on lipid association and lecithin:cholesterol acyltransferase activation. J Biol Chem 262:9389–9396

55. Cramer C, Fici G,Tummala S et al (2006) Effects of a novel synthetic HDL on cholesterol efflux in vitro. XIV international symposium on atherosclerosis, vol P-15, Rome, Italy, p 230

56. Navab M, Anantharamaiah GM, Reddy ST et al (2003) Human apolipoprotein AI mimetic peptides for the treatment of atherosclerosis. Curr Opin Investig Drugs 4:1100–1104

57. Navab M, Reddy ST, Van Lenten BJ et al (2009) The role of dysfunctional HDL in atherosclerosis. J Lipid Res 50:S145–S149

58. Van Lenten BJ, Wagner AC, Anantharamaiah GM et al (2009) Apolipoprotein A-I mimetic peptides. Curr Atheroscler Rep 11:52–57

59. Van Lenten BJ, Wagner AC, Jung CL et al (2008) Anti-inflammatory apoA-I-mimetic peptides bind oxidized lipids with much higher affinity than human apoA-I. J Lipid Res 49:2302–2311

60. Van Lenten BJ, Wagner AC, Anantharamaiah GM et al (2002) Influenza infection promotes macrophage traffic into arteries of mice that is prevented by D-4F, an apolipoprotein A-I mimetic peptide. Circulation 106:1127–1132

61. Van Lenten BJ, Wagner AC, Navab M et al (2004) D-4F, an apolipoprotein A-I mimetic peptide, inhibits the inflammatory response induced by influenza A infection of human type II pneumocytes. Circulation 110:3252–3258

62. Bloedon LT, Dunbar R, Duffy D et al (2008) Safety, pharmacokinetics, and pharmacodynamics of oral apoA-I mimetic peptide D-4F in high-risk cardiovascular patients. J Lipid Res 49:1344–1352

63. Sethi AA, Stonik JA, Demosky SJ et al (2008) Asymmetry in the lipid affinity of bihelical amphipathic peptides. A structural determinant for the specificity of ABCA1-dependent cholesterol efflux by peptides. J Biol Chem 283:32273–32282

64. Sviridov D, Murphy A, Woolard K (2008) High-density lipoprotein reduces the human monocyte inflammatory response through ATP-binding cassette transporter A1. Arterioscler Thromb Vasc Biol 28: e-57, P170

65. Voogt JN, Turner SM, Chang B et al (2008) Effect of the 5A Bi-helical ApoA-I mimetic peptide on cholesterol efflux and global reverse cholesterol transport in vivo. Arterioscler Thromb Vasc Biol 28: e-65, P170

66. Akeefe H, Jo-Ann B, Maltais JB, Murphy A et al (2008) An Apo A-I mimetic peptide LSI-518P exhibits ABCA1-specific efflux and anti-inflammatory properties. Arterioscler Thromb Vasc Biol 28:e-92, P322

67. Bielicki JK, Zhang H, Azhar R et al (2008) A novel synthetic α-Helix peptide that stimulates ABCA1 cholesterol efflux with high efficiency greatly reduces established atherosclerosis in hypercholesterolemic apolipoproteinE null mice. Arterioscler Thromb Vasc Biol 28:e-92, P326

High Density Lipoproteins, Dyslipidemia, and Heart Disease: Past, Present, and Future

Ernst J. Schaefer and Raul D. Santos

Introduction

The standard approach for the physician in assessing lipids in patients is to ask the patient to fast overnight except for water, and then have a fasting lipid profile done. This test provides a measurement of the concentration of total cholesterol, triglyceride, high density lipoprotein (HDL) cholesterol, and calculated low density lipoprotein or LDL cholesterol. A total cholesterol of >240 mg/dl (6.2 mmol/l) has been classified as elevated and associated with increased CHD risk, while a value of <200 mg/dl (5.2 mmol/l) has been classified as optimal [1].

Occasionally, patients will have elevated total cholesterol levels because of increased levels of beta-sitosterol (>225 μmol/mmol of total cholesterol) and campesterol (>270 μmol/mmol of total cholesterol) as in phytosterolemia (treated with ezetimibe to prevent CHD) or elevated cholestanol as in cerebrotendinous xanthomatosis (treated with chenodeoxycholic acid to prevent neurologic disease) [2, 3]. These abnormalities can only be detected by measuring plasma sterols using gas chromatography (see chapter "Introduction to High Density Lipoproteins, Dyslipidemia, and Coronary Heart Disease"). With regard to triglycerides, a value >1,000 mg/dl (11 mmol/l) has been classified as markedly elevated and associated with an increased risk of pancreatitis, while a value >150 mg/dl (1.7 mmol/l) has been classified as increased, and a value <150 mg/dl (1.7 mmol/l) has been classified as optimal [1].

Cholesterol and triglycerides in plasma or serum are measured by automated standardized enzymatic methods that have been standardized by the Centers for Disease Control (Atlanta, GA) [4]. Cholesteryl ester to converted to free cholesterol and then the total free cholesterol is measured. In the triglyceride measurement, all the triglyceride has the fatty acids removed by a lipase, and then total glycerol is measured. Rarely, patients will have elevated free glycerol, without hypertriglyceridemia, due to glycerol kinase deficiency [5] These patients usually present in childhood with episodic vomiting, acidemia, and stupor [5].

Lipoprotein Assessment

Early studies separated lipoproteins by electrophoresis, with chylomicrons migrating at the origin, LDL migrating at the beta position, very low density lipoproteins (VLDL) at the prebeta position, remnant lipoproteins migrating between the prebeta and beta position, and HDL migrating at the alpha position. Barr, Russ, and Eder of New York were the first to document that CHD patients had increases in beta and prebeta migrating lipoproteins, and decreases in alpha migrating lipoproteins [6]. Fredrickson, Levy, and Lees at the National Institutes of Health developed an entire diagnosis and treatment system for lipoprotein disorders based on the measurement of cholesterol and triglyceride and the semi-quantitative determination of plasma lipoproteins by paper electrophoresis with lipid staining [7]. This system had five types of hyperlipoproteinemia: type I (elevated chylomicrons), type IIA (elevated LDL), type IIB (elevations of both LDL and VLDL), type III (elevations of lipoproteins migrating between VLDL and LDL, dysbetalipoproteinemia or elevated remnant lipoproteins), type IV (elevated VLDL), and type V (elevated chylomicrons and VLDL) [7]. It was recognized that patients with type II, III, and IV hyperlipoproteinemia were at increased risk of CHD, while those with types I and V were at increased risk of developing pancreatitis [7].

This terminology is no longer widely used and has been discarded in favor of direct assessment of lipoproteins. Another factor that led to the demise of the typing system was the observation that elevated VLDL, LDL or both could be observed in the same family [8, 9]. Goldstein and colleagues at the University of Washington studied 500 survivors of

E.J. Schaefer (✉)
Lipid Metabolism Laboratory, Tufts University,
711 Washington Street, Boston, MA 02111, USA
e-mail: ernst.schaefer@tufts.edu

E.J. Schaefer (ed.), *High Density Lipoproteins, Dyslipidemia, and Coronary Heart Disease*,
DOI 10.1007/978-1-4419-1059-2_23, © Springer Science+Business Media, LLC 2010

myocardial infarction and their families and documented that 15% had familial combined hyperlipidemia (elevations of either total cholesterol, total triglycerides, or both), and 3% had familial hypercholesterolemia [8, 9].

Lipoprotein Assessment by Ultracentrifugation

Cholesterol and triglyceride along with phospholipids are carried in plasma on lipoproteins (see chapter "Introduction to High Density Lipoprotein, Dyslipidemia, and Coronary Heart Disease"). Lipoproteins were originally characterized by DeLalla and Gofman of Berkeley and by Havel, Bragdon, and Eder at the National Institutes of Health after their separation in the ultracentrifuge [10, 11]. Lipoproteins were separated based on density in the preparative ultracentrifuge. Triglyceride-rich lipoproteins of intestinal origin or chylomicrons were classified as having a density of <0.94 g/ml, while triglyceride-rich lipoproteins of liver origin or very low density lipoproteins (VLDL) were classified as having a density of 0.94–1.006 g/ml. The density of plasma is 1.006 g/ml, slightly greater than that of water which is 1.0 g/ml. Intermediate density lipoproteins (IDL) were classified as having a density of 1.006–1.019 g/ml, LDL as having a density of 1.019–1.063 g/ml, and HDL as having a density of 1.063–1.21 g/ml [11]. LDL was further divided into large

LDL (density 1.019–1.044 g/ml) and small LDL (density 1.044–1.063 g/ml). HDL was further divided into large HDL also known as HDL$_2$ (density 1.063–1.125 g/ml) and small HDL or HDL$_3$ (density 1.125–1.21 g/ml). HDL$_1$ turned out to be lipoprotein(a), whose density was mainly intermediate between small dense LDL and HDL$_2$. An overview of plasma lipoprotein particles is shown in Fig. 1. Gofman and colleagues in Berkeley documented that CHD patients had significantly higher LDL and small dense LDL and significantly lower HDL and large HDL than controls based on the use of the analytical ultracentrifuge [12].

The isolation of lipoproteins by sequential ultracentrifugation was found to be cumbersome and led to substantial losses of material [11]. Therefore, isolation of plasma lipoproteins using single spin gradient ultracentrifugation was developed by Chapman and colleagues in Paris [13]. This methodology was further refined by Patsch and colleagues and by Chung and Segrest at the University of Alabama [14–17]. The latter method using vertical rotor ultracentrifugation was optimized to allow for the measurement of cholesterol concentrations across the entire lipoprotein spectrum, and this is known as the vertical auto profile or (VAP). It provides a measure of cholesterol concentrations in the various lipoprotein fractions including large and small VLDL, large and small LDL, large and small HDL, and an estimate of lipoprotein(a) cholesterol. Doctors can order this VAP profile from Atherotech, a laboratory in Alabama.

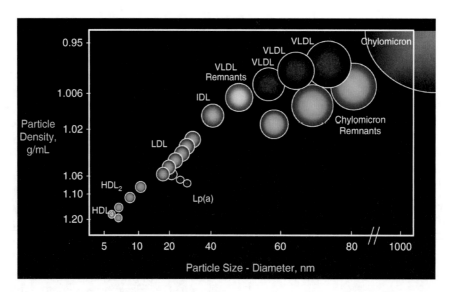

Fig. 1 Plasma lipoproteins are depicted based on their density (vertical axis) and size (diameter in nm). The triglyceride-rich chylomicrons and their remnants as well as triglyceride-rich very low density lipoproteins (VLDL) generally are found at density <1.006 g/ml and have diameters of 50–1,000 nm. Intermediate density and low density lipoproteins are in the density range 1.006–1.063 g/ml and have diameters between 18 and 45 nm. Large and small LDL and Lp(a) are in this density region and size range. High density lipoproteins are in the density range 1.063–1.21 g/ml, and have diameters in the range of 5–12 nm (figure modified from refs. [15–17]). Patients with coronary heart disease often have elevated levels of chylomicron and VLDL remnants, small dense LDL, and Lp(a), and decreased levels of large HDL particles (modified from Chung BH, Segrest JP, Cone JT, Pfau J, Geer JC, Duncan LA. High resolution plasma lipoprotein cholesterol profile by a rapid high volume semi-automated method. J Lipid Res 1981;22:1003–1114)

Lipoprotein Assessment by Gradient Gel Electrophoresis

Another method of assessing lipoproteins has been through the use of gradient gel electrophoresis which can separate LDL and HDL into various sized particles, pioneered by Anderson, Krauss and colleagues of the Donner Laboratory at the University of California, Berkeley [18, 19]. Patients with CHD were shown to have increased amounts of small dense LDL [19]. Physicians can order this testing on their patients through Berkeley Heart Laboratory of California. Patients with a preponderance of small dense LDL and small dense HDL often have elevated triglycerides, and their particles can be optimized by triglyceride lowering [20–23]. Recently, an ion mobility method using gas phase differential electrophoretic macromolecular separation has been developed for assessing LDL and HDL particle size over a range of 17–540 Å [24].

Two dimensional gel electrophoresis allows for the separation of lipoprotein particles by both size in the vertical dimension and charge in the horizontal dimension, and allows for a more precise analysis of HDL particles. The technology was originally developed in the laboratory of Fielding and in the laboratory of Kane at the University of California, San Francisco, and was further optimized by Asztalos and Roheim at Louisiana State University in New Orleans [25, 26]. An overview of these particles is shown in Fig. 2, and is much more fully discussed in the chapters by Dr. Asztalos. The functions of these particles has been defined, as has the apoA-I concentration in these particles in the general population and in CHD patients in studies done by Asztalos and Schaefer at Tufts University in Boston [27, 28]. A diagram showing the interconversions of these HDL particles is shown in Fig. 3.

CHD patients often have elevations of apoA-I in the small prebeta 1 and alpha 4 HDL and decreases in apoA-I in the larger alpha 2 and alpha 1 HDL [28, 29]. These data indicate that they often have decreased conversion of the smaller particles to the larger particles, as well as excess removal of cholesteryl ester from the larger particles to triglyceride-rich lipoproteins via cholesteryl ester transfer protein [28, 29]. Decreased apoA-I levels in large alpha migrating HDL particles (<14 mg/dl in men and <19 mg/dl in women) and increased apoA-I levels in very small prebeta 1 and alpha 4 HDL particles (sum>25 mg/dl) are associated with an increased CHD risk (see Fig. 2). Ideal values are >20 mg/dl in men and >30 mg/dl in women for apoA-I in large alpha 1 HDL and <20 mg/dl for the sum of small prebeta 1 and alpha 4 HDL in both men and women [28–30].

Optimization of these HDL particles with the simvastatin/niacin combination has been associated with the regression of coronary atherosclerosis [30]. Moreover, this HDL particle analysis can be used for the diagnosis of homozygous and heterozygous apoA-I deficiency, Tangier disease, lecithin:cholesterol acyltransferase deficiency, hepatic lipase

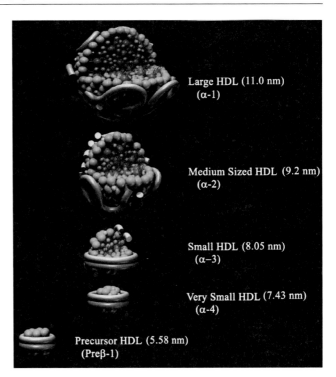

Fig. 2 Models of high density lipoprotein particles as isolated by two dimensional gel electrophoresis are shown as separated by charge (prebeta and alpha mobility) in the horizontal dimension and by size (5.5–11 nm in diameter) in the vertical dimension. Very small discoidal precursor prebeta 1 HDL (5.58 nm in diameter), very small discoidal alpha 4 HDL (7.43 nm in diameter), small spherical alpha 3 HDL (8.05 nm in diameter), medium sized spherical alpha 2 HDL (9.2 nm), and large spherical 1 alpha 1 HDL (11.0 nm) particles are shown. All particles contain apoA-I, but small alpha 3 and medium sized alpha 2 HDL also contain apoA-II. Patients with coronary heart disease often have elevated levels of precursor prebeta 1 and very small alpha 4 HDL, and decreased levels of medium sized alpha 2 and large spherical alpha 1 HDL (see refs. [28, 29]). These abnormalities can be normalized with niacin therapy (see ref. [30]). Patients with apoA-I deficiency have none of these particles, patients with Tangier disease have only prebeta 1 HDL, and patients with lecithin:cholesterol acyl transferase deficiency have only prebeta 1 and alpha 4 HDL, while patients with cholesteryl ester transfer protein deficiency have particles larger than alpha 1 HDL that contain apoA-I, apoA-II, and apoE (see refs. [31–34]). Created by Mr. Martin Jacob. Courtesy of Boston Heart Lab Corporation, Framingham, MA, USA

deficiency, and cholesteryl ester transfer protein deficiency [31–34]. HDL particle analysis by two dimensional gel electrophoresis as well as plasma sterol analysis can be obtained through Boston Heart Laboratory of Massachusetts.

Lipoprotein Assessment by Nuclear Magnetic Resonance

Otvos and colleagues in Raleigh, North Carolina have pioneered this technique which measures plasma liproteins using nuclear magnetic resonance signals, triggered by fatty acids

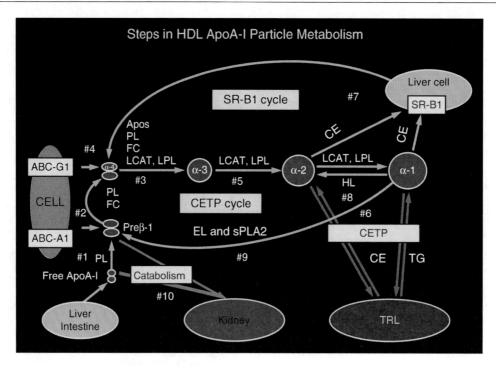

Fig. 3 An overview of HDL particle metabolism documenting the conversion of very small prebeta 1 HDL to larger HDL particles, and the potential for cholesteryl ester on larger HDL to either be transferred to triglyceride-rich lipoproteins (TRL) or to be taken up by the liver via scavenger receptor B1 (SR-B1). The apoA-I can then recycle back to smaller particles or be catabolized via the kidney (see ref. [100])

within the lipids on lipoproteins. This method also provides for an assessment of large and small VLDL, large and small LDL, and large and small HDL. Currently the method is most widely used to assess total LDL particle number, and patients with CHD have elevated levels of this parameter as compared to control subjects [35–37]. These parameters can be used to predict CHD, and can be favorably altered by gemfibrozil, niacin, and statins. It has been documented that this analysis is superior to LDL cholesterol, but does not add information above and beyond that provided by the total cholesterol/ HDL cholesterol ratio [37]. This testing can be obtained through Liposcience Laboratories of North Carolina.

Standard Lipoprotein Assessment Using Precipitation Methods

The previously described methods are all carried out in advanced lipid testing laboratories. Routine laboratories precipitate or remove lipoproteins containing apolipoprotein B (chylomicrons, chylomicron remnants, very low density lipoproteins, LDL, and lipoprotein (a), leaving HDL behind, so that its cholesterol content can be measured. This technique was first developed by Burstein and colleagues in Paris and then in New York in 1969 and 1970 using a variety of polyanions including heparin sodium, magnesium chloride, and dextran sulfate [38–40]. The methodology was standardized by the Lipid Research Clinics program at the National Institutes of Heath using heparin manganese chloride, and also was evaluated by Warnick and Albers of the University of Washington [41, 42]. Warnick and colleagues also optimized the dextran sulfate magnesium precipitation technique [43]. Miller and Miller of London documented that CHD patients had significantly lower HDL cholesterol levels than controls [44]. This finding was subsequently verified in many prospective studies including the Framingham Heart Study [45]. Schaefer, and colleagues at the National Institutes of Health documented that subjects with significant hypertriglyceridemia (types I, IIB, III, IV, and V hyperlipoproteinemia), had marked decreases in HDL cholesterol [46]. Genest, Schaefer and colleagues at Tufts University in Boston studied the families of 500 patients with premature CHD and documented that 20% of families had elevated lipoprotein(a), 15% had dyslipidemia (elevated triglycerides and decreased HDL cholesterol), 14% had combined hyperlipidemia, 4% had isolated low HDL, and 1% had familial hypercholesterolemia [47]. Therefore, low HDL cholesterol is common in families with premature CHD and is usually associated with familial dyslipidemia or familial combined hyperlipidemia [47].

Other investigators have developed other precipitation techniques for non-HDL lipoproteins, including phosphotungstic acid, and polyethylene glycol. These precipitation methods have not been as well standardized, and may not always provide as accurate a measurement of HDL cholesterol. Newer direct online assays from various Japanese companies are now being widely used. We have tested the HDL cholesterol kit being marketed by Roche in the United States and developed by Kyowa Medex of Japan [48]. We have compared the results obtained with this assay and that obtained by the dextran method in participants in the Framingham Offspring Study, and have noted very comparable results (correlation $r^2 = 0.94$) between methods with very similar absolute values) [49]. The value of this methodology is that it does not require manual pretreatment of .the sample, and allows for immediate direct measurement of HDL cholesterol on a high throughput analyzer [49]. An HDL cholesterol <40 mg/dl has been classified as low and is associated with an increased CHD risk, while a value >60 mg/dl has been associated with decreased CHD risk [1]. In Fig. 4, we see these relationships in the Framingham Heart Study for HDL cholesterol values <35 and >60 mg/dl in both men and women as generated by Wilson et al. [50].

After HDL cholesterol is measured, both non-HDL cholesterol (total cholesterol–HDL cholesterol) and LDL cholesterol can be calculated (Friedewald formula, LDL cholesterol=total cholesterol–HDL cholesterol–triglyceride/5) [51]. The Friedewald formula, developed in 1973 by Friedewald, Levy, and Fredrickson at the National Institutes of Health, provides for fairly accurate assessments of LDL cholesterol as compared to new direct measurements after ultracentrifugation or by new homogeneous methods, unless the patient is nonfasting or has triglyceride values over 400 mg/dl [49, 51, 52]. An LDL cholesterol > 160 mg/dl has been classified as elevated, while a value <100 mg/dl has been classified as optimal [1]. In CHD patients, an optional

recommendation has been made to lower LDL cholesterol to <70 mg/dl. Direct homogenous assays for LDL cholesterol have been available for some time and the results obtained correlate very well with those obtained by ultracentrifugation [53, 54].

Lipoprotein Assessment by Specialized Precipitation Methods

Gidez, Miller, Burstein, Eder, and colleagues in New York developed a combined heparin precipitation method and dextran precipitation to measure HDL cholesterol and HDL_3 cholesterol, allowing for the calculation of HDL_2 cholesterol [55]. Using this methodology, it was documented that CHD patients had significantly lower HDL cholesterol levels, especially lower large HDL_2 cholesterol levels, than control subjects [55]. More recently, Hirano and colleagues in Japan using the same principles have developed an even more simplified procedure for measuring the cholesterol concentration in HDL cholesterol and HDL_3 cholesterol, and then calculating HDL_2 cholesterol by difference [56]. This latter test will be available in the future for automated analyzers without pretreatment.

An assay for measuring cholesterol in remnant lipoproteins was developed by Nakajima of Japan and an elevated level of remnant lipoprotein cholesterol >10 mg/dl has been associated with an increased risk of CHD, especially in women [57–60]. These particles can be readily reduced with statins. An assay for measuring Lp(a) cholesterol using lectin affinity was developed by Seman and Schaefer at Tufts University in Boston, and elevated values of >10 mg/dl have been associated with CHD [61, 62]. Elevated Lp(a) cholesterol can be reduced with niacin treatment. In addition Hirano and Ito of Japan have developed an assay for small dense LDL cholesterol, and a value of >40 mg/dl has been associated with an increased CHD risk [63, 64]. An optimal value for small dense LDL cholesterol is <20 mg/dl, and these particles can be effectively lowered with statin therapy. All of these assays require sample pretreatment except for small dense LDL cholesterol, which is now fully automated and homogenous.

**HDL-C as CHD Risk Factor:
Framingham Heart Study
Relative Risk**

HDL-C (mg/dl)	Men	Women
<35	1.46*	2.08*
35-59	1.00	1.00
≥60	0.61*	0.64*

* p < 0.05, Multivariate Analysis

Fig. 4 The relative risk of developing coronary heart disease (CHD) in 2,489 men and 2,856 women, 30–74 years of age who were followed for 12 years. Of these subjects 383 men and 227 women developed CHD over this time period. In men and women, an HDL cholesterol < 35 mg/dl was associated with a significantly increased relative risk of 1.46 and 2.08, respectively as compared to those with values between 35 and 60 mg/dl. In contrast, in men and women, an HDL cholesterol > 60 mg/dl was associated with a relative risk of 0.61 and 0.64, respectively, as compared to those with values between 35 and 60 mg/dl. This analysis controlled for all other risk factors (age, blood pressure, diabetes, smoking, and elevated LDL cholesterol (see ref. [50])

Apolipoproteins

Immunoassays for apoA-I, apoB, and Lp(a) are now widely available and have been reasonably well standardized [65–70]. Some investigators especially Allan Sniderman of Montreal have recommended that apolipoprotein measurement, especially apoB, be more widely used for risk assessment and treatment [65]. ApoA-I is the major protein of HDL, and low values (<120 mg/dl) are associated with an increased risk of CHD [65, 66]. However our own prospective analysis from the Framingham Offspring Study indicated that HDL cholesterol was superior to apoA-I as a CHD prediction variable [66].

ApoB is the integral protein found in chylomicron and their remnants, VLDL, LDL, and Lp(a). However apoB-48, the form of apoB made in the intestine, only contributes a very small amount to total apoB (approximately 0.5–2.0 mg/dl), and therefore can be ignored in terms of total plasma measurements which are usually about 100-fold higher [71, 72]. Elevated levels of apoB > 120 mg/dl have been associated with premature CHD, and have been found to be better predictors of CHD than LDL cholesterol, and even non-HDL cholesterol [37, 65–68]. An ideal apoB value is <80 mg/dl [65]. In our analysis from Framingham, the total cholesterol/HDL cholesterol ratio provided identical information to that provided by the apoB/apoA-I ratio [66] (see Fig. 5).

Lp(a) is a lipoprotein containing apoB-100 with another protein attached to it known as apo(a) (see chapter "Introduction to High Density Lipoprotein, Dyslipidemia, and Coronary Heart Disease"). There are two ways to measure Lp(a) in the clinical laboratory. One can use commercially available immunoassays to measure apo(a), and generate an estimated value for total Lp(a). The alternative is to measure the cholesterol content of Lp(a) either after ultracentrifugation as is done in the VAP profile by Atherotech using the vertical rotor procedure, or after binding Lp(a) with a lectin based procedure, as was pioneered by Seman and

colleagues in our laboratory [61, 62]. At this point in time, the immunoassays are the most widely used, and Marcovina of the University of Washington has standardized apoA-I, apoB, and Lp(a) immunoassays [65]. The advantage of Lp(a) cholesterol (about 33% of total Lp(a)) is that the value can be used to calculate a true LDL cholesterol (true LDL cholesterol = total LDL cholesterol – Lp(a) cholesterol). It is important to know this information, because those patients who have elevated LDL cholesterol only because of elevated Lp(a) are best treated with niacin instead of a statin, since statins have no effect on Lp(a) levels. Patients with total Lp(a) values >30 mg/dl or Lp(a) cholesterol values >10 mg/dl are at increased risk of CHD, and high Lp(a) has clearly been shown to be an independent risk for both heart disease and stroke [70]. Niacin is the treatment of choice for elevated levels of Lp(a). In our view, the measurement of apoA-I, apoB, and Lp(a) is worthwhile for optimization of therapy in high risk patients or those with CHD, but only Lp(a) is important in screening [70].

Inflammatory Markers

There are many inflammatory markers. However, the two markers that are most widely used are C reactive protein (CRP) and lipoprotein associated phospholipase A_2 (LpPLA$_2$) (see Fig. 6). Moreover, both of these markers are now commercially available and can be run on automated analyzers without sample pretreatment. For CRP, it is important to use

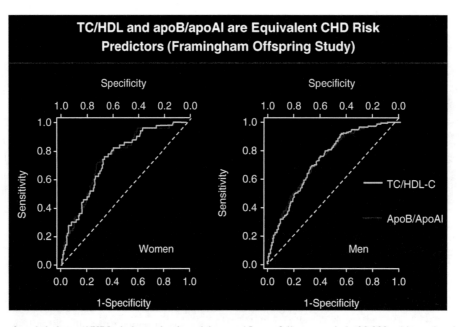

Fig. 5 A comparison of total cholesterol/HDL cholesterol ratio and the apoB/apoA-I ratio in women (*left panel*) and in men (*right panel*) in terms of their sensitivity in predicting new coronary heart disease over a 15 year followup period of 3,322 subjects showing virtual identity of the two ratios. This analysis controlled for the standard risk factors (age, blood pressure, diabetes, and smoking) (see ref. [66])

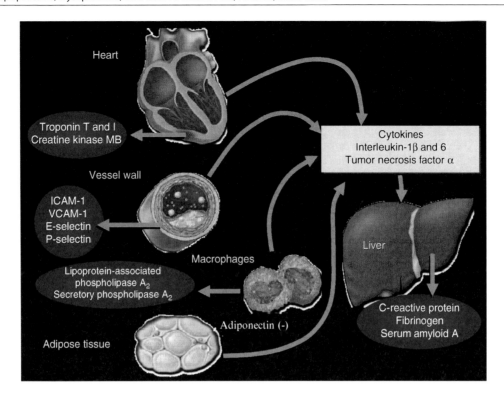

Fig. 6 The interplay of inflammatory markers linked to coronary heart disease is shown. The most widely used marker is C reactive protein (CRP), which is made in the liver in response to excess liver lipid along with two other acute phase proteins fibrinogen and serum amyloid A. Lipoprotein associated phospholipase A_2 (LpPLA$_2$) is made in monocytes and macrophages in response to excess cellular cholesterol. Elevated levels of both of these markers have been associated with an increased risk of coronary heart disease and stroke (see refs. [73–75])

the high sensitivity assay. CRP is made by the liver in response to excess triglyceride storage, while LpPLA$_2$ is made by macrophages in response to excess cholesterol storage. Elevated CRP levels >3 mg/l using a high sensitivity assay and elevated LpPLA$_2$ values >270 ng/ml have been associated with an increased CHD risk. Ideal values for CRP are <2 mg/l and for LpPLA$_2$ are <200 ng/ml [73, 74]. A panel has recommended that if LpPLA$_2$ is elevated, one should consider lowering the LDL cholesterol goal by 30 mg/dl [74]. There is a strong interrelationship between elevated inflammatory markers, insulin resistance, central adiposity, and dyslipidemia [75].

Weight loss, treatment of insulin resistance, and statins will all lower levels of CRP and LpPLA$_2$ [73, 75–77]. Ridker of Boston has advocated for a wider use of high sensitivity CRP, and the large amount of data that he and his colleagues have generated justify this approach. The most compelling data comes from the JUPITER Trial, of which Ridker was the principal investigator. In the JUPITER Trial subjects without CHD, an LDL cholesterol <130 mg/dl, but having a CRP>2.0 mg/l, were selected as participants. Rosuvastatin at a dose of 20 mg/day lowered CHD risk by 55% if an LDL cholesterol of <70 mg/dl was achieved, by 62% if a CRP of <2.0 mg/l was achieved, by 65% if both these goals were achieved, and by 79% if an LDL cholesterol of <70 mg/dl

and a CRP of <1.0 mg/l were both achieved [73]. This study justifies CRP measurement and goals of therapy as <2.0 mg/l, optimally <1.0 mg/l.

Coronary Heart Disease Risk Assessment

There are many ways to assess CHD risk. There is a time honored saying in our field that: "The best predictor of future heart disease is the presence of disease." Plaque in coronary arteries has been associated with calcification [78–80]. It has been documented that quantitating the amount of calcium in the heart using computer tomography (CT) (see Fig. 7) is a very powerful predictor of future CHD risk and mortality. Greenland and colleagues, Vliegenthart and colleagues, and Detrano and colleagues have all documented in prospective studies that a cardiac calcium score of over 300 is associated with more than a threefold increased CHD risk [78–80]. Folsom and associates reported that cardiac calcium score was superior to carotid wall thickness as a measure of future cardiac outcome, with each one standard deviation increase resulting in more than a twofold increased future CHD risk [81]. Budoff and colleagues carried out a study, in which 25,253 subjects had a baseline cardiac calcium score done

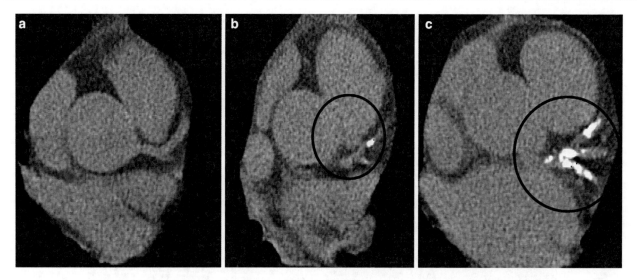

Fig. 7 Images of cardiac calcium based on computed tomographic (CT) scanning are shown with no calcium (**a**), modest amounts of calcium (**b**), and high amounts of cardiac calcium (**c**). The finding in **c** is associated with a very significant increased risk of heart disease and mortality (see refs. [78–84])

and were followed for 6.8 years for death [82]. Cardiac calcium scores of 11–100, 101–299, 300–399, 400–699, 700–999, and >1,000, respectively were associated with hazard ratios of 2.2, 4.5, 6.4, 9.2, 10.4, and 12.5 versus those with no detectable cardiac calcium [82]. Boyar has developed a risk assessment tool that combines standard Framingham risk factors with cardiac calcium score to provide a very precise estimate of future cardiac endpoints [83]. According to Budoff and colleagues, absolute cardiac calcium scoring is preferable to age and gender adjusted values for risk assessment [84].

At the same time, one measures cardiac calcium assessment, one can also inject contrast material if indicated and do CT angiography to image calcified and noncalcified soft plaque in the coronary arteries provided one is using a 64 or a 320 slice CT scanner (see Fig. 8). In our view, this latter technology is very useful in patients with rare inborn errors of lipid metabolism such as homozygous familial hypercholesterolemia or homozygous apolipoprotein A-I deficiency for assessing whether significant CHD is present (Fig. 9a and b). [31, 85–88]. It does appear that homozygous familial hypercholesterolemia (FH) is mainly associated with atherosclerosis in the aorta and very proximally in the coronary arteries. In Fig. 9a, we see the CT angiogram of a 19 year old male patient with homozygous familial hypercholesterolemia, who despite therapy with a statin, ezetimibe and LDL apheresis, had a severely calcified aorta, ostial plaque in his left main coronary artery, and who had required a bypass graft to his left anterior descending coronary artery, and an internal mammary graft to his right coronary artery, which was occluded at its origin (see Fig. 9a and ref. [85]). In contrast, the 39 year old patient with homozygous familial apolipoprotein A-I deficiency and an HDL cholesterol of 2 mg/dl had an unaffected aorta, had

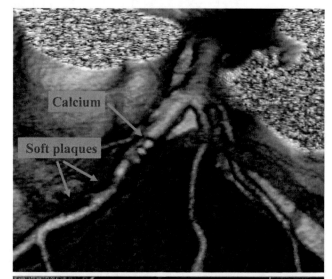

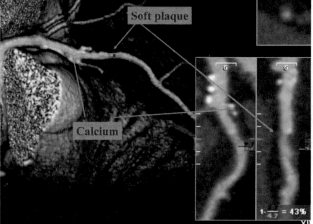

Fig. 8 CT angiography images using a 64 slice scanner are shown documenting the presence of soft non-calcified and calcified coronary plaques (courtesy Dr. Melvin Clouse, Department of Radiology, Beth Israel Deaconness Medical Center, Boston)

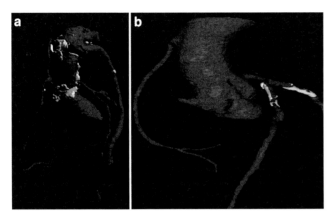

Fig. 9 Modeling of CT angiographic images are shown. Calcified plaque are *white*, while lipid-rich plaques are *green* or *yellow*. The modeling was carried out by Dr. David Chen of Medical Metrx Corporation of Lebanon, NH, based on images supplied by Dr. Raul Santos, INCOR, Sao Paulo, Brazil. (**a**) In the *left panel*, we see the CT angiogram of a 19-year male with homozygous familial hypercholesterolemia, being treated with a statin, ezetimibe, and LDL apheresis every 2 weeks. Despite this therapy this patient has a severely calcified aorta, ostial plaque in his left main coronary artery, but almost no plaques in his distal coronary arteries. He also has required a bypass graft to his left anterior descending coronary artery, and an internal mammary graft to his right coronary artery, which is occluded at its origin (see ref. [85]). (**b**) In the *right panel*, we see modeling of a CT angiogram from a 39-year-old patient with undetectable plasma apolipoprotein A-I, marked high density lipoprotein deficiency (HDL cholesterol of 2 mg/dl), and premature coronary artery age at age 39 years. His aorta was not affected, but he had plaques in the left anterior descending coronary artery and the diagonal branches, and his right coronary artery was totally obstructed, with a vein graft to the distal right coronary artery (see refs. [31, 85, 87])

plaques in the left anterior descending coronary artery and the diagonal branches, with a totally occluded right coronary artery, with a vein graft to the distal right coronary artery (see refs. [31, 87]). Therefore, in this latter case with severe HDL deficiency, the coronary atherosclerosis that was observed was more typical of what one sees in the general population (see Fig. 9b).

Framingham Risk Assessment

The Framingham Heart Study was begun in 1948 to identify risk factors for heart disease and stroke. This long term prospective study has been extremely successful in this regard. One can calculate the 10 year CHD risk using the point system as shown in ref. [1], and developed by D'Agostino and many other investigators at the Framingham Heart Study and Boston University [1]. One only needs to know the gender, the age, the systolic blood pressure, smoking status, the total cholesterol, and the HDL cholesterol in order to calculate the 10 year risk of CHD [1]. The third

Adult Treatment Panel of the National Cholesterol Education Program (NCEP) established LDL cholesterol goals of treatment based on this 10 year CHD risk [1]. Risk assessment with this algorithm can easily be accessed on the web at http://www.framinghamheartstudy.org . In subjects with CHD, diabetes, or where the 10 year CHD risk is >20%, the LDL cholesterol goal is < 100 mg/dl, in those in whom this value is 10–20%, the LDL cholesterol goal is <130 mg/dl, and in those with low risk (<10%), the LDL cholesterol goal is <160 mg/dl [1]. In 2004, the NCEP established an optional goal for LDL cholesterol of >70 mg/dl in patients with CHD [89]. Most recently Framingham Heart Study investigators have published their algorithm for assessing 30 year risk of CHD using gender, age, systolic blood pressure, smoking, diabetes, total cholesterol, and HDL cholesterol as developed by Pencina, D'Agostino and colleagues [90].

Reynolds Risk Score and PROCAM Risk Prediction

An alternative risk engine is the Reynold Risk Score for men and women developed for US populations by Ridker and colleagues in Boston [91, 92]. This risk assessment tool also uses gender, age, systolic blood pressure, smoking, diabetes, total cholesterol, and HDL cholesterol, but adds family history of CHD prior to age 60 years, and CRP [91, 92]. This data base is more recent and is based on a larger number of subjects and CHD cases, and it is our preference to use this risk engine. It can easily be accessed at http://www.reynoldsriskscore.org. A third alternative risk engine is the Prospective Cardiovascular Muenster (PROCAM) Study scoring system developed by Assmann and colleagues in Muenster, Germany which uses the same variables as the Reynolds risk score, except that it adds triglyceride levels and does not use CRP, and can be accessed at http://www.chd-taskforce.com [93]. However, this algorithm has not been tested or calibrated for a US population. Many doctors do not use these risk assessment tools, but rather treat aggressively if CHD or diabetes is present, or if the patient is male and over 45 years of age with two more risk factors (hypertension, smoking, diabetes, low HDL) or if female and over age 55 years with two or more risk factors (based on the original guidelines of the National Cholesterol Education Program.

Our preference is for the Reynolds Risk Score because it allows for the use of CRP and family history, and because it is based on a very large number of individuals and a large number of events. It is especially valuable for women, where neither Framingham or PROCAM have sufficient numbers of CHD cases. However, the Framingham scoring system will probably continue to be used in the national cholesterol guidelines. Moreover Framingham has now published an algorithm allowing for the calculation of a 30 year risk of CHD [90]. When the Framingham risk score was evaluated in a very large population in China, it was found that the risk score functions very well, except that the absolute risk was substantially overestimated [94]. Moreover, it has been documented that the substantial increase in cardiovascular mortality observed in Beijing between 1984 and 1999 could be related to increases in total cholesterol in the population over that time period due to "westernization of the diet" [95]. All of these risk algorithms assume that doctors will actually use them, and treat patients according to risk. However, unfortunately this is rarely the case.

The INTERHEART Experience

Worldwide, most of the cases of coronary heart disease (CHD) occur in lower and middle income groups. Yusuf and colleagues of Canada collected data on 15,152 men and women with CHD, and 14,820 age and gender matched controls in 52 countries from all six inhabited continents in lower and middle income groups [96]. Nine risk factors accounted for 90% of the risk in men and 94% of the risk in women. The significant positive risk factors were: (1) elevated apoB/apoA-I ratio (relative risk 3.25), (2) smoking (relative risk 2.87), (3) psychosocial stress (relative risk 2.67), (4) diabetes (relative risk 2.37), (5) hypertension (relative risk 1.91), and 6) obesity (relative risk 1.62), while the three significant negative risk factors were (1) daily intake of vegetable and fruits (relative risk 0.70), (2) regular physical activity (relative risk 0.86), and alcohol intake (relative risk 0.91) [96]. The data suggest that intervention to modify these factors is clearly warranted. It should be noted that this was a case-control study and not a prospective study; however, the data does provide valuable insights for the development of strategies to decrease the global burden of cardiovascular disease.

The Polypill

An alternative strategy, advocated by Wald and Law of the United Kingdom, is the use of a polypill which has the potential according to the authors to reduce CHD by 80% or more in persons over the age of 55 [97]. Such an approach was used and the effects of a daily pill containing three antihypertensive agents (12.5 mg of hydrochlorothiazide, 50 mg of atenolol, and 5 mg of ramipril), a statin (simvas-tatin 20 mg), and 100 mg of aspirin was evaluated. This polypill reduced systolic blood pressure by 6 mmHg and LDL cholesterol by 27 mg/dl, and was well tolerated in 412 subjects over a 12 week period as part of a randomized, blinded trial [98].

Secondary Causes of Lipid Abnormalities

To rule out secondary causes of lipid abnormalities, the physician should order the following blood tests after an overnight fast: glucose, creatinine, alkaline phosphatase, liver transaminases, alkaline phosphatase, and thyroid stimulating hormone. Diabetes and renal insufficiency are both associated with elevated triglycerides, increased small dense LDL, and decreased HDL cholesterol. Hypothyroidism and obstructive liver disease with elevated levels of alkaline phosphatase are both often associated with elevated LDL cholesterol. Hepatocellular disease with elevated transaminases are often observed in patients with hypertriglyceridemia. Oral estrogens and alcohol intake can significantly raise triglyceride levels, while anabolic steroids usually markedly lower HDL cholesterol levels. If no secondary causes are present, then a familial disorder may be present, and measuring lipids in first degree relatives is warranted especially when CHD runs in the family [47].

Common Genetic Forms of HDL Deficiency

Rare HDL deficiency states are covered in the chapters in apoA-I deficiency, apoA-I variants, Tangier disease, and LCAT deficiency, while common genetic variants affecting HDL levels are covered in the chapter by Dr. Brousseau. Common genetic lipoprotein disorders associated with premature coronary heart disease and low HDL include familial combined hyperlipidemia (elevated low density lipoproteins and TRL) and familial dyslipidemia (elevated TRL, low HDL), each observed in about 15% of families with premature CHD, while familial hypoalphalipoproteinemia (isolated low HDL cholesterol) is only observed in about 5% of such families [47]. When men with CHD and low HDL were selected for the Veteran Affairs HDL Intervention Trial, they were generally overweight or obese and had elevated insulin levels [99]. Therefore, adiposity and insulin resistance are major factors predisposing to low HDL cholesterol in the general population. Moreover, patients with combined hyperlipidemia, elevated triglycerides, and insulin resistance generally have increased CETP activity causing more cholesteryl ester to be transferred to remnant lipoproteins or VLDL. This situation leads to low

HDL cholesterol and lack of large alpha 1 HDL, because of enhanced cholesteryl ester transfer to triglyceride-rich lipoproteins (TRL) [100] (see Fig. 3).

Diet and Lifestyle Modification

The effects of diet and exercise on HDL metabolism are covered in greater detail in the chapter by Dr. Schaefer, and the effects of alcohol on HDL are covered in the chapter by Dr. Brinton. Lifestyle represents the cornerstone of therapy for lipid disorders. In hypercholesterolemic patients and high risk patients, it is recommended that dietary saturated fat be restricted to <7% of calories, trans fats be minimized, dietary cholesterol be restricted to <200 mg/day, animal fats be replaced by vegetable oils, and fish intake be increased [1]. This is best accomplished by: (1) replacing butter with soft margarine (including high plant sterol margarines) and vegetable oils (especially soybean and canola oils); (2) replacing whole milk and cream with 1% low-fat or skim milk; (3) replacing red meat with chicken, turkey (white meat) or fish; and (4) replacing high fat/high sugar desserts, with fruits, vegetables, and whole grains Increased physical activity (at least 30 min/day of walking, riding on an exercise, or some other activity) as well as weight control are very important for optimizing HDL levels [1, 101]. These two latter requirements are particularly important for raising HDL cholesterol and large alpha 1 HDL particles, along with weight loss in obese subjects [76]. Moreover, replacing animal fat with vegetable oil has been shown to be an extremely powerful modality to reduce CHD risk, and polyunsaturated oils increase reverse cholesterol transport by upregulating SR-B1 [101].

Pharmacologic Agents

Statins

Statins, originally discovered in Tokyo by Akira Endo, and first developed in Japan and by Merck in the United States, are the cornerstone of therapy for LDL control after lifestyle change, and have clearly been shown to reduce CHD risk and stroke risk [1]. In addition to lowering LDL and triglyceride, these agents have a very beneficial effect on HDL particles. Rosuvastatin and atorvastatin are not only very effective at lowering LDL cholesterol and small dense LDL cholesterol, but also raise HDL cholesterol modestly. Please see Dr. Lamon-Fava's chapter on the effects of statins on HDL metabolism. Rosuvastatin and atorvastatin significantly lower very small prebeta 1 HDL by 40%, and increase large

alpha 1 HDL by 12–25% [102, 103]. Rosuvastatin is significantly more effective in raising HDL cholesterol and large alpha 1 HDL than is atorvastatin, especially in those with low HDL [103]. It is known that statins do not significantly affect HDL apoA-I production, therefore for prebeta 1 HDL to decline markedly, these statins must increase the conversion of prebeta 1 HDL to alpha 4 HDL, and then on to larger alpha 1 HDL particles [102–105] (see Figs. 2 and 9). The strikingly beneficial effects of rosuvastatin have been well documented in the JUPITER Trial [73].

Statins induce cellular inhibition of cholesterol synthesis and upregulation of LDL receptor activity, probably increases ABCA1 activity, resulting in a greater amount of cellular cholesteryl efflux onto small prebeta 1 HDL causing them to be converted to alpha migrating HDL [102–105]. Please refer chapter on statins by Dr. Lamon-Fava. Rosuvastatin may be more effective than other statins in raising large HDL cholesterol because it has greater renal metabolism, and may cause a decrease in the renal clearance of very small discoidal prebeta 1 or alpha 4 HDL (see Fig. 9). In addition statins are known to decrease CETP activity, resulting in larger HDL particles because of less cholesteryl ester transfer to triglyceride-rich lipoproteins under these circumstances. In a posthoc analysis of the Scandinavian Simvastatin Survival Study, benefit was associated not only with LDL lowering, but also with HDL raising [106]. In the meta-analysis of intravascular ultrasound studies of coronary artery atheroma by Nicholls et al., it was concluded that the beneficial effects of statins on coronary atherosclerosis were related both to LDL lowering and HDL raising [107]. The authors concluded that in order for a patient to get regression of coronary atheroma, the LDL cholesterol must be <88.5 mg/dl, and the HDL cholesterol needed to be raised by at least 7.5% [107].

Fibrates

The effects of fibrates on HDL metabolism are covered in much greater depth in the chapter by Dr. Watts and colleagues. Fibrates are most useful and effective as triglyceride lowering agents. Two fibrates are currently in use: gemfibrozil and fenofibrate. These agents are peroxisomal proliferation activation receptor alpha (PPAR alpha) agonists and increase lipoprotein lipase, apoA-I and apoA-II gene expression, and decrease apoC-III gene expression, resulting in up to 50% reductions in triglycerides, very slight LDL cholesterol reductions, and modest increases in HDL cholesterol [108]. The use of these agents has been shown to increase the synthesis of apoA-I and apopA-II, but also to significantly enhance the fractional catabolism of apoA-I, resulting in virtually no change in apoA-I concentration, but about a 20% increase in plasma apoA-II levels [109–114]. The net effect is to increase intermediate sized HDL particles namely alpha 2 and alpha 3 HDL, both of which contain apoA-I and apoA-II, with no significant effect on the large protective alpha 1 HDL [109, 110].

Gemfibrozil reduced CHD risk prospectively by 34% in approximately 5,000 healthy men with non-HDL cholesterol above 200 mg/dl or 5.2 mmol/l (Helsinki Heart Study, organized by Nikkila, Frick, Manninen and others in Helsinki) [115] The greatest benefit was in those with low HDL. In this trial, benefit was associated with the approximate 10% LDL cholesterol lowering as well as the approximate 10% HDL cholesterol raising [115]. In the Veterans Affairs HDL Intervention Trial (VA HIT) organized by Rubins and Robins in Boston, 2,561 men with CHD, HDL cholesterol below 40 mg/dl, and LDL cholesterol below 140 mg/dl had a significant 22% CHD risk reduction with gemfibrozil (600 mg orally twice daily) versus placebo over a 5 year period, related in part to a modest 6% increase in HDL cholesterol [116]. The greatest benefit in CHD risk reduction was observed in those with plasma insulin levels above 25 μmol/l [99].

Fenofibrate is currently the most widely used fibrate, and has the benefit of not having any interactions with statins in contrast to gemfibrozil. Steiner and colleagues reported in the Diabetes Atherosclerosis Intervention Study (DAIS) in 416 diabetics, that fenofibrate at a dose of 160 mg/day reduced triglyceride levels by 30%, raised HDL cholesterol by 6%, and significantly reduced coronary atherosclerosis progression by 22%, versus placebo over a 2 year period of time [117]. In FIELD (Fenofibrate Intervention and Lipid Lowering Trial in Diabetes) Keech and colleagues of Sydney, Australia that in 9,795 patients with diabetes, fenofibrate lowered CHD (fatal and nonfatal myocardial infarction) by a nonsignificant 11%, but it significantly lowered all cardiovascular events by 14% and nonfatal MI by 24%, the need for laser treatment for retinopathy by more than 50%, and the need for lower extremity amputation by 46% [118–120]. Therefore, fenofibrate in this study was associated with very large and significant benefits in reducing evidence of microvascular disease in patients with diabetes mellitus [119, 120].

Niacin

Please refer the chapter by Dr. Lamon-Fava on the effects of niacin on HDL metabolism. Niacin is the most effective agent currently available for HDL raising. The most widely used form of niacin has been reformulated as an extended release product (Niaspan), which causes less flushing than immediate release niacin or other forms of extended release niacin. Niaspan at a dose of 2 g/day taken at bedtime decreases LDL cholesterol by about 10–20%, triglycerides

by about 30%, and Lp(a) by about 25%, while increasing HDL cholesterol by approximately 25–30%. Side effects may include flushing, gastric irritation, and elevations of uric acid, glucose, and liver enzymes in some patients. Niacin should not be used in patients with liver disease or a history of an ulcer. Daily aspirin taken prior to niacin administration will minimize flushing.

In the Coronary Drug Project organized by the National Institutes of Health, 8,341 men with CHD, aged 30–64 years, were placed on placebo, niacin 2 g/day, clofibrate, high and low dose estrogen, and D-thyroxine. No benefit was noted with clofibrate, and the estrogen and D-thyroxine arms had to be discontinued because of adverse effects. Only niacin was found to reduce CHD risk by 20% and nonfatal myocardial infarction by 28% at the end of the 5 year trial [121]. After discontinuation of the trial, there continued to be followup for a mean of 9 years, Canner and colleagues reported that the niacin group (n = 1,119) had a significantly lower total mortality (11% lower with 52.0% mortality in the niacin group and 58.2% mortality in the placebo group, p < 0.0001) as compared to the placebo group [121, 122]. In addition, groups of patients with either diabetes or metabolic syndrome also got very significant benefit from niacin treatment [123, 124].

Brown and colleagues in Seattle documented that niacin plus statin promoted regression of coronary atherosclerosis and a marked reduction in CHD clinical events as compared to placebo in the HDL Atherosclerosis Treatment Study (HATS) in 160 CHD patients with low HDL [125]. In this study, we documented that coronary regression was related to niacin induced increases in large alpha 1 HDL particles [30]. Large scale studies are currently underway to determine whether niacin will reduce CHD risk above and beyond the effects of a statin. Niaspan, an extended release formulation, is currently being tested versus placebo in a trial of over 3,000 heart disease patients with HDL cholesterol below 40 mg/dl all on simvastatin therapy. Niacin, together with a flushing inhibitor laropiprant, is currently also being tested versus placebo in a trial of over 20,000 patients all on simvastatin therapy. These trials will be completed in 2012, and in our opinion will provide hard evidence for the benefits of niacin in HDL cholesterol raising and Lp(a) lowering.

We have recently documented that niacin in humans increases HDL because of increases in apoA-I synthesis, while reducing the levels of triglyceride-rich lipoprotein and Lp(a) by enhancing their fractional clearance [126]. Moreover, niacin doubles the levels of adiponectin, an effective anti-inflammatory compound [126]. We now have data from monkey and hamster studies indicating that niacin significantly increases liver apoA-I and ABCA1 mRNA levels. These finding are consistent with the observation that niacin increases HDL cholesterol more than twice as much as apoA-I levels, and suggests that niacin significantly enhances cellular cholesterol efflux. Moreover, the doubling of adiponectin that we have observed with niacin, suggests that this agent has a very beneficial effect on fat tissue [126]. Niacin at present is the most effective available agent for HDL raising. As newer and better tolerated niacin agents become available, niacin will become a more widely used lipid modifying agent for HDL raising and Lp(a) lowering.

Ezetimibe

Ezetimibe is a second line agent for cholesterol lowering, and was developed by Harry Davis and colleagues at Schering in New Jersey. Ezetimibe blocks intestinal cholesterol absorption, and lowers LDL C by 18% [127]. This agent is generally well tolerated, and is especially helpful in hyporesponders to statins (see chapter "Introduction to High Density Lipoprotein, Dyslipidemia, and Coronary Heart Disease"). It has minimal effects on HDL cholesterol, but potentiates the effects of statins not only for LDL lowering, but also for the lowering of CRP [128]. No prospective studies have clearly shown clinical benefit at this point. In our view, the large study (IMPROVE-IT) testing ezetimibe plus simvastatin versus simvastatin alone in over 18,000 patients with acute coronary syndrome, will document additional significant clinical benefit of ezetimibe above and beyond statin therapy alone. The statin/ezetimibe combination is ideal for getting patients to their LDL cholesterol goal [128].

Anion Exchange Resins

Anion exchange resins bind bile acids in the intestine, increase the conversion of liver cholesterol to bile acids, and upregulate LDL receptors in liver, decreasing plasma LDL by about 15–20%. Side effects can include bloating and constipation, elevation of triglycerides, and interference with the absorption of digoxin, tetracycline, D-thyroxine, phenylbutazone, and Coumadin. In the Lipid Research Clinics Coronary Primary Prevention Trial (LRC-CPPT) carried out by Robert I. Levy of the National Institutes of Health and many collaborators in over 7,000 men with elevated LDL cholesterol levels, the use of cholestyramine was associated with 11% lower LDL cholesterol levels, 3% higher HDL cholesterol levels, and a significant 19% reduction in CHD risk over a 7 year period as compared to placebo [129]. Benefit was associated with both the LDL lowering and the HDL raising [129]. A new resin, colesevelam is available in tablet form and is given at a dose of six 625 mg tabs per day, and has been shown to lower LDL cholesterol by 16–18%, and also improves glycemic control in patients with diabetes [130]. This agent can

be used together with ezetimibe, especially in statin intolerant patients to get them to their LDL cholesterol goals.

Fish Oil Capsules

High doses of fish oil as well as diets very high in oily fish have long been known to significantly lower triglyceride levels based on studies carried out by Connor and colleagues in Portland, Oregon [131]. Based on our own work in Boston, high dose fish oil or high fish diets also suppress the immune response by decreasing monocyte production of interleukins 1 and 6 and tumor necrosis factor alpha, as well as by decreasing helper T cells and delayed hypersensitivity response as determined by skin testing [132, 133]. Over the counter fish oil capsules are available, as is a prescription form of concentrated fish oil known as LOVAZA given as two 1 g capsules twice daily (total dose is 1,860 mg of eicosapentaenoic acid or EPA and 1,500 mg of docosahexaenoic acid or DHA). This formulation given at this dose will substantially lower triglycerides levels especially in patients with hypertriglyceridemia [134]. The same effect can be obtained with regular fish oil capsules at a far lower cost, but three 1 g capsules twice daily need to be taken. Fish oil at this dose not only lowers triglyceride levels, but can raise the levels of large alpha 1 HDL particles substantially, but only raises HDL cholesterol modestly by 5–10%. Their major effect is to decrease the secretion of VLDL triglyceride and apoB [135]. These agents can also lower levels of $LpPLA_2$.

In the Diet and Reinfarction Trial Burr and associates in the United Kingdom reported that two fish oil capsules daily reduced mortality by 29% in heart disease patients as compared to usual care, but this was not confirmed in the followup study [136, 137]. In the large Gruppo Italiano per lo Studio della Sopravvivenza nell' Infarto Miocardico (GISSI) study, 11,323 post myocardial infarction patients were randomized to one capsule per day of concentrated fish oil (Omacor or LOVAZA containing 465 mg of EPA and 375 mg of DHA), 300 units of vitamin E, the combination, or placebo [137, 138]. Marchioli and colleagues in Italy noted no benefit with vitamin E, and no effect of the fish oil on lipids was noted. However over a 3.5 year period, those that received the fish oil had a significant 20% reduction in fatal myocardial infarction as compared to the control group [137]. In addition, in the first 4 months of the study, there was a significant 53% decrease in sudden death as compared to the group that did not receive fish oil [138].

More recently, investigators have carried out the Japan EPA Lipid Intervention Study (JELIS) in 18,645 hypercholesterolemic patients all placed on statin and then equally randomized to 1,800 mg of eicosapentaenoic acid (EPA) or usual care [138]. Over a 4.6 year followup period, the use of EPA was associated with a significant 19% reduction in the primary endpoint of major cardiac events (fatal and nonfatal myocardial infarction, sudden death, unstable angina, angioplasty, or coronary artery bypass surgery) [139]. There was no significant effect on sudden death, with the major benefit being due to a reduction in nonfatal myocardial infarction [139]. In addition, no reduction in stroke was noted in those without prior stroke, but a significant 20% reduction (6.8% vs. 10.5%) in stroke was observed in those with a prior stroke in the EPA group [140]. In a subanalysis of patients with no prior cardiovascular disease, those with triglycerides >150 mg/dl and HDL cholesterol <40 mg/dl had a 71% increase in relative risk of cardiac events versus those not in this category. In addition, subject in this group receiving EPA had a 54% reduction in cardiac events as compared to those not receiving EPA [141].

Brouwer and colleagues of Amsterdam have done a pooled analysis and summarized the results of three trials, in which fish oil capsules have been tested versus placebo in patients with implanted cardioverter defibrillators [142]. In these studies, there is no convincing evidence that this therapy has any significant benefit in such patients [142]. Overall, the data suggest that EPA has immunologic effects, while DHA is more likely to have lipid modifying effects and effects on membrane fluidity. There is also data suggesting the fish intake associated with increased plasma phospholipid DHA decreases the risk of dementia and Alzheimer's disease [143]. It does appear the low dose fish oil (one to two capsules per day) will decrease the risk of death in the first year after myocardial infarction, and that a supplement containing 1,800 mg of EPA will reduce CHD risk especially in those with high triglycerides and low HDL. Moreover, it is also clear that high dose fish oil (four capsules per day of LOVAZA or six or more regular fish oil capsules per day) will significantly lower triglyceride levels. Fish oil can be safely given together with statin therapy [134].

Therapies Under Development

Two HDL raising therapies are currently underdevelopment. The use of reconstituted HDL with apoA-I Milano or normal apoA-I has been associated with regression of coronary artery disease based on studies by Nissen of Cleveland and Tardif of Montreal [144, 145]. The chapter by Dr. Brewer covers this form of therapy, and it is clearly a promising area for the treatment of significant coronary atherosclerosis. CETP inhibition is another form of therapy currently under development, which also has great promise, and is covered in the chapter by Dr. Schaefer. CETP inhibition is a very powerful way to raise HDL cholesterol and large HDL particles, and to prevent the transfer of cholesteryl ester from HDL to triglyceride-rich lipoproteins. In our view, both these forms of therapy hold great promise.

Conclusions

In this book and atlas, we have provided the reader with an overview of HDL particle metabolism, HDL deficiency states, and the use of various strategies for HDL raising. In our view, risk assessment, in addition to the standard markers, will include cardiac calcium scoring, and measurements of CRP, LpPLA$_2$, Lp(a), lipoprotein subspecies analysis including HDL particle assessment, and plasma sterol analysis in high risk individuals, especially those who are not at their LDL cholesterol target. The most effective currently available HDL raising strategies include lifestyle modification, weight loss if indicated, and niacin therapy. A meta analysis of 23 lipid modifying trials indicates that for every 1% decrease in LDL cholesterol, there is an approximate 1% decrease in CHD risk, and for every 1% increase in HDL cholesterol there is an approximate 1% decrease in CHD risk [146] (see Fig. 10).

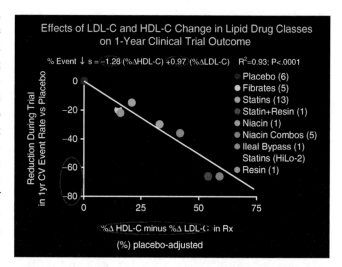

Fig. 10 Figure based on a meta-analysis of 23 lipid trials documenting independent benefit in CHD risk reduction of both LDL cholesterol lowering and HDL cholesterol raising (see ref. [146])

In the future, in our view better niacin preparations, CETP inhibitors and HDL infusion therapy will all become available, and these modalities will provide the physician with powerful HDL raising treatments, especially for the secondary prevention of CHD. In the future in high risk and CHD patients in addition to goals for LDL cholesterol lowering (goal of LDL cholesterol<70 mg/dl), there will be the following goals to optimize therapy: apoB<80 mg/dl, small dense LDL cholesterol<20 mg/dl, non HDL cholesterol<100 mg/dl, triglycerides<150 mg/dl, Lp(a)<30 mg/dl, and CRP<2 mg/l, ideally<1 mg/l. In addition in the future, we will have an HDL cholesterol goal of >60 mg/dl, and in our view apoA-I levels in large alpha 1 HDL should be >20 mg/dl if coronary atherosclerosis regression is desired (see Fig. 11). Lifestyle modifi-

Ideal Goals of Therapy for CHD Risk Reduction

- No Smoking
- Systolic BP < 130 mmHg
- Glycosylated Hemoglobin < 7.0%
- CRP < 2.0 mg/L , ideally < 1.0 mg/L
- LDL C < 70 mg/dl (sdLDL C < 20 mg/dl)
- Non HDL C < 100 mg/dl, and TC/HDL-C < 4.0
- ApoB < 80 mg/dl
- Lp(a) < 30 mg/dl or 74 nmol/L and/or Lp(a) C < 10 mg/dl
- Triglyceride < 150 mg/dl and remnant lipoprotein C< 10 mg/dl
- HDL C > 60 mg/dl (large HDL apoA-I > 20 mg/dl)

Fig. 11 Our view of optimals goal of therapy in high risk and CHD patients are shown. Smoking cessation, control of blood pressure and glycosylated hemoglobin are all very important. Optimal lowering of LDL cholesterol, small dense LDL cholesterol, Lp(a), triglycerides, remnant lipoprotein cholesterol, and CRP, as well as raising of HDL cholesterol and apoA-I in large HDL are critical for preventing CHD events

cation is critical for CHD risk reduction, but statins, niacin preparations, ezetimibe, resins, fibrates, and fish oil all have their place in lipid modification and CHD risk reduction. In 2012 in our view, clinical trials will show that niacin preparations, ezetimibe, and CETP inhibitors will all have significant clinical benefit when added to statin therapy.

References

1. Expert Panel (2001) Executive summary of the third report of the National Cholesterol Education Program (NCEP) Expert Panel on Detection, Evaluation, and Treatment of High Blood Cholesterol in Adults (Adult Treatment Panel III). J Am Med Assoc 285: 2486–2497
2. Patel MD, Thompson PD (2006) Phytosterols and vascular disease. Atherosclerosis 186:12–19
3. Keren Z, Falik-Zaccel TC (2009) Cerebrotendinous xanthomatosis (CTX), a treatable lipid storage disorder. Pediatr Endocrinol Rev 7:6–11
4. McNamara JR, Schaefer EJ (1987) Automated enzymatic standardized lipid analyses for plasma and lipoprotein fractions. Clin Chim Acta 166:1–8
5. Ginns EI, Barranger JA, McClean SW, Sliva C, Young R, Schaefer EJ, Goodman SI, McCabe RB (1984) A juvenile form of glycerol kinase deficiency with episodic vomiting, acidemia, and stupor. J Pediatr 5:736–739
6. Barr DP, Russ E, Eder HA (1951) Protein-lipid relationships in human plasma. II. In atherosclerosis and related conditions. Am J Med 1:480–493
7. Fredrickson DS, Levy RI, Lees RS (1967) Fat transport in lipoproteins – an integrated approach to mechanisms and disorders. N Engl J Med 276:34–42, 94–103, 148–156, 215–225, 273–281 (five part review article)
8. Goldstein JL, Hazzard WR, Schrott HG, Bierman EL (1973) Hyperlipidemia in coronary heart disease. I. Lipid levels in 500 survivors of myocardial infarction. J Clin Invest 52:1533–1543
9. Goldstein JL, Hazzard WR, Schrott HG, Bierman EL (1973) Hyperlipidemia in coronary heart disease. II. Genetic analyses of lipid levels in 176 families and delineation of a new inherited disorder, combined hyperlipidemia. J Clin Invest 52:1544–1568
10. DeLalla OF, Elliott HA, Gofman JW (1954) Ultracentrifugal studies of high density serum lipoproteins in clinically healthy subjects. Am J Physiol 179:333–337
11. Havel RJ, Eder HA, Bragdon JH (1955) The distribution and chemical composition of ultracentrifugally separated lipoproteins in human serum. J Clin Invest 34:1345–1353
12. Gofman JW, Young W, Tandy R (1966) Ischemic heart disease, atherosclerosis, and longevity. Circulation 34:679–697
13. Chapman MJ, Goldstein S, Lagrange D, Lapaud PM (1981) A density gradient ultracentrifugal procedure for the isolation of the major lipoprotein density classes from human serum. J Lipid Res 22:339–358
14. Patsch JR, Sailer S, Kostner G, Sandhofer F, Holasek A, Braunsteiner H (1974) Seperation of the main lipoprotein density classes from human plasma by rate zonal ultracentrifugation. J Lipid Res 15: 356–366
15. Chung BH, Wilkinson T, Geer JC, Segrest JP (1980) Preparative and quantitative isolation of plasma lipoproteins: rapid single density gradient ultracentrifugation in a vertical rotor. J Lipid Res 21:284–291
16. Chung BH, Segrest JP, Cone JT, Pfau J, Geer JC, Duncan LA (1981) High resolution plasma lipoprotein cholesterol profile by a rapid high volume semi-automated method. J Lipid Res 22:1003–1114
17. Kulkarni KR, Marcovina SM, Krauss RM, Garber DW, Glasscock AM, Segrest JP (1997) Quantitation of HDL_2 and HDL_3 cholesterol by the vertical auto-profile-II (VAP-II) methodology. J Lipid Res 38:2353–2364
18. Anderson DW, Nichols AV, Forte TM, Lindgren FT (1977) Particle distribution of human serum high density lipoproteins. Biochim Biophys Acta 493:55–68
19. Austin MA, Breslow JL, Hennekens CH, Buring JE, Willett WC, Krauss RM (1988) Low density lipoprotein subclass patterns and risk of myocardial infarction. JAMA 260:1917–1921
20. Campos H, Genest JJ, Blijlevens E, McNamara JR, Jenner J, Ordovas JM, Wilson PWF, Schaefer EJ (1992) Low density lipoprotein particle size and coronary artery disease. Arterioscler Thromb 12:187–195
21. Campos H, Blijlevens E, McNamara JR, Ordvoas JM, Wilson PWF, Schaefer EJ (1992) LDL particle size distribution: results from the Framingham Offspring Study. Arterioscler Thromb 12:1410–1419
22. McNamara JR, Jenner JL, Li Z, Wilson PWF, Schaefer EJ (1992) Change in low density lipoprotein particle size is associated with change in plasma triglyceride concentration. Arterioscler Thromb 12:1284–1290
23. Li Z, McNamara JR, Ordovas JM, Schaefer EJ (1994) Analysis of high density lipoproteins by a modified gradient gel electrophoresis method. J Lipid Res 35:1698–1711
24. Caulfield MP, Li S, Lee G, Blanche PJ, Salameh WA, Benner WH, Reitz RE, Krauss RM (2008) Direct determination of lipoprotein particle sizes and concentrations by ion mobility analysis. Clin Chem 54:1307–1316
25. Chau P, Nakamura Y, Fielding CJ, Fielding PE (2006) Mechanisms of pre-beta HDL formation and activation. Biochemistry 45:3981–3987
26. Asztalos BF, Sloop CH, Wong L, Roheim PS (1993) Two dimensional electrophoresis of plasma lipoproteins: recognition of new apoA-I containing subpopulations. Biochim Biophys Acta 1169:291–300
27. Asztalos BF, De la Llera-Moya M, Dallal GE, Horvath KV, Schaefer EJ, Rothblat GH (2005) Differential effects of HDL subpopulations on cellular ABCA1 and SRB1-mediated cholesterol efflux. J Lipid Res 46:2246–2253

28. Asztalos BF, Cupples LA, Demissie S, Horvath KV, Cox CE, Batista MC, Schaefer EJ (2004) High-density lipoprotein subpopulation profile and coronary heart disease prevalence in male participants in the Framingham Offspring Study. Arterioscler Thromb Vasc Biol 24:2181–2187

29. Asztalos BF, Collins D, Cupples LA, Demissie S, Horvath KV, Bloomfield HE, Robins SJ, Schaefer EJ (2005) Value of high density lipoprotein (HDL) subpopulations in predicting recurrent cardiovascular events in the Veterans Affairs HDL Intervention Trial. Arterioscler Thromb Vasc Biol 25:2185–2191

30. Asztalos BF, Batista M, Horvath KV, Cox CE, Dallal GE, Morse JS, Brown GB, Schaefer EJ (2003) Change in alpha 1 HDL concentration predicts progression in coronary artery stenosis. Arterioscler Thromb Vasc Biol 23:847–852

31. Santos RD, Schaefer EJ, Asztalos BF, Polisecki E, Hegele RA, Martinez L, Miname M, Coimbra SR, Da Luz P, Rochitte CE, Maranhao R (2008) Characterization of high density lipoprotein particles in familial apolipoprotein A-I deficiency with premature coronary atherosclerosis, corneal arcus and opacification, and tuboeruptive and planar xanthomas. J Lipid Res 49:349–357

32. Asztalos BF, Brousseau ME, McNamara JR, Horvath KV, Roheim PS, Schaefer EJ (2001) Subpopulations of high-density lipoproteins in homozygous and heterozygous Tangier disease. Atherosclerosis 156:217–225

33. Asztalos BF, Schaefer EJ, Horvath KV, Yamashita S, Miller M, Franceschini G, Calabresi L (2007) Role of LCAT in HDL remodeling: an investigation in LCAT deficiency states. J Lipid Res 48: 592–599

34. Asztalos BF, Horvath KV, Kajinami K, Nartsupha C, Cox CE, Batista M, Schaefer EJ, Inazu A, Mabuchi H (2004) Apolipoprotein composition of HDL in cholesteryl ester transfer protein deficiency. J Lipid Res 45:448–455

35. Otvos JD, Collins D, Freedman DS, Shalaurova I, Schaefer EJ, McNamara JR, Bloomfield HE, Robins SJ (2006) Low density and high density lipoprotein particle subclasses predict coronary events and are favorably changed by gemfibrozil therapy in the Veteran Affairs High Density Lipoprotein Intervention Trial. Circulation 113:1556–1563

36. Cromwell WC, Otvos JD, Keyes MJ, Pencina MJ, Sullivan L, Vasan RS, Wilson PW, D'Agostino RB (2007) LDL particle number and risk of future cardiovascular disease in the Framingham Offspring Study – Implications for LDL Management. J Clin Lipidol 1:583–592

37. Mora S, Otvos JD, Rifai N, Rosenson RS, Buring JE, Ridker PM (2009) Lipoprotein particle profiles by nuclear magnetic resonance compared with standard lipid and apolipoproteins in predicting incident cardiovascular disease in women. Circulation 119:931–939

38. Burstein M, Morfin R (1969) Precipitation des lipoproteins seriques et par des polysaccharide sulfates en presence de chlorure manganese. Nouv Rev Fr Hematol 9:231–244

39. Burstein M, Scholnick HR, Morfin R (1970) Rapid method for the isolation of lipoproteins from human serum by precipitation with polyanions. J Lipid Res 11:583–595

40. Burstein M, Scholnick HR (1973) Lipoprotein-polyanion-metal interactions. Adv Lipid Res 11:67–108

41. Manual of Laboratory Operations. Lipid Research Clinics Program (1975) Lipid and lipoprotein analysis. DHEW Pub (NIH) 75–628

42. Warnick GR, Albers JJ (1978) A comprehensive evaluation of the heparin-manganese precipitation procedure for estimating high density lipoprotein HDL cholesterol. J Lipid Res 19:65–76

43. Warnick GR, Benderson J, Albers JJ (1982) Dextran sulfate-Mg^{2+} precipitation procedure for quantitation of high-density lipoprotein cholesterol. Clin Chem 28:1379–1388

44. Miller GJ, Miller NE (1975) Plasma high density lipoprotein concentration and the development of ischemic heart disease. Lancet 1:16–19

45. Castelli WP, Doyle JT, Gordon T, Hames CG, Hjortland MC, Hulley SB, Kagan A, Zukel WJ (1977) HDL cholesterol and other lipids in coronary heart disease. The Cooperative Lipoprotein Phenotyping Project. Circulation 55:767–772

46. Schaefer EJ, Levy RI, Anderson DW, Danner RN, Brewer HB Jr, Blackwelder WC (1978) Plasma-triglycerides in regulation of HDL-cholesterol levels. Lancet 2:391–393

47. Genest JJ, Martin-Munley S, McNamara JR, Ordovas JM, Jenner J, Meyers R, Wilson PWF, Schaefer EJ (1992) Prevalence of familial lipoprotein disorders in patients with premature coronary artery disease. Circulation 85:2025–2033

48. Sugiuchi H, Uji Y, Okabe H, Irie T, Uekama K, Kayahara N, Miyauchi K (1995) Direct measurement of high-density lipoprotein cholesterol in serum with polyethylene glycol-modified enzymes and sulfated alpha-cyclodextrin. Clin Chem 41:717–723

49. Otokozawa S, Ai M, Asztalos BF, White CC, Demissie-Banjaw S, Cupples LA, Nakajima K, Wilson PW, Schaefer EJ (in press). Direct assessment of plasma low density lipoprotein and high density lipoprotein cholesterol. Atherosclerosis

50. Wilson PW, D'Agostino RA, Levy D, Belanger AM, Silbershatz H, Kannel W (1998) Prediction of coronary heart disease using risk factor categories. Circulation 97:1837–1847

51. Friedewald WT, Levy RI, Fredrickson DS (1972) Estimation of the concentration of low density lipoprotein cholesterol in plasma, without use of the preparative ultracentrifuge. Clin Chem 18:499–502

52. McNamara JR, Cohn JS, Wilson PWF, Schaefer EJ (1990) Calculated values for low-density lipoprotein cholesterol in the assessment of lipid abnormalities and coronary disease risk. Clin Chem 36:36–42

53. McNamara JR, Cole TG, Contois JH, Ferguson CA, Ordovas JM, Schaefer EJ (1995) Immunoseparation method for measuring low-density lipoprotein cholesterol directly from serum evaluated. Clin Chem 41:232–240

54. Sugiuchi H, Irie T, Yoshinori U, Ueno T, Chaen T, Uekama K, Okabe H (1998) Homogeneous assay for measuring low-density lipoprotein cholesterol in serum with triblock copolymer and alpha-cyclodextrin. Clin Chem 44:522–531

55. Gidez LI, Miller GJ, Burstein M, Slagle S, Eder HA (1982) Seperation and quantitation of subclasses of plasma high density lipoproteins by a simple precipitation procedure. J Lipid Res 23:1206–1223

56. Hirano T, Nohtomi K, Koba S, Muroi A, Ito Y (2008) A simple and precise method for measuring HDL cholesterol subfractions by a single precipitation followed by homogeneous HDL-C assay. J Lipid Res 49:1130–1136

57. McNamara JR, Shah PK, Nakajima K, Cupples LA, Wilson PWF, Ordovas JM, Schaefer EJ (1998) Remnant lipoprotein cholesterol and triglyceride reference ranges from the Framingham Heart Study. Clin Chem 44:1224–1232

58. McNamara JR, Shah PK, Nakajima K, Cupples LA, Wilson PWF, Ordovas JM, Schaefer EJ (2001) Remnant-like particle (RLP) cholesterol is an independent cardiovascular disease risk factor in women: results from the Framingham Heart Study. Atherosclerosis 154:229–236

59. Schaefer EJ, Audelin MC, McNamara JR, Shah PK, Tayler T, Daly JA, Augustin JL, Seman LJ, Rubenstein JL (2001) Comparison of fasting and postprandial plasma lipoproteins in subjects with and without coronary heart disease. Am J Cardiol 88:1129–1133

60. Schaefer EJ, McNamara JR, Shah PK, Nakajima K, Cupples LA, Ordovas JM, Wilson PWF (2002) Elevated remnant-like particle cholesterol and triglyceride levels in diabetic men and women in the Framingham Offspring Study. Diabetes Care 25:989–994

61. Seman LJ, Jenner JL, McNamara JR, Schaefer EJ (1994) Quantification of lipoprotein (a) in plasma by assaying cholesterol in lectin bound plasma fraction. Clin Chem 40:400–403

62. Seman LJ, DeLuca C, Jenner JL, Cupples LA, McNamara JR, Wilson PWF, Castelli WP, Ordovas JM, Schaefer EJ (1999) Lipoprotein(a)-cholesterol and coronary heart disease in the Framingham Heart Study. Clin Chem 45(7):1039–1046

63. Hirano T, Ito Y, Saegusa H, Yoshino G (2003) A novel and simple method for quantification of small dense LDL. J Lipid Res 44:2193–2220

64. Koba S, Yokota Y, Hirano T, Ito Y, Ban Y, Tsunoda F, Sato T, Shoji M, Suzuki H, Geshi E, Kobayashi Y, Katgiri T (2008) Small LDL-cholesterol is superior to LDL-cholesterol for determining severity of coronary atherosclerosis. J Atheroscler Thromb 15:350–360

65. Sniderman AD, Marcovina SM (2006) Apolipoprotein AI and B. Clin Lab Med 26:733–750

66. Ingelsson E, Schaefer EJ, Contois JH, McNamara JR, Sullivan L, Keyes MJ, Pencina MJ, Schoonmaker C, Wilson PW, D'Agostino RB, Vasan RS (2007) Clinical utility of different lipid measures for prediction of coronary heart disease in men and women. JAMA 298:776–785

67. Avogaro P, Bob GB, Cazzolato G, Quinci GB (1979) Are apolipoproteins better discriminators than lipids for atherosclerosis. Lancet 1:101–103

68. Sniderman AD, Wolfson C, Teng B, Franklin FA, Bachorik PS, Kwiterovich PO Jr (1982) Association of hyperapobetalipoproteinemia with endogenous hypertriglyceridemia and atherosclerosis. Ann Intern Med 97:833–839

69. Schaefer EJ, Lamon-Fava S, Jenner JL, Ordovas JM, Davis CE, Lippel K, Levy RI (1994) Lipoprotein(a) levels predict coronary heart disease in the lipid research clinics coronary prevention trial. JAMA 271:999–1003

70. Erqou S, Kaptoge S, Perry PC, DiAngelantino E, Thompson A, White IR, Marcovina SM, Collins R, Thompson SG, Danesh J; Emerging Risk Factors Collaboration (2009) Lipoprotein(a) as a risk factor for coronary heart disease and stroke. JAMA 302:412–423

71. Otokozawa S, Ai M, Asztalos BF, Tanaka A, Stein E, Jones PH, Schaefer EJ (2009) Effects of maximal atorvastatin and rosuvastatin therapy on apolipoprotein B-48 and remnant lipoprotein cholesterol levels. Atherosclerosis 205:197–201

72. Otokozawa S, Ai M, Diffenderfer M, Asztalos BF, Lamon-Fava S, Schaefer EJ (2009) Fasting and post-prandial apolipoprotein B-48 levels in healthy, obese, and hyperlipidemic subjects. Metabolism 58:1136–1142

73. Ridker PM, Danielson E, Fonseca FA, Genest J, Gotto AM Jr, Kastelein JJ, Koenig W, Libby P, Lorenzatti AJ, MacFayden JG, Nordestgaard BG, Shepherd J, Willerson JT, Glynn RJ; JUPITER Trial Study Group (2009) Reduction in C reactive protein and LDL cholesterol and cardiovascular event rates after initiation of rosuvastatin: a prospective study of the JUPITER trial. Lancet 373:1175–1182

74. Davidson MH, Corson MA, Alberts MJ, Anderson JL, Gorelick PB, Jones PH, Lerman A, McDonnell JP, Weintraub HS (2008) Consensus panel recommendation for incorporating lipoprotein-associated phospholipase A$_2$ testing into cardiovascular disease risk assessment guidelines. Am J Cardiol 101:51F–57F

75. Rader DJ (2007) Effect of insulin resistance, dyslipidemia, and intraabdominal adiposity on the development of cardiovascular disease and diabetes mellitus. Am J Med 20:S12–S18

76. Asztalos BF, Swarbrick MM, Schaefer EJ, Dallal GE, Horvath KV, Ai M, Stanhope KL, Austrheim-Smith J, Wolfe BM, Ali M, Havel PJ (2009) Effects of weight loss, induced by gastric bypass surgery, on HDL remodeling in obese women. J Lipid Res

77. Schaefer EJ, McNamara JR, Asztalos BF, Tayler T, Daly JA, Gleason JL, Seman LJ, Ferrara A, Rubenstein JL (2005) Effects of atorvastatin versus other statins on fasting and post-prandial C-reactive protein and lipoprotein associated phospholipase A2 in patients with coronary artery disease versus control subjects. Am J Cardiol 95:1025–1032

78. Greenland P, LaBree L, Azen SP, Doherty TM, Detrano R (2004) Coronary calcium score combined with Framingham risk score for risk prediction in asymptomatic individuals. JAMA 291:210–215

79. Vliegenthart R, Oudkerk M, Hofman A, Oei HH, van Dijck W, van Rooij FC, Witteman JC (2005) Coronary calcification improves cardiovascular risk prediction. Circulation 112:572–577

80. Detrano R, Guerci AD, Carr JJ, Bild DE, Burke G, Folsom AR, Liu K, Shea S, Szklo M, Bluemke DA, O'Leary DH, Drely R (2008) Coronary calcification as a predictor of coronary events in 4 racial or ethnic groups. New Engl J Med 358:1336–1345

81. Folsom AR, Kronmal RA, Detrano RA, Detrano RC, O'Leary DH, Bild DE, Bluemke DA, Budoff MJ, Liu K, Shea S, Szklo M, Tracy RP, Watson KE, Burke GL (2008) Coronary artery calcification as compared with carotid intimal medial thickness in the prediction of cardiovascular disease incidence: the Multi-Ethnic Study of Atherosclerosis (MESA). Arch Intern Med 168:1333–1339

82. Budoff MJ, Shaw LJ, Liu ST, Weinstein SR, Mosier TP, Tseng PH, Flores FR, Callister TQ, Raggi P, Berman DS (2007) Long term prognosis associated with coronary calcification: observations from a registry of 25,253 patients. J Am Coll Cardiol 49:1860–1870

83. Boyar A (2006) Creating a web application that combines Framingham risk with electron beam CT coronary calcium score to calculate a new event risk. J Thorac Imaging 21:91–96

84. Budoff MJ, Nasir K, McClelland RL, Detrano R, Wong N, Blumenthal RS, Kondos G, Kronmal RA (2009) Coronary calcium predicts events even better with absolute calcium score than age, sex, race, ethnic percentiles. J Am Coll Cardiol 53:345–352

85. Santos RD, Miname MH, Martinez LR, Rochitte CE, Chacra AP, Nakandakare ER, Chen D, Schaefer EJ (2008) Non-invasive detection of aortic and coronary atherosclerosis in homozygous familial hypercholesterolemia by 64 slice multi-detector row computed tomography angiography. Atherosclerosis 197:910–915

86. Sprecher DS, Schaefer EJ, Kent K, Gregg RE, Zech LA, Hoeg JM, McManus B, Roberts D, Brewer HB Jr (1984) Cardiovascular features of homozygous familial hypercholesterolemia: analysis of 16 patients. Am J Cardiol 54:20–30

87. Santos RD, Miname L, Asztalos BF, Polisecki E, Schaefer EJ (2008) Clinical presentation, laboratory values, and coronary heart disease risk in marked high density lipoprotein deficiency states. J Clin Lipidol 2:237–247

88. Schaefer EJ, Heaton WH, Wetzel MG, Brewer HB Jr (1982) Plasma apolipoprotein A-I absence associated with marked reduction of high density lipoproteins and premature coronary artery disease. Arteriosclerosis 2:16–26

89. Grundy SM, Cleeman JI, Merz CN, Brewer HB Jr, Clark LT, Hunninghake DB, Paternak RC, Smith SC Jr, Stone NJ (2004) Implications of recent clinical trials for the National Cholesterol Education Adult Treatment Panel III guidelines. Circulation 110:227–239

90. Pencina MJ, D'Agostino RB, Larson MG, Massaro JM, Vasan RS (2009) Predicting the 30-year risk of cardiovascular disease. The Framingham Study. Circulation 119:3078–3084

91. Ridker PM, Buring JE, Rifai N, Cook NR (2007) Development and validation of improved algorithms for the assessment of global cardiovascular risk in women. The Reynolds Risk Score. JAMA 297:611–619

92. Ridker PM, Paynter NP, Rifai N, Gaziano JM, Cook NR (2008) C-reactive protein and parental history improve global risk prediction: the Reynolds Risk Score for men. Circulation 118:2243–2251

93. Assman G, Schulte H, Cullen P, Sedorf U (2007) Assessing risk of myocardial infarction and stroke; new data from the Prospective Cardiovascular Muenster (PROCAM) Study. Eur J Clin Invest 37:925–932

94. Liu J, Hong Y, D'Agostino RB Sr, Wu Z, Wang W, Sun J, Wilson PW, Kannel WB, Zhao D (2004) Predictive value for the Chinese population of the Framingham coronary heart disease risk assessment tool as compared with the Chinese Multi-Provincial Cohort Study. JAMA 291:2491–2599

95. Critchley J, Liu J, Zhao D, Wei W, Capewell S (2004) Explaining the in increase in coronary heart disease mortality in Beijing between 1984 and 1999. Circulation 110:1236–1244

96. Yusuf S, Hawken S, Ounpuu S, Dans T, Avezum A, Larras F, McQueen M, Budaf A, Pais P, Varigos J, Lishery L; Interheart

Study Investigators (2004) Effect of potentially modifiable risk factors associated with myocardial infarction in 52 countries (the INTERHEART Study) case-control study. Lancet 364:937–952

97. Wald NJ, Law MR (2003) A strategy to reduce cardiovascular disease by more than 80%. BMJ 326:1419–1420

98. The Indian Polycap Study (2009) Effects of a polypill (Polycap) on risk factors in middle-aged individuals withouts cardiovascular disease (TIPS): a phase II, double blind, randomized trial. Lancet 373:1341–1351

99. Rubins HB, Robins SJ, Collins D, Nelson DB, Elam MB, Schaefer EJ, Faas FH, Anderson JW; VA-HIT Study Group (2002) Diabetes, plasma insulin, and cardiovascular disease. Subgroup analysis from the Department of Veterans Affairs High-Density Lipoprotein Intervention Trial (VA-HIT). Arch Intern Med 162:2597–2604

100. Schaefer EJ, Asztalos BF (2007) Increasing high density lipoprotein cholesterol, inhibition of cholesteryl ester transfer protein, and heart disease risk reduction. Am J Cardiol 100:S25–S31

101. Schaefer EJ (2002) E.V. McCollum Award Lecture: lipoproteins, nutrition, and heart disease. Am J Clin Nutr 75:191–212

102. Asztalos BF, Horvath KV, McNamara JR, Roheim PS, Rubenstein JJ, Schaefer EJ (2002) Comparing the effects of five different statins on the HDL subpopulation profiles of coronary heart disease patients. Atherosclerosis 164:361–369

103. Asztalos BF, Horvath KV, McNamara JR, Roheim PS, Rubenstein JJ, Schaefer EJ (2002) Effects of atorvastatin on the HDL subpopulation profile of coronary heart disease patients. J Lipid Res 43:1701–1707

104. Asztalos BF, LeMaulf F, Dallal GE, Stein E, Jones PH, Horvath KV, McTaggert F, Schaefer EJ (2007) Comparison of the effects of high doses of rosuvastatin versus atorvastatin on the subpopulations of high density lipoproteins. Am J Cardiol 99:681–685

105. Lamon-Fava S, Diffenderfer MR, Barrett PH, Buchsbaum A, Matthan NR, Lichtenstein AH, Dolnikowski GG, Horvath K, Asztalos BF, Zago V, Schaefer EJ (2007) Effects of different doses of atorvastatin on human apolipoprotein B-100, B-48, and A-I metabolism. J Lipid Res 48:1746–1753

106. Pedersen TR, Olsson AG, Faergeman O et al (1998) Lipoprotein changes and reduction the incidence of major coronary heart disease events in the Scandinavian Simvastatin Survival Study (4S). Circulation 97:1453–1460

107. Nicholls SJ, Tuzxu EM, Sipathi I, Grasso AW, Schoenhagen P, Hu T, Wolski K, Crowe T, Desai MY, Hazen SL, Kapadia SR, Nissen SE (2007) Statins, high-density lipoprotein cholesterol and regression of coronary atherosclerosis. JAMA 297:499–508

108. Staels B, Dallongeville J, Auwerx J, Schoonjans K, Leitersdorf E, Fruchart JC (1998) Mechanisms of action of fibrates on lipid and lipoprotein metabolism. Circulation 98:2088–2093

109. Schaefer EJ, Lamon Fava S, Cole T, Sprecher DL, Cilla DD Jr, Balagtas CC, Rowan JP, Black DM (1996) Effects of regular and extended-release gemfibrozil on plasma lipoproteins and apolipoproteins in hypercholesterolemic patients with decreased HDL cholesterol levels. Atherosclerosis 127:113–122

110. Asztalos BF, Collins D, Horvath KV, Bloomfield HE, Robins SJ, Schaefer EJ (2008) Relation of gemfibrozil treatment and high-density lipoprotein subpopulation profile with cardiovascular events in the Veterans Affairs High-Density Lipoprotein Intervention Trial. Metabolism 57:77–83

111. Saku K, Gartside PS, Hynd BA, Kashyap MI (1985) Mechanism of action of gemfibrozil on lipoprotein metabolism. J Clin Invest 75:1702–1712

112. Watts GF, Barrett PH, Ji J, Serone AP, Chan DC, Croft KD, Loehrer F, Johnson AG (2003) Differential effects of atorvastatin and fenofibrate on lipoprotein kinetics in subjects with the metabolic syndrome. Diabetes 52:803–811

113. Chan DC, Watts GF, Ooi EM, Rye KA, Ji J, Jophnson AG, Barrett PH (2009) Regulatory of the effects fenofibrate and atorvastatin on

lipoprotein A-I and lipoprotein A-I:A-II in the metabolic syndrome. Diabetes Care 32(11):2111–2113

114. Millar JS, Dufy D, Gadi R, Bloedon LT, Dunbar RL, Wolfe ML, Mowa R, Shah A, Fuki IV, McCoy M, Harris CJ, Wang MD, Howey DC, Rader DJ (2009) Potent and selective PPAR alpha agonist LY51867 upregulates both apoA-I production and catabolism in human subjects with the metabolic syndrome. Arterioscler Thromb Vasc Biol 29:140–146

115. Manninen V, Elo O, Frick HH et al (1988) Lipid alterations and decline in the incidence of coronary heart disease in the Helsinki Heart Study. J Am Med Assoc 260:641–651

116. Robins SJ, Collins D, Wittes JT, Papademetriou V, Deedwania PC, Schaefer EJ, McNamara JR, Kashyap ML, Hershman JM, Wexler LF, Rubins HB (2001) for the VA-HIT Study Group. Relation of gemfibrozil treatment and lipid levels with major coronary events. VA-HIT: a randomized controlled trial. J Am Med Assoc 285:1585–1591

117. The DAIS Investigators (2001) Effect of fenofibrate on the progression of coronary artery disease in type 2 diabetes: the Diabetes Atherosclerosis Intervention Study (DAIS): a randomized trial. Lancet 357:1890–1895

118. Keech AC, Simes RJ, Barter P, Best J, Scott R, Taskinen MR, Forder P, Pillai A, Davis T, Glasziou P, Drury P, Kesaniemi YA, Sullivan D, Hunt D, Colman P, d'Emden M, Whiting M, Ehnholm C, Laakso M; FIELD Investigators (2005) Effects of long term fenofibrate therapy on cardiovascular events in 9795 people with type 2 diabetes mellitus (the FIELD study): a randomized controlled trial. Lancet 366:1849–1861

119. Keech AC, Mitchell P, Summanen PA, O'Day J, Davis TM, Moffitt MS, Taskinen MR, Simes RJ, Tse D, Williamson E, Merrifield A, Laatikainen LT, d'Emden MC, Crimet DC, O'Connell RL, Colman P; FIELD Study Investigators (2007) Effect of fenofibrate on the need for laser treatment for diabetic retinopathy (FIELD Study): a randomized controlled trial. Lancet 370:1687–1697

120. Rajamani K, Colman PG, Li LP, Best JD, Voysey M, D'Emden MC, Laakso M, Baker JR, Keech AC (2009) Effect of fenofibrate on amputation events in people with type 2 diabetes mellitus (FIELD study): a prespecified analysis of a randomised controlled trial. Lancet 373:1780–1788

121. Canner PL, Berge KG, Wenger NK, Stamler J, Freedman L, Prineas RJ, Friedewald W (1986) Fifteen year mortality in Coronary Drug Project patients: long term benefits with niacin. J Am Coll Cardiol 8:1245–1255

122. Berge KG, Canner PL (1991) Coronary drug project: experience with niacin. Coronary Drug Project Research Group. Eur J Clin Pharm 40(Suppl 1):S49–S51

123. Canner PL, Furberg CD, Terrin ML, McGovern ME (2005) Benefits of niacin by glycemic status in patients with healed myocardial infarction. From the Coronary Drug Project. Am J Cardiol 95:254–257

124. Canner PL, Furberg CD, McGovern ME (2006) Benefits of niacin in patients with versus without the metabolic syndrome and healed myocardial infarction; from the Coronary Drug project. Am J Cardiol 97:477–479

125. Brown GB, Zhao XQ, Chait A, Fisher LD, Cheung M, Morse JS, Dowdy AA, Marino EK, Bolson EL, Alaupovic P, Frohlich J, Albers JJ (2001) Simvastatin and niacin, antioxidant vitamins, or the combination for the prevention of coronary artery disease. N Engl J Med 345:1583–1592

126. Lamon-Fava S, Diffenderfer MR, Barrett PHR, Buchsbaum A, Nyaku M, Horvath K, Asztalos BF, Otokozawa S, Ai M, Matthan NR, Lichtenstein AH, Dolnikowski GG, Schaefer EJ (2008) Extended-release niacin alters the metabolism of plasma apolipoprotein (apo) A-I and apoB-containing lipoproteins. Arterioscler Thromb Vasc Biol 28:1672–1678

127. Sudhop T, Lutjohann D, Kodal A, Igel M, Tribble DL, Shah S, Perevozskaya I, von Bergmann K (2002) Inhibition of intestinal

cholesterol absorption by ezetimibe in humans. Circulation 106: 1943–1948

128. Pearson TA, Ballantyne CM, Veltri E, Shah A, Bird S, Lin J, Rosenberg E, Tershakovec AM (2009) Pooled analysis of effects on C reactive protein and low density lipoprotein cholesterol in placebo controlled trials of ezetimibe or ezetimibe added to base-line statin therapy. Am J Cardiol 103:369–374

129. The Lipid Clinics Coronary Primary Prevention Trial results: II. (1984) The relationship of reduction in incidence of coronary heart disease to cholesterol lowering. J Am Med Assoc 251:365–374

130. Fonseca VA, Rosenstock J, Wang K, Truitt KE, Jones MR (2008) Colesevelam HCL improves glycemic control and lowers LDL-C in patients with inadequate control of type II diabetes on sulfony-lurea therapy. Diabetes Care 31:1479–1484

131. Phillipson BE, Rothrock DW, Connor WE, Harris WS, Illingworth DR (1985) Reduction of plasma lipids, lipoproteins, and apolipo-proteins by dietary fish oils in patients with hypertriglyceridemia. N Engl J Med 312:1210–1216

132. Endres S, Ghorbani R, Kelley VE, Georgilis K, Lonneman G, Van Der Meer JWM, Cannon JG, Klempner M, Schaefer EJ, Wolff SM, Dinarello CA (1989) Dietary n-3 polyunsaturated fatty acids suppress synthesis of interleukin-1 and tumor necrosis factor. N Eng J Med 320:265–271

133. Meydani SN, Lichtenstein AH, Cornwall S, Meydani M, Goldin BR, Rasmussen H, Dinarello CA, Schaefer EJ (1993) Immunologic effects of National Cholesterol Panel Step 2 diets with and without fish derived omega 3 fatty acid enrichment. J Clin Invest 92:105–113

134. Davidson MH, Stein EA, Bays HE, Maki KC, Doyle RT, Shalwitz RA, Ballantyne CM, Ginsberg HN (2007) Combination prescrip-tion omega 3 fatty acids with simvastatin (COMBOS). Clin Ther 29:1354–1367

135. Chan DC, Watts GF, Mori TA, Barrett PH, Redgrave TG, Beilin LJ (2003) Randomized controlled trial of the effects of n-3 fatty acid supplementation on the metabolism of apolipoprotein B-100 and chylomicron remnants in men with visceral adiposity. Am J Clin Nutr 77:300–307

136. Burr ML, Gilbert JF, Rogers S, Holliday RM, Sweetnam PM, Elwood PC, Deadman NM (1989) Effects of changes in fat, fish, and fibre intakes on death and myocardial infarction. Lancet 2:757–761

137. Burr ML (2007) Secondary prevention of coronary heart disease in UK men: the Diet and Reinfarction Trial and its sequel. Proc Nutr Soc 66:9–15

138. Gissi Prevenzione Investigators (1999) Dietary supplementation with n-3 polyunsaturated fatty acids and vitamin E after myocar-dial infarction: results of the Gissi Prevenzione Trial. Lancet 354:447–455

139. Yokoyama M, Oryasa H, Matzuzaki M, Matsuzawa Y, Saito Y, Ishikawa Y, Oikawa S, Sasaki J, Hishida H, Itakura H, Kita T, Kitabatake A, Nakaya N, Sakata T, Shimada K, Shirato K; Japan EPA lipid intervention study (JELIS) investigators (2007) Effects of eicosapentaenoic acid on major coronary events in hypercholes-terolemic patients (JELIS): a randomized open label, blinded end-point analysis. Lancet 370:1090–1098

140. Tanaka K, Ishikawa Y, Yokoyama M, Oryasa H, Matsusaki M, Saito Y, Matsuzawa Y, Sasaki J, Oikawa S, Hishida H, Kakura H, Kita T, Kitabatake A, Nakaya N, Sakata T, Shimada K, Shirato K; JELIS Investigators Japan (2008) Reduction in the recurrence of stroke by EPA for hypercholesterolemic patients:subanalysis of the JELIS trial. Stroke 39:2052–2058

141. Saito Y, Yokohama M, Oryasa H, Matsuzaki M, Matsuzawa Y, Ishikawa Y, Oikawa S, Sasaki J, Hishida H, Hakura H, Kita T, Kitabatake A, Nakaya N, Sakata T, Shimada K, Shirato K; JELIS Investigators Japan (2008) Effects of EPA on coronary artery disease in hypercholesterolemic patients with multiple risk factors: sub-analysis of primary prevention cases from the Japan EPA Lipid Intervention Study (JELIS). Atherosclerosis 200:135–140

142. Brouwer IA, Riatt MH, Dallemeijjer C, Kraemer DF, Zock PL, Morris C, Katan MB, Connor WE, Camm JA, Schouten EJ, McAnulty J (2009) Effect of fish oil on ventricular tachyarrhyth-mia in 3 studies in patients with implantable cardioverter defibril-lators. Eur Heart J 30:820–826

143. Schaefer EJ, Bongard V, Beiser AS, Tucker KL, Kyle DJ, Wilson PWF, Wolf PA (2006) Plasma phosphatidylcholine docosa-hexaenoic acid content, and risk of dementia and Alzheimer's dis-ease: The Framingham Study. Arch Neurol 63:1545–1550

144. Nissen SE, Tsunoda T, Tuzcu EM, Schoenhagen P, Cooper CJ, Yasin M, Eaton GM, Lauer MA, Sheldon WS, Grines CL, Halpern S, Crowe T, Blankenship JC, Kerensky R (2003) Effect of recom-binant ApoA-I Milano on coronary atherosclerosis in patients with acute coronary syndromes: a randomized controlled trial. JAMA 290:2292–2300

145. Tardif JC, Grégoire J, L'Allier PL, Ibrahim R, Lesperance J, Heinonen TM, Kouz S, Berry C, Basser R, Lavoie MA, Guertin MC, Rodes-Cabau J; Effect of rHDL on Atherosclerosis-Safety and Efficacy (ERASE) Investigators (2007) Effects of reconsti-tuted high-density lipoprotein infusions on coronary atherosclero-sis: a randomized controlled trial. JAMA 297:1675–1682

146. Brown BG, Stukowsky KH, Zhao XQ (2006) Simultaneous low-density lipoprotein-C lowering and high-density lipoprotein-C elevation for optimum cardiovascular disease prevention with various drug classes, and the combination: a meta-analysis of 23 randomized lipid trials. Curr Opin Lipidol 17:631–636

Index